Pathology of Glomerular Diseases

Pallav Gupta • Ramesh K. Gupta

Pathology of Glomerular Diseases

Atlas of Clinical Case Studies

Springer

Pallav Gupta
Consultant Renal Pathologist
Department of Histopathology
Sir Ganga Ram Hospital
New Delhi, India

Ramesh K. Gupta
Former Head of Department Pathology
Sanjay Gandhi Postgraduate Instutute of Medical Sciences
Lucknow, India

ISBN 978-981-19-1429-4 ISBN 978-981-19-1430-0 (eBook)
https://doi.org/10.1007/978-981-19-1430-0

This Springer imprint is published by the registered company Springer Nature Singapore Pte Ltd.
The registered company address is: 152 Beach Road, #21-01/04 Gateway East, Singapore 189721, Singapore

This book is dedicated to my mother Dr. Sushma Gupta for her encouragement and support.

—Pallav Gupta

Foreword

It's a matter of pleasure for me to write this foreword for a book entitled "*Pathology of Glomerular Diseases—Atlas of Clinical Case Studies*" authored by Professor R K Gupta and Dr. Pallav Gupta. Professor Gupta has more than 30 years of experience in renal pathology and has significantly contributed to the development of Renal and Transplant Pathology in India. Dr. Pallav Gupta has specialized in renal pathology and has more than 10 years of experience in the field.

Over the past few decades, the practice of nephrology has advanced offering optimal therapeutic measures for patients with renal diseases. Renal biopsy diagnosis is crucial for proper management of these cases. Proper identification of morphological alterations, as may be observed on evaluation of renal biopsy is a challenging task both in terms of technical skills and interpretation requiring sufficient expertise in the field. Besides the use of various staining procedures, the application of immunofluorescence techniques and electron microscopy have significantly contributed to better diagnosis of renal diseases. Still there are closely resembling/overlapping morphological lesions encountered on evaluation of renal biopsy, which at times may be difficult to opine with absolute certainty. Timely diagnosis of underlying kidney diseases is essential not only for proper management of these patients but also to minimize the development of chronic kidney disease and renal failure in them.

The authors, applying their experience and expertise in the field, have included in this publication a large number of illustrative photomicrographs of various glomerular lesions, supplementing succinct descriptions of pathological findings. This "Illustrative Atlas on Pathology of Glomerular Diseases" should benefit renal pathologists, nephrologists, and postgraduates, enabling prompt identification of glomerular lesions on histopathological examination.

Parmjeet Randhawa

President Renal Pathology Society
Professor Department of Pathology
Division of Transplantation Pathology
The Thomas E Starzl Transplantation Institute
University of Pittsburgh, Montefiore Hospital
Pittsburgh, PA, USA
May 2021

Preface

Global annual prevalence of renal diseases is estimated to be 15 million and that of CKD to be 87 thousand per million populations. Whereas in India, the prevalence of CKD is approximately 95 thousand per million populations and the burden of CKD in India is estimated to be 115 million. Globally 8.5 lakh people die of kidney diseases every year constituting 12th most important cause of death world over.

Morphological assessment of kidney biopsy is not only essential for proper diagnosis of underlying renal disease but also for guiding appropriate therapeutic management, follow-up, and prognosis of these patients. Proper assessment of kidney biopsy requires high technical skills and expertise on the part of reporting renal pathologist. At times the morphological appearances of various kidney lesions may be overlapping requiring clear understanding and interpretation of these changes so as to achieve appropriate morphological diagnosis.

This atlas provides for morphological appearances of various glomerular lesions encountered in a wide range of kidney diseases involving renal glomeruli. More than 60 different renal diseases predominantly involving glomeruli with more than 375 high quality colored photomicrographs and about 75 EM images have been included in this publication. Various renal diseases have been grouped in different chapters. Each chapter has a brief text with relevant references for further reading and multiple colored microphotographs of light microscopic and IF/IHC appearances depicting the distinctive morphological features of glomeruli as may be encountered in these diseases. EM images have also been provided wherever required. Each case has a descriptive legend providing complete clinical history with lab workup and other relevant investigations along with renal biopsy findings as considered essential for proper evaluation of the patient. In view of the detailed clinical and lab workup, along with renal biopsy assessment for each glomerular disease, the book provides for systemic approach for proper clinico-pathological correlation and diagnosis of the underlying disease conditions.

It is believed that eyes do not see what mind does not know. The visual understanding of the glomerular pathology so gained will help the early career renal pathologists, histopathologist, and nephrologists to have a clear understanding of underlying renal disease thus helping in proper evaluation and appropriate therapeutic management of the patient. It may also guide to predict the likely prognostic outcome of the patient. This book besides being of use to renal pathologists and nephrologists will also provide a good resource material for clear understanding of the glomerular lesions to the beginners and postgraduates in nephrology, renal pathology, and allied specialties.

Your comments and suggestions are most welcome.

New Delhi, India
Lucknow, India
July 2021

Pallav Gupta
Ramesh K. Gupta

Acknowledgments

We are grateful to Dr. Parmjeet Randhawa, President, Renal Pathology Society and Professor, Department of Pathology, Division of Transplantation Pathology, The Thomas E Starzl Transplantation Institute, University of Pittsburgh, Montefiore Hospital, Pittsburgh, USA, for kindly writing the foreword for this book.

Majority of the cases included in this atlas are from the own experience of the authors, while some cases have been contributed by friends and colleagues from other institutes both within the country and abroad.

We gratefully acknowledge the contribution of the interesting cases by contributing authors Dr. Helen Liapis, Professor of Pathology and Immunology and Internal Medicine (Renal) retired, Washington University School of Medicine, Saint Louis, MO, USA; Dr. Joris J. Roelofs, Department of Pathology, Amsterdam University Medical Centers, Amsterdam, The Netherlands; Dr. Geetika Singh, Additional Professor, Department of Pathology, All India Institute of Medical Sciences, New Delhi, India; Dr. Megha Uppin, Associate Professor, Department of Pathology, Nizam's Institute of Medical Sciences, Hyderabad, India; Dr. V. Gnanapriya, Assistant Professor, Department of Pathology, St. John's Medical College, Bangalore, India; and Dr. Bhavna Asit Mehta, Senior Consultant histoanatomic and nephropathologist, Head of Histoanatomic Pathology Department, Supratech Micropath Laboratory (a Neuberg Associate), Neuberg Supratech Reference Laboratory, Ahmedabad, India.

The authors are also grateful to Dr. D. S. Rana, Chairman, Board of Management; Dr. A. K. Bhalla, Chairman, Department of Nephrology; Dr. Ashwani Gupta, Co-chairman, Department of Nephrology; Dr. Manish Malik, Senior Consultant, Department of Nephrology; Dr. Vinant Bhargava, Consultant, Department of Nephrology; Dr. Anurag Gupta Senior Consultant, Department of Nephrology; Dr. P. K. Pruthi, Senior Consultant, Department of Pediatric Nephrology; and Dr. Kanav Anand, Consultant, Department of Pediatric Nephrology, Ganga Ram Institute of Postgraduate Medical Education and Research (GRIPMER) and Sir Ganga Ram Hospital, New Delhi, India, for providing clinical workup of their cases.

We sincerely thank Dr. Lorraine C. Racusen, Former Professor, Department of Pathology, The Johns Hopkins University, School of Medicine, Baltimore, Maryland, USA; Dr. Surya V. Seshan, Professor, Department of Pathology and Laboratory Medicine, Weill Cornell Medical Center-New York-Presbyterian Hospital, New York, USA; and Dr. Swarnalata Gowrishankar, Senior Consultant, Department of Histopathology, Apollo Hospitals, Jubilee Hills, Hyderabad, India, for consenting to peer review this book.

We are also grateful to all our colleagues and friends extending all possible support in compilation of this book. We also are thankful to unconditional support of our family members Dr. Sushma Gupta, Former Professor and Head Physiology, GSVM Medical College, Kanpur; Dr. Surbhi Gupta, Kushagra Gupta and Seedhita Gupta.

We are also thankful to the technical staff, Department of Pathology, Sir Ganga Ram Hospital, New Delhi, India for their dedication and hard work without which this manuscript would not have been possible.

The authors are thankful to the publishers M/s Springer Science + Business Media Singapore Pte Ltd, Singapore, for so meticulously publishing and making the book presentable.

Contents

1 Evaluation of Renal Biopsy

Direct examination of the tissue is the most effective diagnostic procedure. Kidney biopsy is an indispensable tool for the diagnosis of underlying disease conditions. However, renal biopsy is a challenge in terms of both, technique and interpretation, requiring adequate laboratory setup and trained renal pathologists.

The first open surgical renal biopsy was performed in 1923 and the first percutaneous kidney biopsy was performed in 1934. Since the 1950s, percutaneous renal biopsies are being routinely performed world over. It is a safe procedure and the complications are rare. Although microscopic hematuria for a couple of days is not infrequent, gross hematuria is uncommon; rarely hematuria may be severe enough to warrant nephrectomy (1 in 2000–5000). The use of ultrasound imaging and biopsy gun have added further to the safety of the procedure. Biopsy core obtained by biopsy gun is shown in (Fig. 1.1).

Renal biopsy is undertaken to achieve certain objectives:

(a) Diagnosis of underlying renal disease
(b) Assess the severity or staging of the disease
(c) Guide therapy and assess prognosis

Kidney biopsy is essential for the diagnosis of:

(a) Nephrotic syndrome in adults
(b) Asymptomatic proteinuria and/or hematuria
(c) Acute renal failure
(d) Renal involvement in systemic diseases (SLE, Vasculitis)
(e) Renal allograft dysfunction (Rejection)
(f) Chronic renal failure

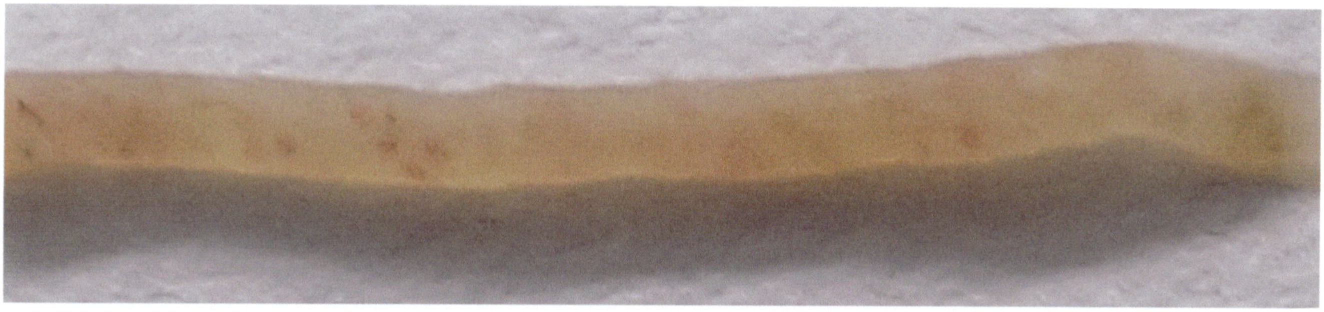

Fig. 1.1 Gross appearance of a renal biopsy core. Glomeruli appear as tiny raised dots. The biopsy should be examined under a stereoscopic microscope or a hand lens for adequacy at the biopsy site

P. Gupta, R. K. Gupta, *Pathology of Glomerular Diseases*, https://doi.org/10.1007/978-981-19-1430-0_1

1.1 Laboratory Procedure

Availability of the following facilities would essentially constitute adequate laboratory setup for workup of renal biopsies:

(a) Thin paraffin sections (2–3 μ)
(b) Special staining procedures (HE, PAS, MT, Silver Methanamine, Orcein, Congored)
(c) Cryostat sections
(d) Immunofluorescence and immunostaining procedures
(e) Ultramicrotomy and Electron microscopy

If light microscopy, immunofluorescence, and electron microscopy are together indicated, at least two biopsy cores should be obtained (Fig. 1.2) and if possible three cores 1 each in 10% buffered formalin, normal saline and 3% glutaraldehyde. Sufficient care is exercised during handling so as the tissue is not compressed (avoid using forceps, needle or sharp objects; rather use soft wooden stick or soft hair brush). The adequacy of the biopsy should be ascertained at the biopsy site, cortex being darker showing glomeruli as tiny red dots visualized under a hand lens or stereoscopic microscope. For further processing, the tissue needs to be fixed as per requirement. For light microscopy, apart from 10% formaldehyde or neutral formal saline, other fixatives viz. 4% paraformaldehyde for in situ hybridization, and Helly's fluid (for juxtaglomerular apparatus), Duboscq-Brasil/Alcoholic Bouin's, have also been recommended. After routine overnight processing, the biopsy should be embedded in paraffin wax of higher melting point or preheated paraffin wax or paraffin wax with ceresin or beeswax, so as to obtain 2–3 μ thick sections. At times, such as in post-transplant biopsies, rapid microwave processing is undertaken by shortening fixation to 30 min, dehydration and clearing to 10–20 min; sections are thus available within 4 h.

Apart from hematoxylin and eosin stain, periodic acid schiff (PAS) is the most essential and most informative stain especially for basement membrane, mesangium and to demonstrate protein reabsorption droplets in tubules. Periodic acid silver methenamine (PSM) stain clearly reveals membranous changes like epimembranous spikes and holes within glomerular capillary basement membrane in membranous glomerulonephritis and duplication of the capillary basement membrane in MPGN. Masson's trichrome (MT) stain is useful for the demonstration of fibrin thrombi and immune deposits and in the evaluation of interstitial fibrosis. Other stains like orcein for elastic fibers, congored and thioflan T for amyloid, phosphotungstic acid hematoxylin for fibrin and Perl's stain for hemosiderin are used as and when required.

1.2 Histopathological Evaluation

Microscopically, a biopsy containing at least ten glomeruli for light microscopy and at least 1 glomeruli each for DIF and EM is considered adequate. However, at times, a definitive diagnosis can be offered by examination of a single glomerulus in typical lesions such as amyloidosis or membranous glomerulonephritis.

A systemic approach to examining different compartments (glomerular, tubular, interstitial, and vascular) for the distribution and severity of various lesions is essential for the proper evaluation of renal biopsies.

1.3 Glomerular Lesions

For glomerular lesions, term focal refers to involvement of few glomeruli (<50%), while diffuse refers to the involvement of majority of glomeruli (>50%). Segmental and global

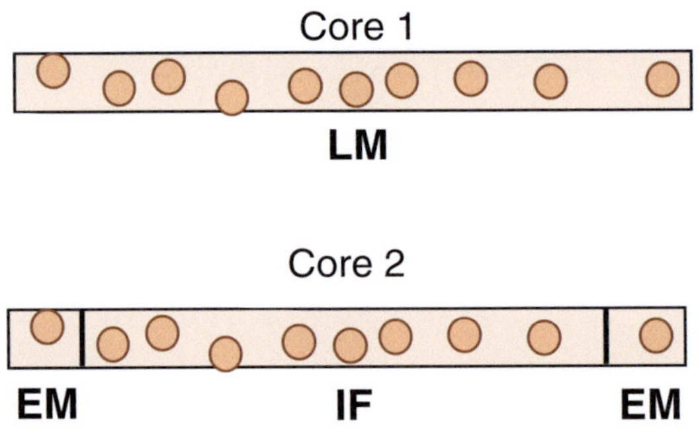

Fig. 1.2 Schematic representation of the divisions of two core renal biopsies for light microscopy (LM), immunofluorescence (IF), and electron microscopy (EM). One core is processed for LM. Another core is divided into three parts using a sharp knife; sufficient care is taken not to damage the biopsy core. The pieces from two ends containing at least one glomerulus are preserved/processed for EM, and the central portion of the biopsy core is processed for IF

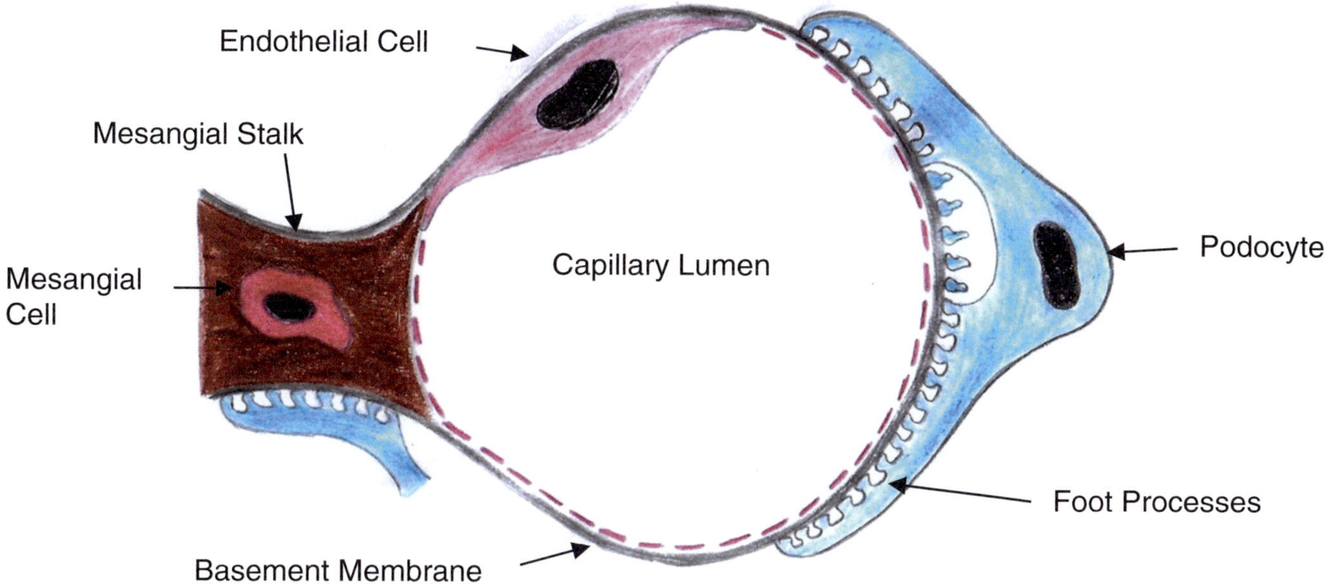

Fig. 1.3 Schematic representation of the structure of a glomerular capillary loop (Contributor: Dr. Surbhi Gupta)

glomerular involvements refer to the involvement of part (<50%) or major part/whole (≥50%) of the glomerulus, respectively.

In adults, glomeruli are 170–220 μ in size; juxtamedullary glomeruli are larger than outer cortical glomeruli. Schematic diagram of normal glomerular capillary loop is shown in (Fig. 1.3). Larger glomeruli are seen in proliferative and infiltrative lesions; reduced size of the glomeruli is due to collapse or sclerosis of glomerular capillary tuft which may be vascular or obstructive in origin. More than 20% of completely obsolescent glomeruli are considered abnormal for patients between 2 and 60 years of age. The percentage of globally sclerosed glomeruli present in a biopsy normally as a part of aging can roughly be assessed using the formula: age/2−10. Few authors have provided upper reference limit to derive age adjusted global glomerulosclerosis in a biopsy based on age of patient and number of glomeruli and is more reliable method for calculating the same.

A glomerulus in 2–3 μ section shows 4–5 ill-defined lobules and 40–60 cells. Each mesangial area contains 2–3 cells. Mesangial hypercellularity is characterized by the presence of four or more mesangial cells surrounded by a matrix in one or more mesangial areas. The perihilar region should be disregarded when accessing mesangial hypercellularity. Although not strictly defined, the presence of more than four leukocytes in a glomerulus is considered abnormal. Endocapillary hypercellularity is characterized by luminal narrowing or occlusion of capillary lumen due to an increase in the cells within lumen. The glomerular cellularity may be increased due to the proliferation of mesangial, endothelial or epithelial cells or due to infiltration of leucocytes. Accentuated lobulation is usually seen in MPGN; reduced lobulation with or without mesangiolysis may be seen in cases of thrombotic microangiopathy.

Glomerular sclerosis refers to an increased extracellular matrix with or without obliteration of capillary loops, the lesions could be segmental or global.

Glomerular necrosis could be focal and segmental or may cause complete destruction of glomerulus, common causes include lupus nephritis, thrombotic microangiopathy, Anti-GBM disease (Goodpasture's syndrome), pauci-immune small vessel vasculitides.

On light microscopy, glomerular immune deposits are best identified with Masson's trichrome (MT) stain. Electron microscopic evaluation demonstrates electron-dense immune deposits to be located in mesangial, intramembranous, subepithelial, or subendothelial location in different glomerular diseases. Large subepithelial deposits (humps) are characteristic of post-streptococcal glomerulonephritis, multiple small subepithelial deposits are seen in membranous glomerulonephritis, subendothelial deposits are seen in immune complex-mediated MPGN (previous term type I MPGN) and highly electron-dense intramembranous deposits in dense deposit disease-DDD (previous term type II MPGN). In lupus, nephritis deposits can be seen in subendothelial, subepithelial, and mesangial locations within the glomerulus.

Normal adult glomerular capillary basement membrane is 200–400 nm in thickness. It may be thickened due to deposition of immune complexes, substances such as amyloid, due to microangiopathy or due to age related changes. It can be thickened in membranous nephropathy, diabetes and MPGN. Wrinkling of capillary basement membrane may be seen in ischemic collapse as in hypertension and in HUS.

Bowman's space may be obliterated by exudates, synechiae, or crescents; the space may be cystically dilated in congenital nephrotic syndrome or in cases with the ischaemic collapse of glomerular tuft.

Capsular basement membrane may be fragmented in Wegener's granulomatosis and Goodpasture's syndrome and the capsule may be thickened due to deposits or pericapsular fibrosis.

1.4 Renal Tubules

Tubules may reveal atrophy, hypertrophy, or abnormalities of lining epithelium. Various degenerative changes like cytoplasmic vacuolation, pigmentation, calcification, nuclear inclusions, or multinucleation may be encountered. Protein reabsorption droplets and lipid droplets can be seen in patients with heavy proteinuria. Many different forms of tubular casts including granular casts, WBC casts, RBC casts, epithelial cell casts, myoglobin casts, and fractured casts (light chain cast nephropathy) can be seen.

1.5 Renal Interstitium

Normal renal biopsy shows minimal interstitial tissue. Interstitial fibrosis needs to be differentiated from edema. Interstitial inflammatory infiltrate in a majority of cases may not be indicative of definitive etiology except in the case of infiltrate chiefly comprising of neutrophils, which is indicative of infective pathology. Granulomatous inflammation can be seen in the interstitium. Besides tuberculosis, epithelioid cell granulomas may also be seen in drug-induced interstitial nephritis, sarcoidosis, and pauci-immune crescentic glomerulonephritis.

1.6 Renal Vessels

Both large and small size renal arteries and arterioles should be evaluated for the presence of intimo-medial changes including endothelial cell swelling, edema, mucoid change, sclerosis, fibroelastosis, hyalinosis, and medial hyperplasia. Fibrinoid necrosis of the vessel wall may be seen in malignant hypertension and vasculitic disorders.

1.7 Immunofluorescence and Immunohistochemistry

Immunostaining has proved essential for primary diagnosis of conditions like Goodpasture's syndrome, IgA nephropathy, membranous glomerulonephritis, C3 glomerulopathy, immune complex-mediated glomerulonephritis including post-infectious glomerulonephritis, MPGN, and lupus nephritis. The commonly employed panel includes a demonstration of immunoglobulins (IgG, IgM, and IgA), immunoglobulin light chains (kappa and lambda), complement components (C3 and C1q), albumin, and fibrinogen. Interpretation of results depends upon distribution, pattern, and intensity of immunostaining.

1.8 Electron Microscopy

In the USA and many European countries, EM studies on renal biopsy are done in routine. Wherever possible immuno-electron microscopy can also be carried out. However, EM is essential for the diagnosis of only a few conditions like minimal change disease, basement membrane abnormalities of Alport's syndrome and thin basement membrane disease. It is extremely useful in glomerular diseases with organized deposits like fibrillary and immunotactoid glomerulonephritis, monoclonal immunoglobulin deposition disease, etc.

Although EM studies greatly enhance the diagnostic scope, for logistic reasons, they are essential only infrequently and well-conducted light microscopic evaluation along with immunofluorescence (IF) are adequate in the majority of cases.

1.9 Renal Biopsy Reporting

Renal biopsy report should record the presence of cortical and medullary tissue along with total number of glomeruli seen in the biopsy and the number of completely sclerosed glomeruli. Changes in different compartments (glomerular, tubular, interstitial, and vascular) should be recorded noting the relative severity and distribution of lesions. An attempt should also be made to assess the activity and chronicity of lesions which might determine the therapeutic benefit and prognostic outcome. The diagnosis should preferably be in morphological terms with a suggestion of etiological factors, clinical terms, and differential diagnosis wherever possible.

1.10 Distribution of Lesions in Renal Biopsy (Fig. 1.4)

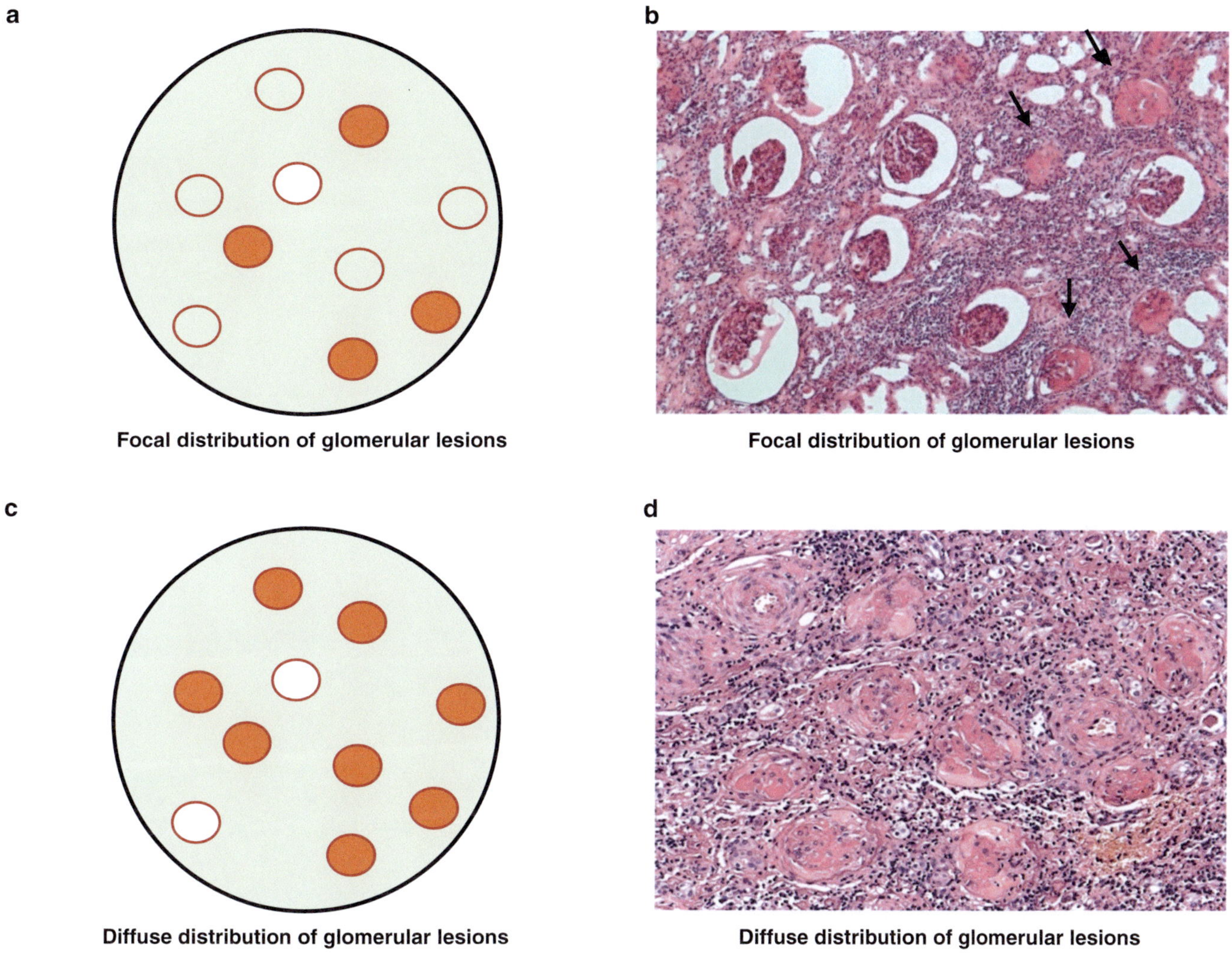

Fig. 1.4 Commonly used terms in describing the morphological distribution of lesions in renal biopsy. Lesions are described as focal when involving <50% of glomeruli and diffuse when involving ≥50% glomeruli. (**a**) Schematic representation of focal lesions in a renal biopsy where only 4/10 glomeruli are involved and (**b**) microphotograph showing similar focal nature of the involvement where only 4/11 glomeruli (arrows) are involved. (**c**) Schematic representation of diffuse lesions in a renal biopsy where 8/10 glomeruli are involved and (**d**) microphotograph showing that all the glomeruli (100%) are globally sclerosed

1.11 Tubular Changes (Fig. 1.5)

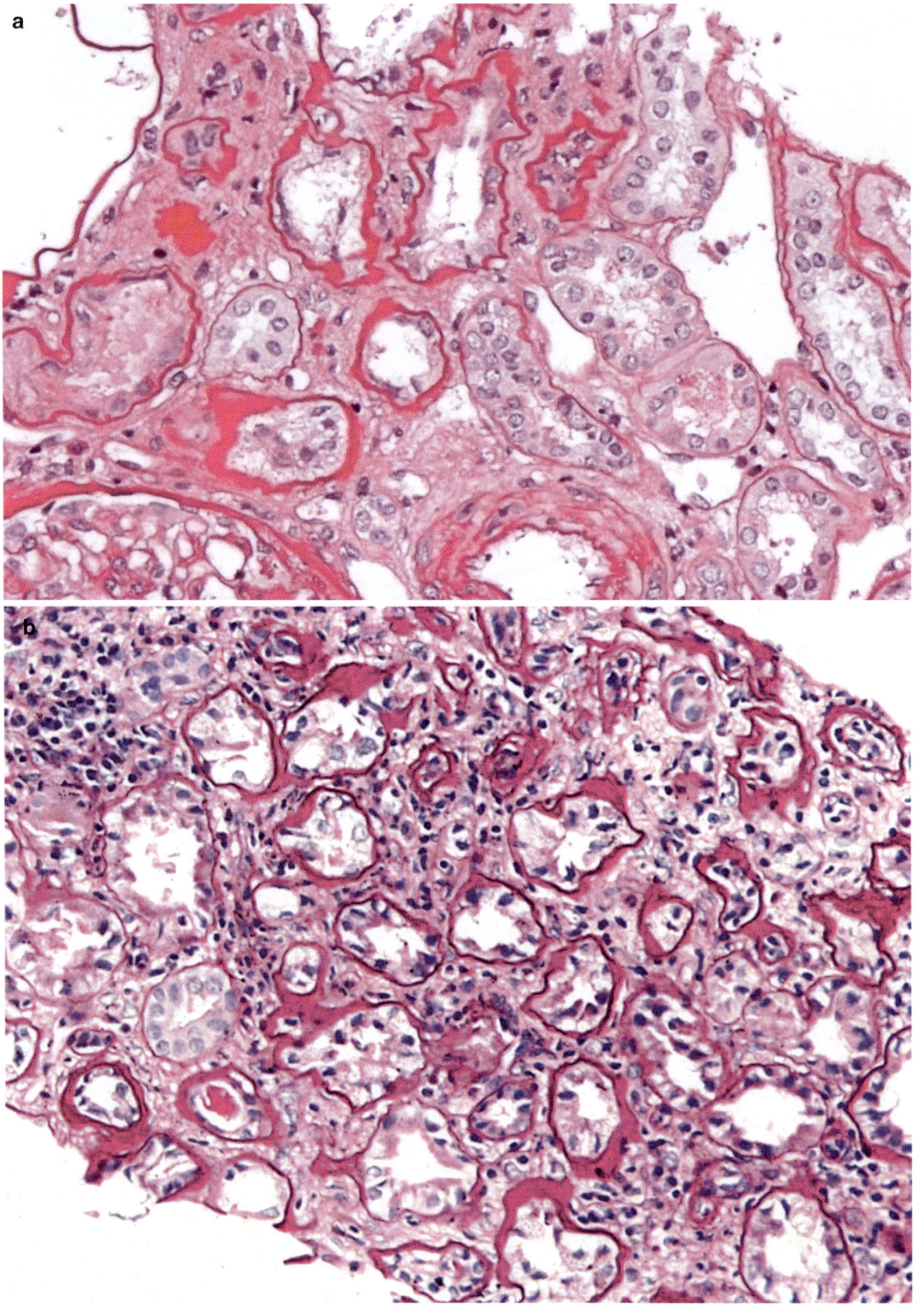

Fig. 1.5 Microphotographs showing mild and severe tubular atrophy. (**a**) Only few proximal convoluted tubules are showing atrophy, therefore the lesion is mild/focal. (**b**) Shows that almost all (>50%) proximal convoluted tubules are showing atrophy, therefore the lesion is severe/diffuse. (**a**) PAS ×400, (**b**) PAS ×200

1.12 Extent of Glomerular Involvement (Fig. 1.6)

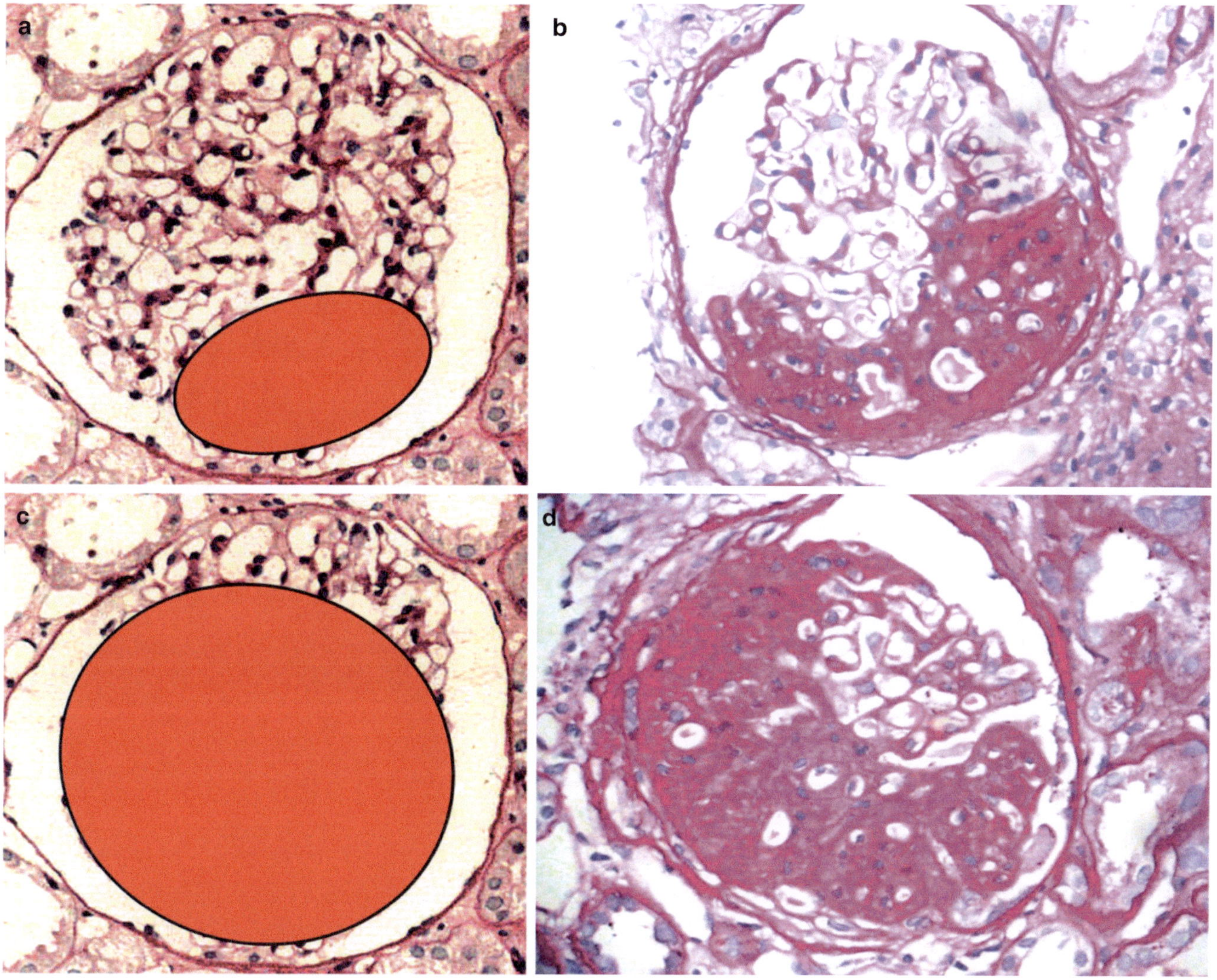

Fig. 1.6 Representation of the extent of glomerular involvement by semi-schematic diagrams and microphotographs of glomerular lesions explaining segmental and global glomerular lesions. The extent of glomerular involvement is called segmental when involving <50% of the glomerular tuft. (**a**) The semi-schematic diagram and (**b**) the microphotograph showing the segmental glomerular sclerosis which is involving <50% of the glomerulus. The extent of glomerular involvement is global when ≥50% of the glomerular tuft is involved. (**c**) The semi-schematic diagram and (**d**) the microphotograph showing the global glomerulosclerosis involving ≥50% of the glomerular tuft

1.13 Morphology of Normal Glomerulus (Fig. 1.7)

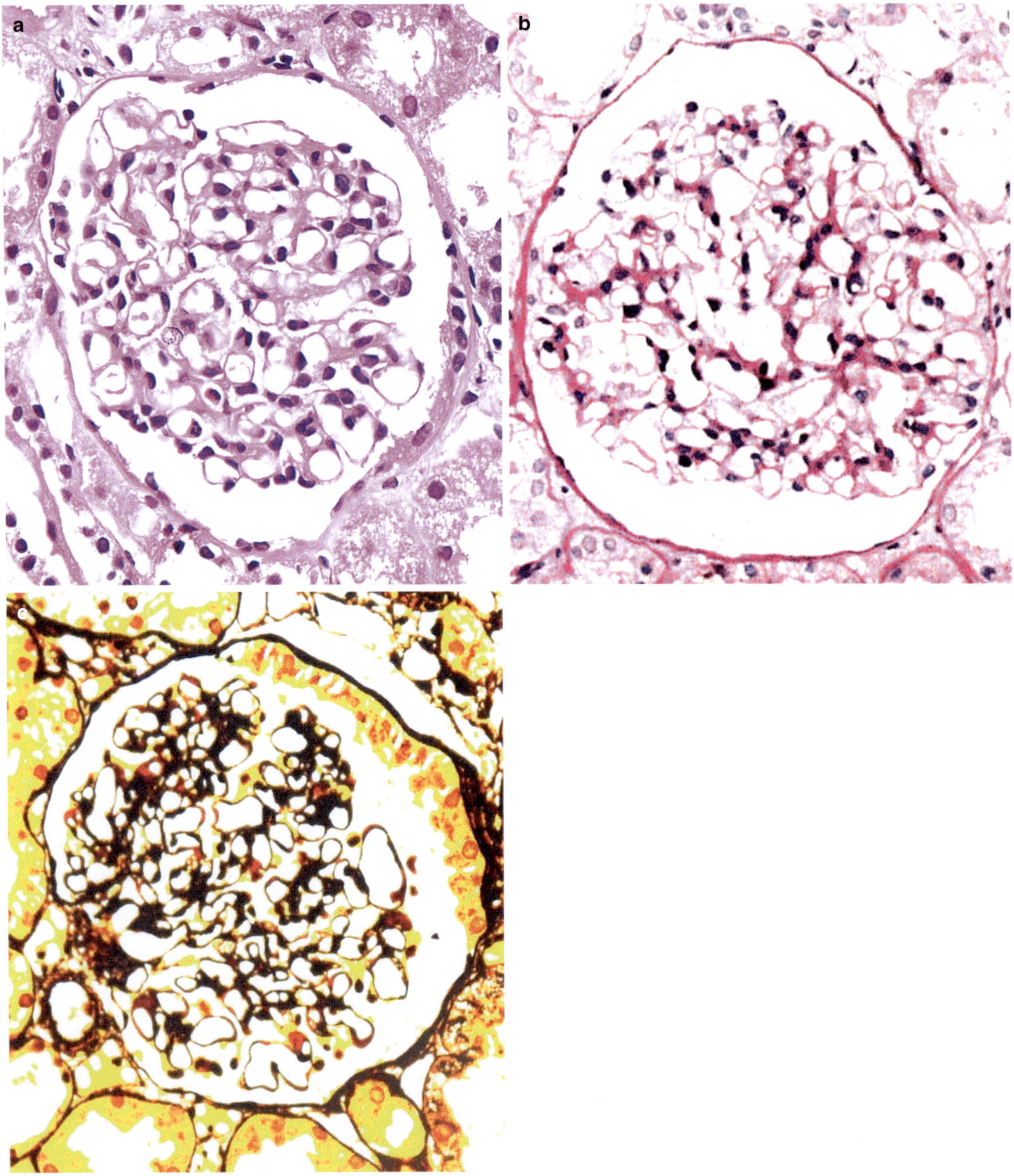

Fig. 1.7 Morphlogical appearance of the normal glomerulus. The glomeruli are spherical in shape and about 200 ± 20 μ in size. A glomerulus has 4–5 ill-defined lobules of glomerular tuft of capillaries lined by endothelial cells. On the outer aspect of glomerular capillaries podocytes can be seen. The capillary basement membrane is thin, smooth, and uniform and the mesangium contains only 1–2 cells/stalk. The Bowman's capsule is thin and uniform and completely surrounds the glomerulus, parietal epithelial cells line the Bowman's capsule; the Bowman's space is clear. (**a**) HE ×400, (**b**) PAS ×400, and (**c**) PSM ×400

1.14 Common GBM Alterations in Diseases Involving Glomeruli (Fig. 1.8)

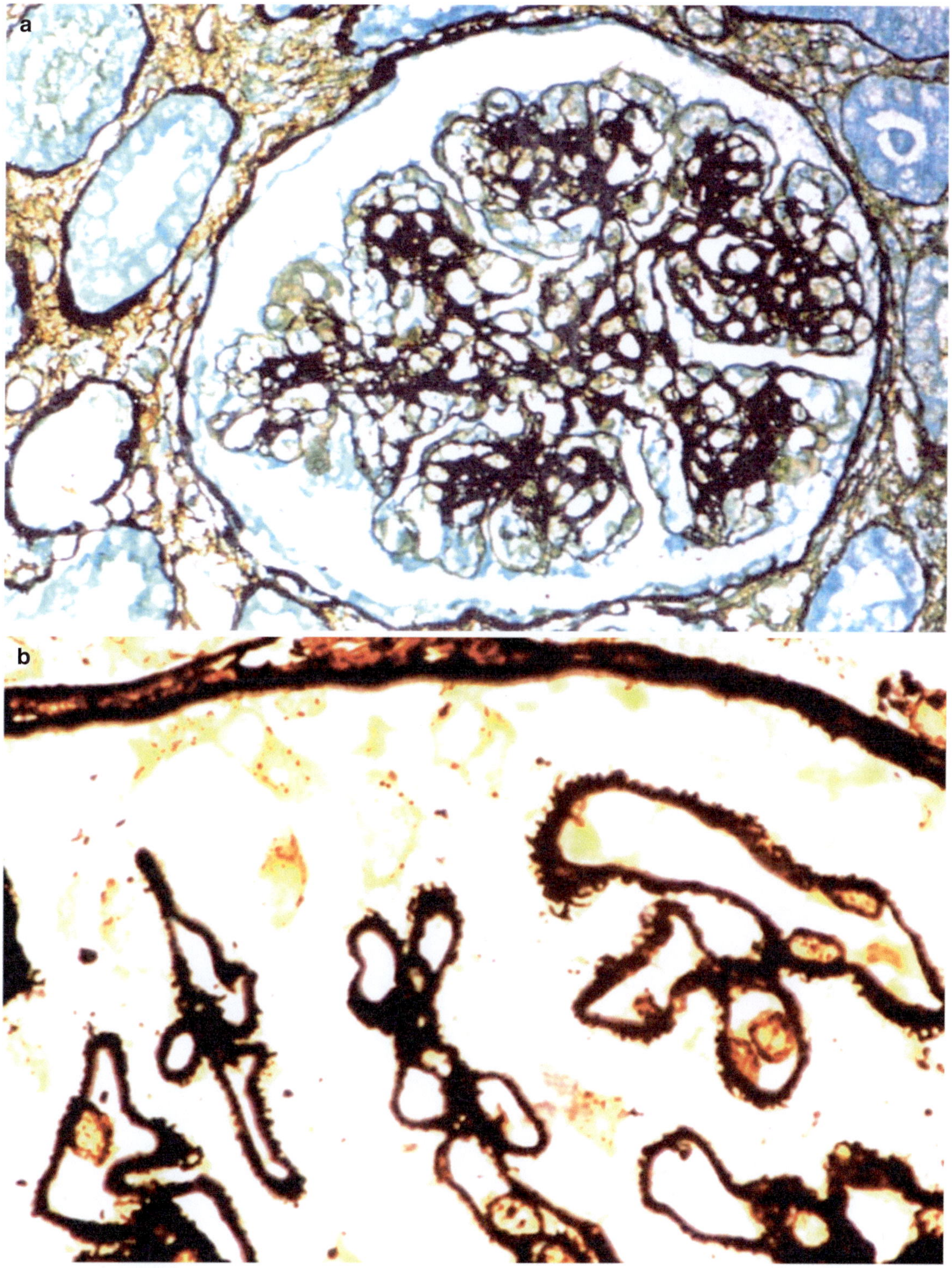

Fig. 1.8 Common GBM alterations in diseases involving glomeruli. (**a**) Wide splitting of GBM with interpositioning of mesangium. The GBM has a double contour with mesangium (greenish material) between two layers of GBM; its best identified in the peripheral glomerular capillary loops (PSM ×400). This morphological appearance is due to subendothelial immune deposits and mesangial interposition as in MPGN. (**b**) Epimemranous spikes, the outer surface of the GBM shows saw-like projections. It is also best seen in the peripheral glomerular capillary loops (PSM ×1000). It is due to intervening projections of basement membrane between subepithelial immune deposits as in membranous glomerulopathy

1.15 Location of Immune Deposits in GBM (Fig. 1.9)

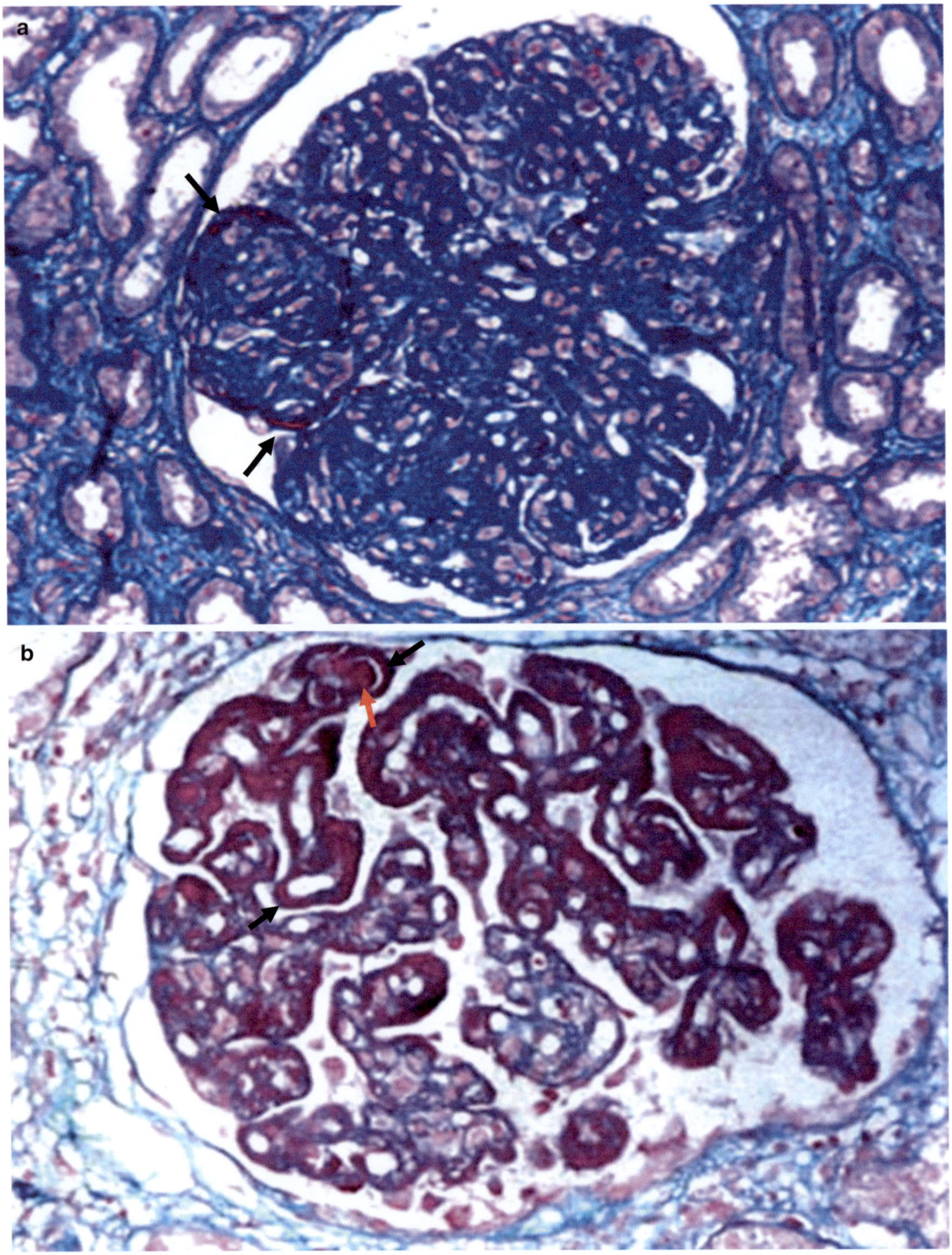

Fig. 1.9 Location of immune deposits in GBM. (**a**) Intramembranous and subendothelial deposits of immune complexes can be observed in MPGN, in MT stain these deposits give fuchsinophilic appearance (arrow, MT ×400). It is best observed in peripheral capillary loops. (**b**) Predominantly subendothelial deposition of immune complexes (Fuchsinophilic staining) is observed in class III and class IV lupus nephropathy. Due to immune complex deposition, the glomerular capillary loops become thick and stiff (similar to inoculating wire loops) which is why these lesions are called wire loop lesions (black arrow). These lesions are best observed in peripheral capillary loops (MT ×400); intraluminal fibrin thrombi are also seen in this glomerulus (red arrow)

1.16 Fibrin Thrombi and Segmental Fibrinoid Necrosis (Fig. 1.10)

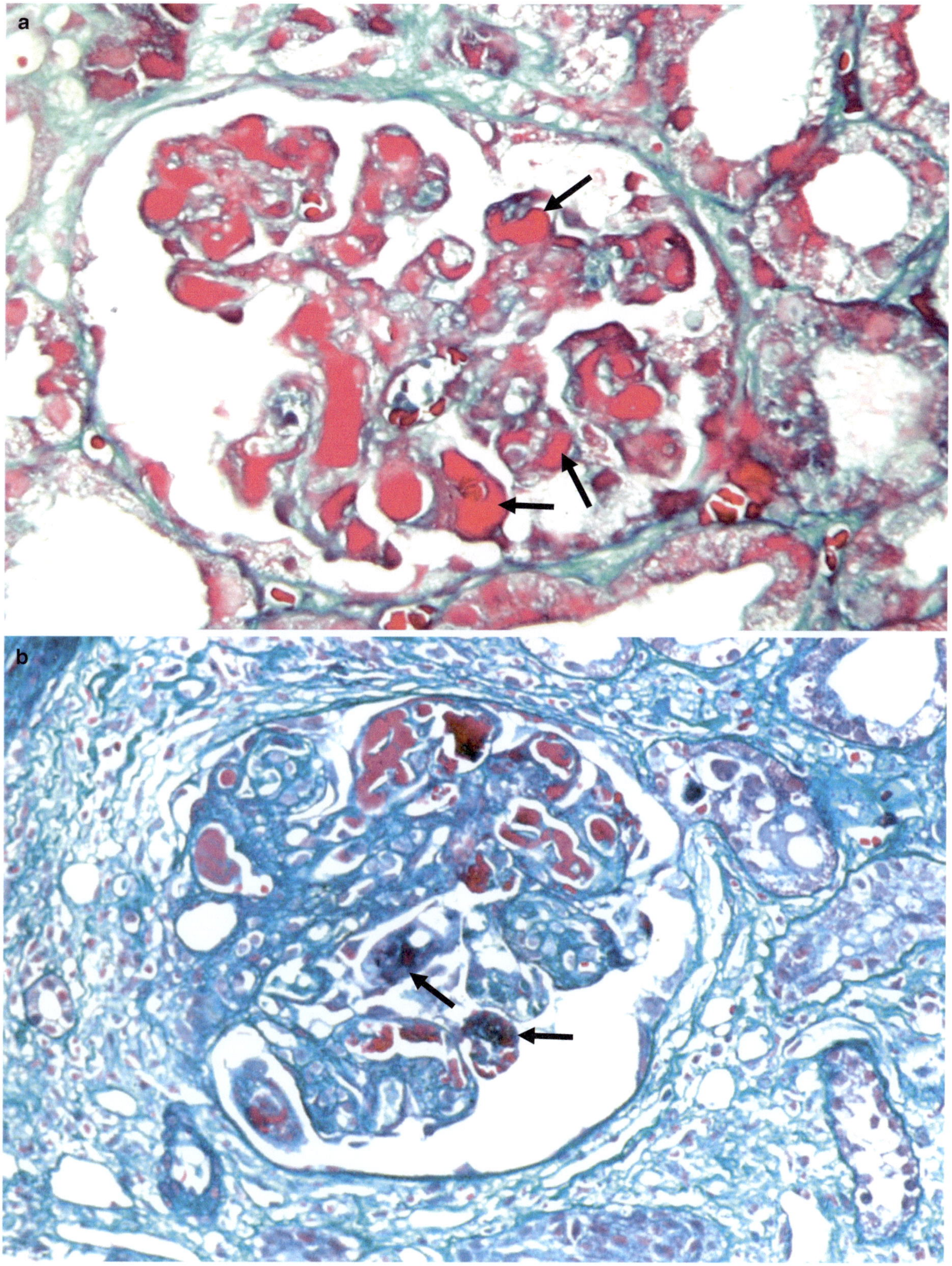

Fig. 1.10 Intracapillary fibrin thrombi (**a**) are observed in certain glomerular lesions such as TMA. They are located in the lumen of glomerular capillary loops and appear as fuchsinophilic intraluminal deposits in MT stain (arrows, MT ×400). Segmental glomerular necrosis (**b**) can be observed in several glomerular diseases including lupus nephritis. It can be demonstrated by MT stain (arrows, MT ×400)

1.17 **Crescents** (Fig. 1.11)

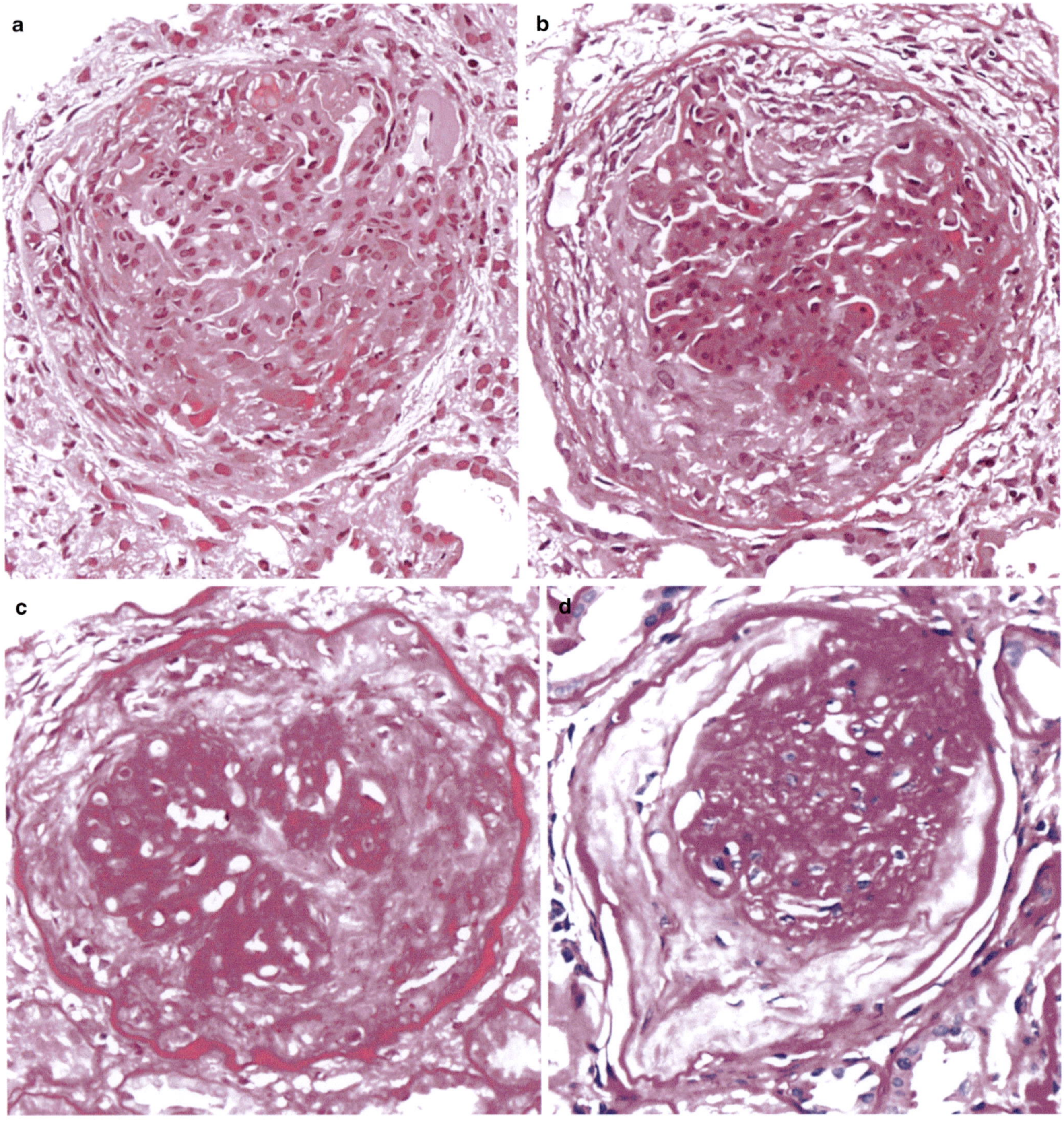

Fig. 1.11 Microphotographs showing cellular (**a** and **b**), fibrocellular (**c**) and fibrous crescents (**d**). Crescents are found in several primary and secondary glomerular diseases. (**a** and **b**) HE ×400, (**c** and **d**) PAS ×400

2 Minimal Change Disease (MCD)

Minimal change disease (MCD) is the most common cause of nephrotic syndrome in children and the third most common cause in adults. Edema including pedal and periorbital is the most common presenting symptom in children and young adults whereas renal dysfunction and hypertension may be presenting symptoms in elderly patients. Light microscopic examination of renal biopsy shows almost normal-appearing glomeruli or in some cases mild mesangial prominence may be seen. Immunofluorescence is usually negative; however, at times, low-intensity mesangial IgM deposits may be seen. On electron microscopy, diffuse effacement of podocyte foot process is observed without any electron-dense deposits. In the mesangial hypercellularity variant of MCD >4 cells per mesangial region affecting at least 80% glomeruli may be present (Fig. 2.1).

P. Gupta, R. K. Gupta, *Pathology of Glomerular Diseases*, https://doi.org/10.1007/978-981-19-1430-0_2

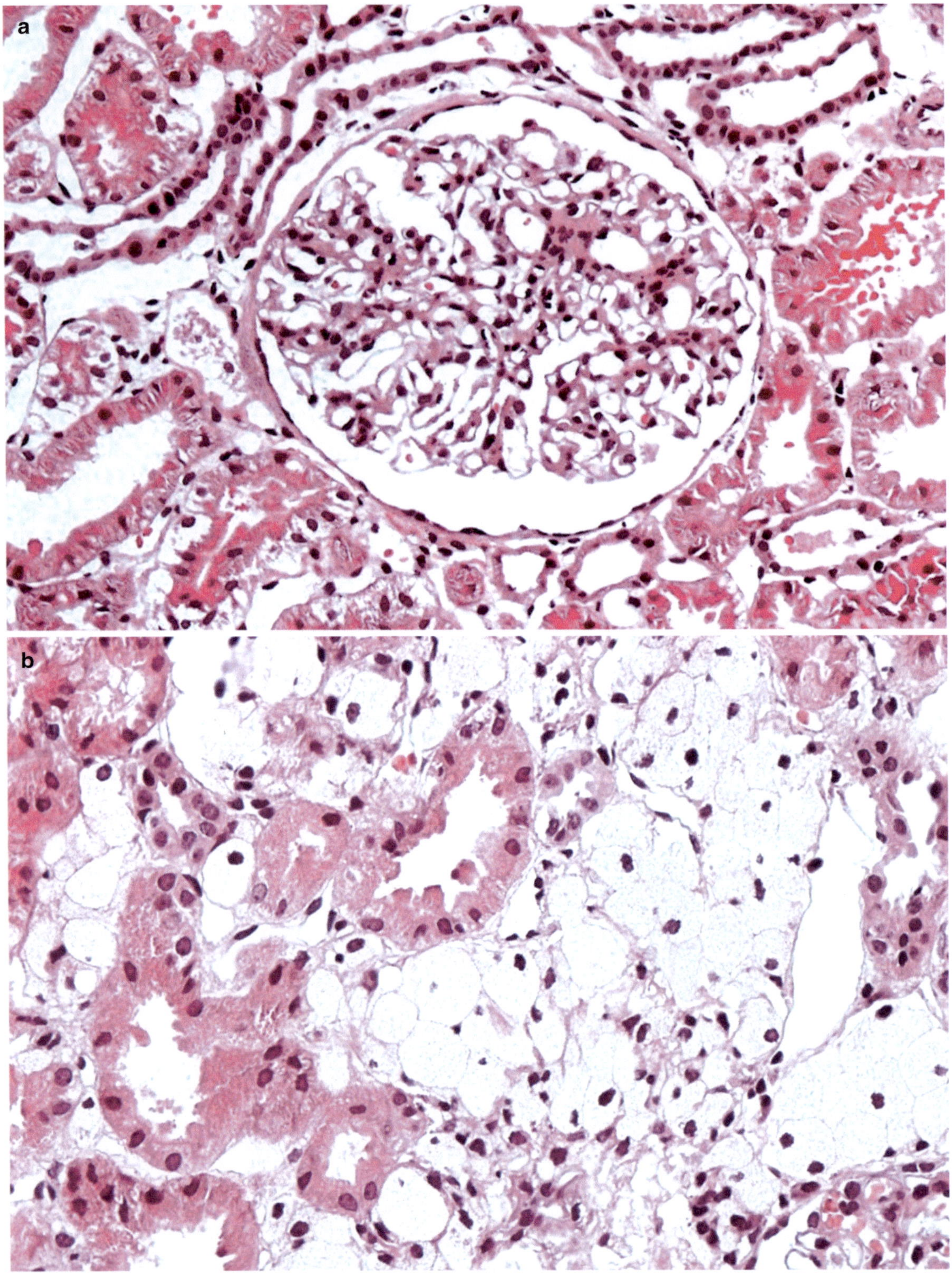

Fig. 2.1 **Minimal Change Disease** A 10-years female child presented with steroid-resistant nephrotic syndrome. She was normotensive and had no hematuria. Urinary protein was 4+ with bland urinary sediment; 24 h urinary protein was 4.2 g. Her serum albumin was 1.2 g/dL, serum cholesterol was 394 mg/dL, and serum creatinine was 0.15 mg/dL. Serum complement C3 was within normal limits and ANA and HbsAg were negative. Renal biopsy had 17 glomeruli, on light microscopy none of them had any morphological abnormality; interstitium had plenty of foam cells. Renal tubules and blood vessels were also unremarkable. EM showed diffuse effacement and flattening of foot processes of podocytes. No electron-dense deposits were seen. (**a** and **b**) HE ×400, (**c**) PAS ×400, (**d**) PSM ×400 and (**e**) EM (identity of the patient has been concealed)

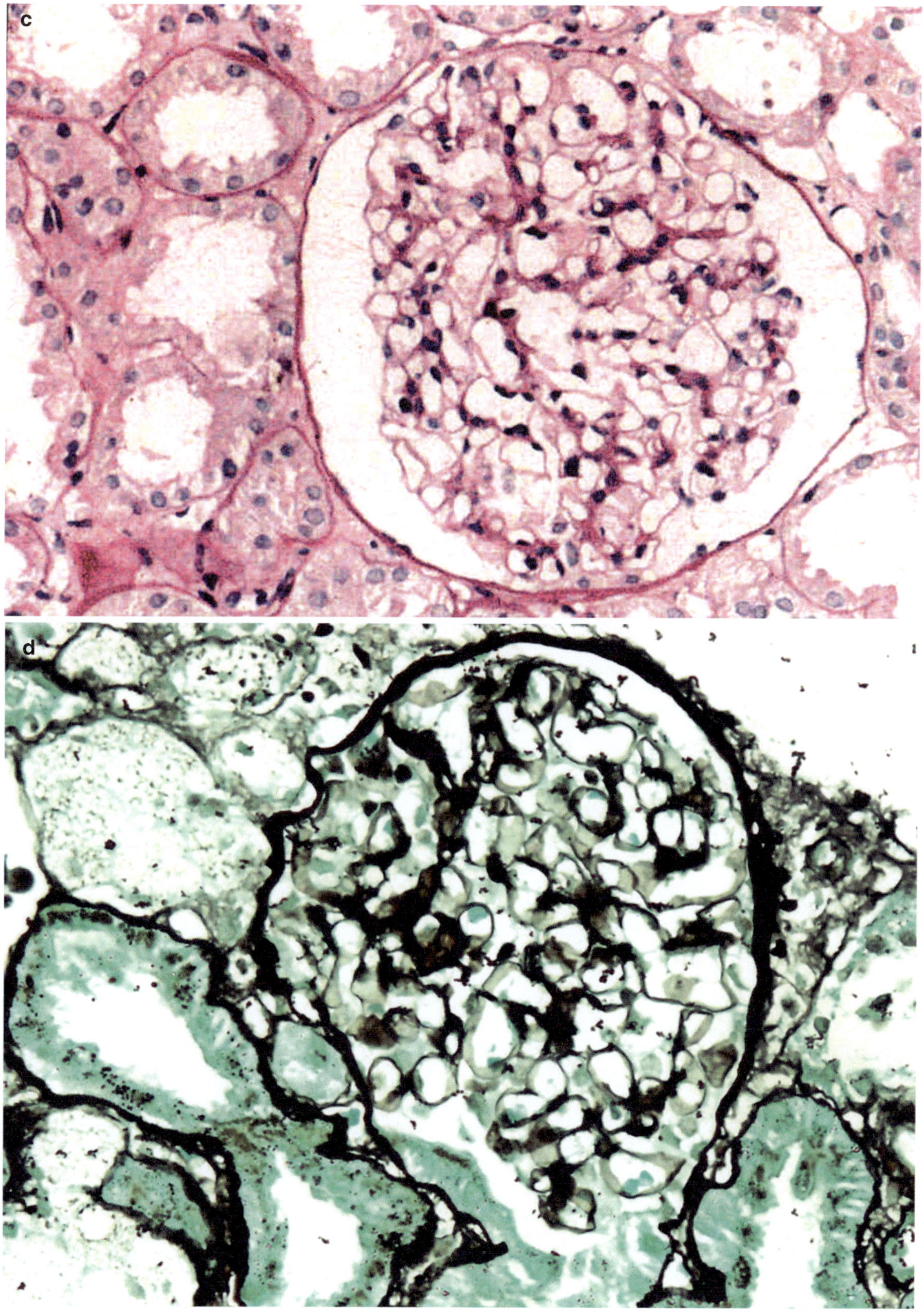

Fig. 2.1 (continued)

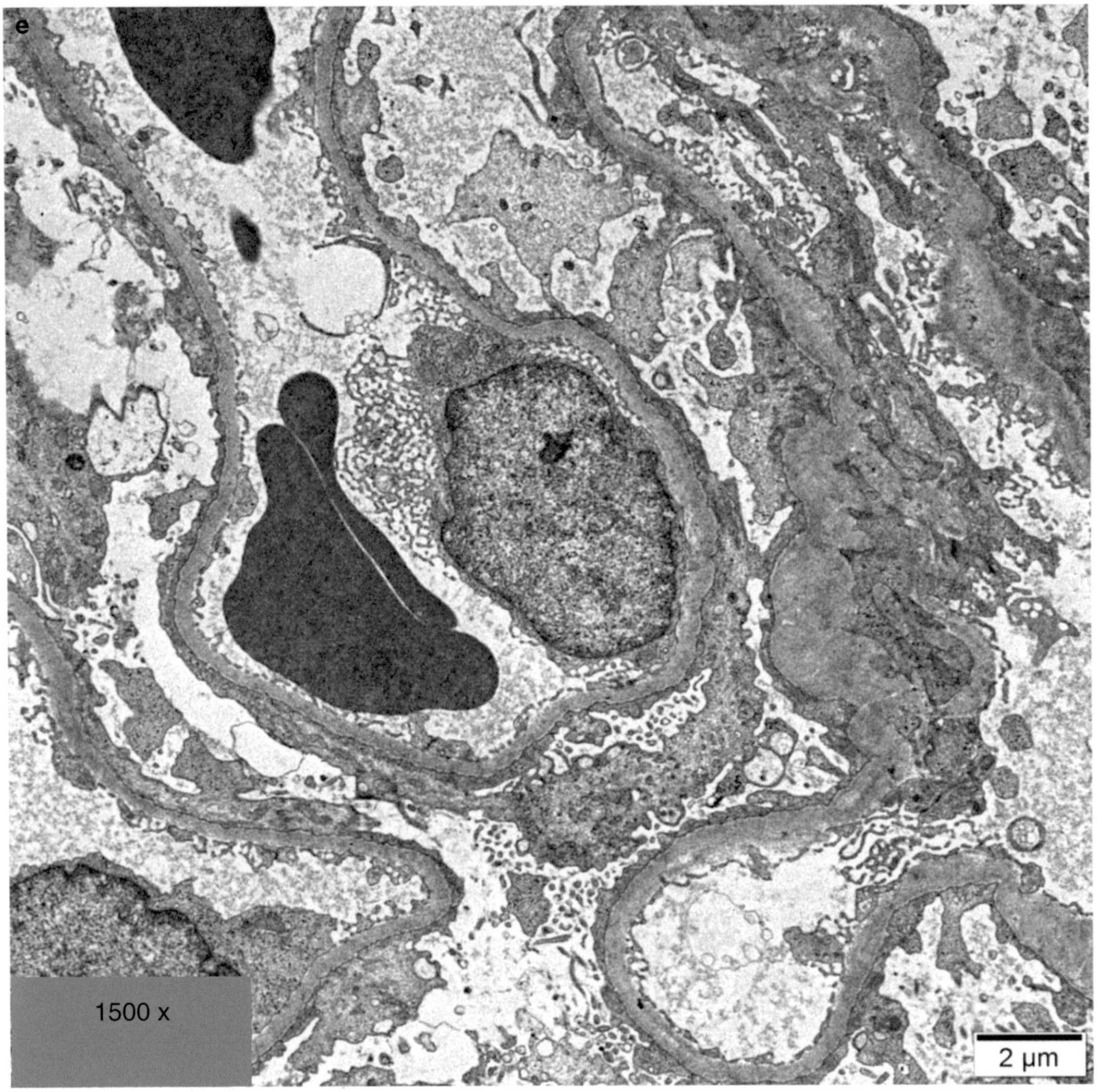

Fig. 2.1 (continued)

Further Reading

Brenner BM, Nachman PH, Jennette JC, Falk RJ. Primary glomerular disease. In: Brenner BM, editor. The kidney. 8th ed. Philadelphia: Saunders Elsevier; 2008. p. 987–1066.

Cameron JS. The nephrotic syndrome and its complications. Am J Kidney Dis. 1987;10:157–71.

Eddy AA, Symons JM. Nephrotic syndrome in childhood. Lancet. 2003;362:629–39.

Gulati S, Gupta RK. Do current recommendations of kidney biopsy in nephrotic syndrome need modifications? Pediatr Nephrol. 2002;17:404–8.

Gulati S, Sural S, Sharma RK, Gupta A, Gupta RK. Spectrum of adolescent onset nephrotic syndrome in Indian children. Pediatr Nephrol. 2001;16:1045–8.

Pardo V, Riesgo I, Zilleruelo G, Strauss J. The clinical significance of mesangial IgM deposits and mesangial hypercellularity in minimal change nephrotic syndrome. Am J Kidney Dis. 1984;3:264–9.

Ranganathan S. Pathology of podocytopathies causing nephrotic syndrome in children. Front Pediatr. 2016;4:32.

Waldman M, Crew RJ, Valeri A, Busch J, Stokes B, Markowitz G, D'Agati V, Appel G. Adult minimal-change disease: clinical characteristics, treatment, and outcomes. Clin J Am Soc Nephrol. 2007;2:445–53.

3 Focal Segmental Glomerulosclerosis (FSGS)

Focal segmental glomerulosclerosis is a type of podocytopathy characterized by a focal and segmental increase in the mesangial matrix with scarring and obliteration of the glomerular capillary lumen. According to Columbia classification, various morphological variants such as NOS, perihilar, collapsing, tip, and cellular have been identified. The prognostic significance of these variants is debatable. Based on etiopathogenesis, FSGS has also been classified into primary and secondary FSGS. The secondary FSGS could be associated with various conditions such as maladaptive as in obesity, drug induced, viral infections, and genetic forms (autosomal dominant, recessive, X-linked) or mitochondrial. FSGS can also be encountered in post-transplant settings, both recurrent and de novo forms have been recognized. Primary FSGS is thought to be the result of a circulating factor that causes podocyte injury and patients have nephrotic syndrome. It shows diffuse podocyte foot process effacement and responds well to steroids, plasmapheresis, or immunomodulatory agents. Secondary FSGS shows focal foot process effacement; it usually has subnephrotic proteinuria which requires renin–angiotensin–aldosterone inhibitors and resolution of an offending agent like virus or drugs.

3.1 FSGS (NOS)

It is the most common pattern of FSGS. It is characterized by segmental obliteration of the glomerulus by increased extracellular matrix resulting in consolidation of the glomerular capillary tuft. Adhesion of sclerosed tuft to Bowman's capsule can be seen. Podocyte hypertrophy or hyperplasia may also be appreciated. Intraglomerular foam cells and hyalinosis can be seen. Patchy focal tubular atrophy and interstitial fibrosis are usually present. Other variants of FSGS have to be excluded to make this diagnosis (Fig. 3.1).

P. Gupta, R. K. Gupta, *Pathology of Glomerular Diseases*, https://doi.org/10.1007/978-981-19-1430-0_3

a

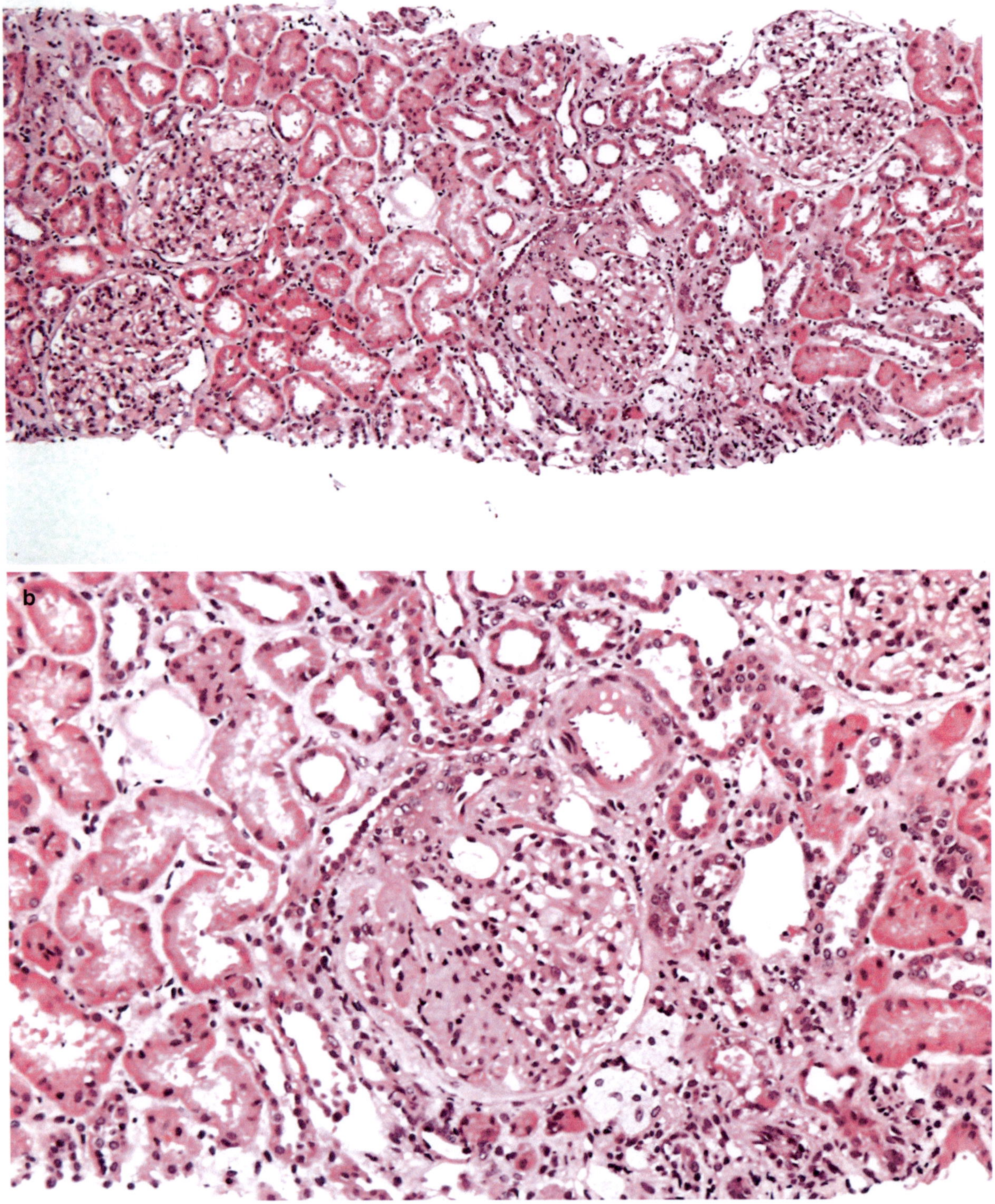

Fig. 3.1 **FSGS (NOS)** A 30-years female patient presented with an increased frequency of micturition since 2–3 months. On clinical examination she was found to have pedal edema; her systemic examination was wnl. On laboratory workup she was found to have nephrotic range proteinuria with urinary protein 3+ and bland urinary sediment; 24 h urinary protein was 4.8 g. Serum cholesterol and serum creatinine were wnl. Serum C3 and C4 were normal being 970 mg/L and 340 mg/L. HBsAg and ANA were negative. Renal biopsy had ten glomeruli; one glomerulus was globally sclerosed and one had segmental sclerosis; foam cells were present in the glomeruli as well as in interstitium. Focal tubular atrophy and focal interstitial fibrosis were present. IF showed IgM deposits in sclerotic mesangial areas. EM showed diffuse effacement and focal microvillous transformation of foot processes. (**a**) HE ×100, (**b**) HE ×200, (**c**) and (**d**) HE ×400, (**e**) and (**f**) PAS ×400, (**g**) PSM ×400; (**h**) IF ×400, (**i**) and (**j**) EM (identity of patient has been concealed)

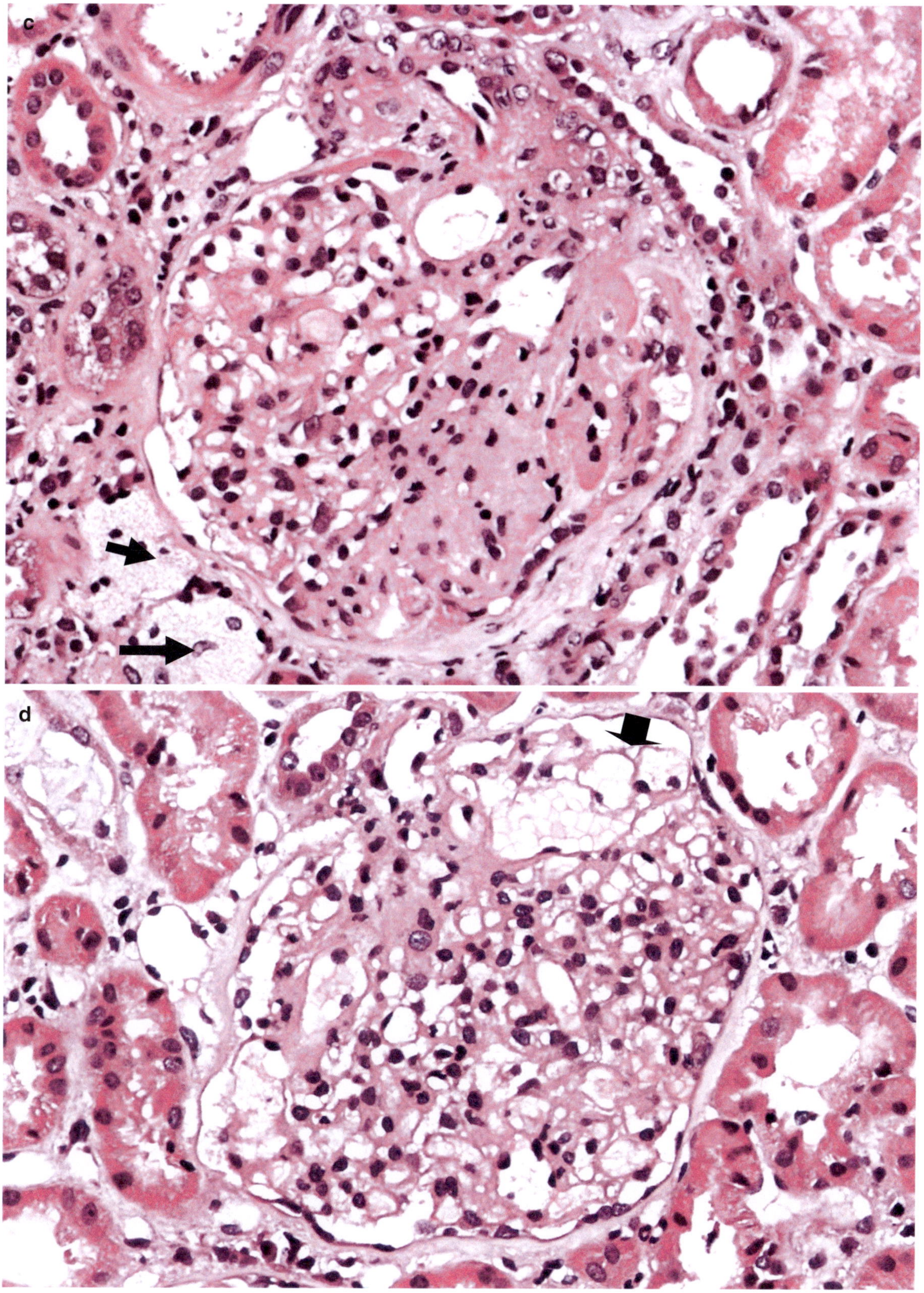

Fig. 3.1 (continued)

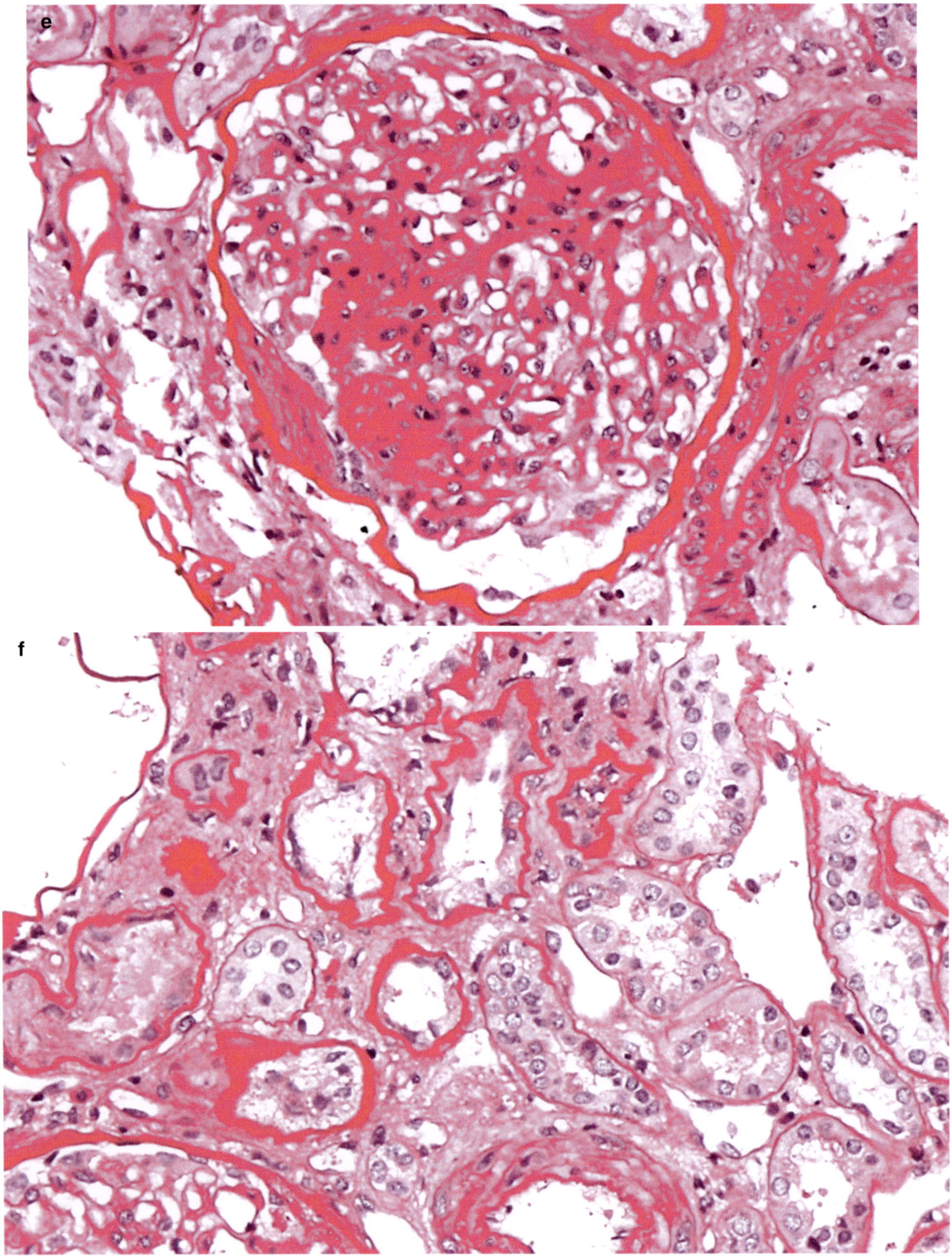

Fig. 3.1 (continued)

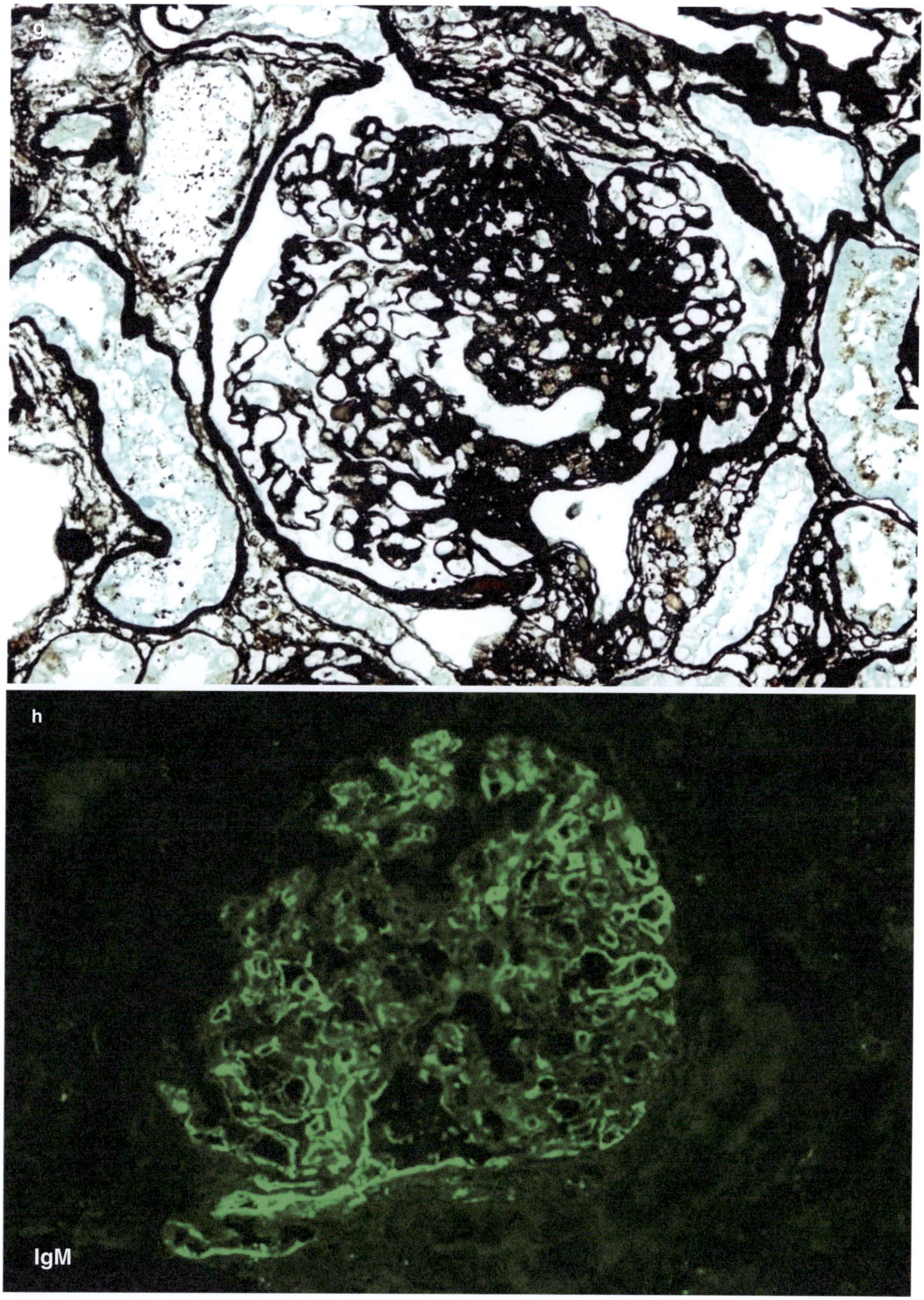

Fig. 3.1 (continued)

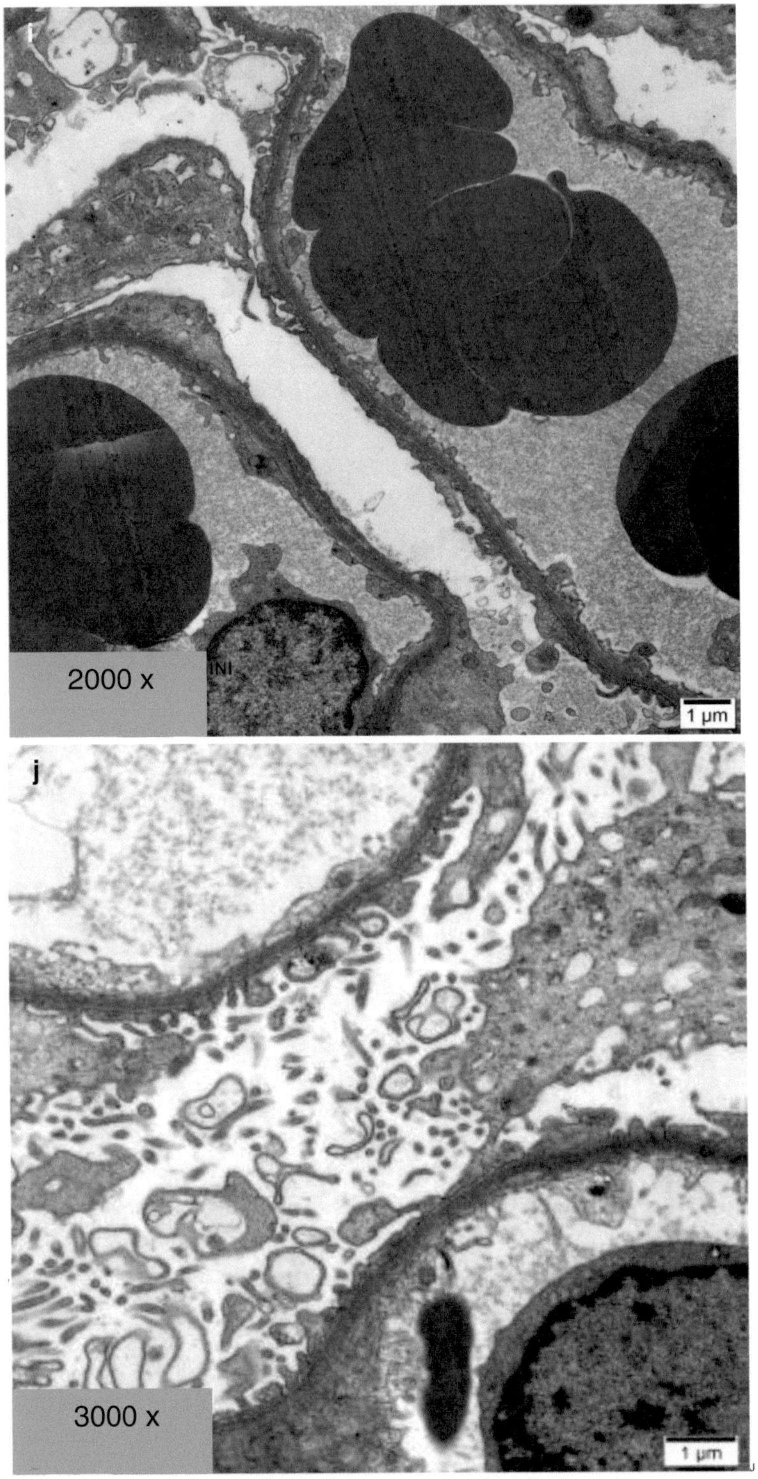

Fig. 3.1 (continued)

3.2 FSGS (Perihilar Variant)

In this morphologic type, segmental sclerosis and hyalinosis are seen in the perihilar region involving >50% of segmentally sclerotic glomeruli. Glomerulomegaly and intraglomerular foam cells can be seen. This variant is commonly seen in maladaptive FSGS as in patients with obesity, renal agenesis, and reflux nephropathy, but can also be seen in primary FSGS (Fig. 3.2).

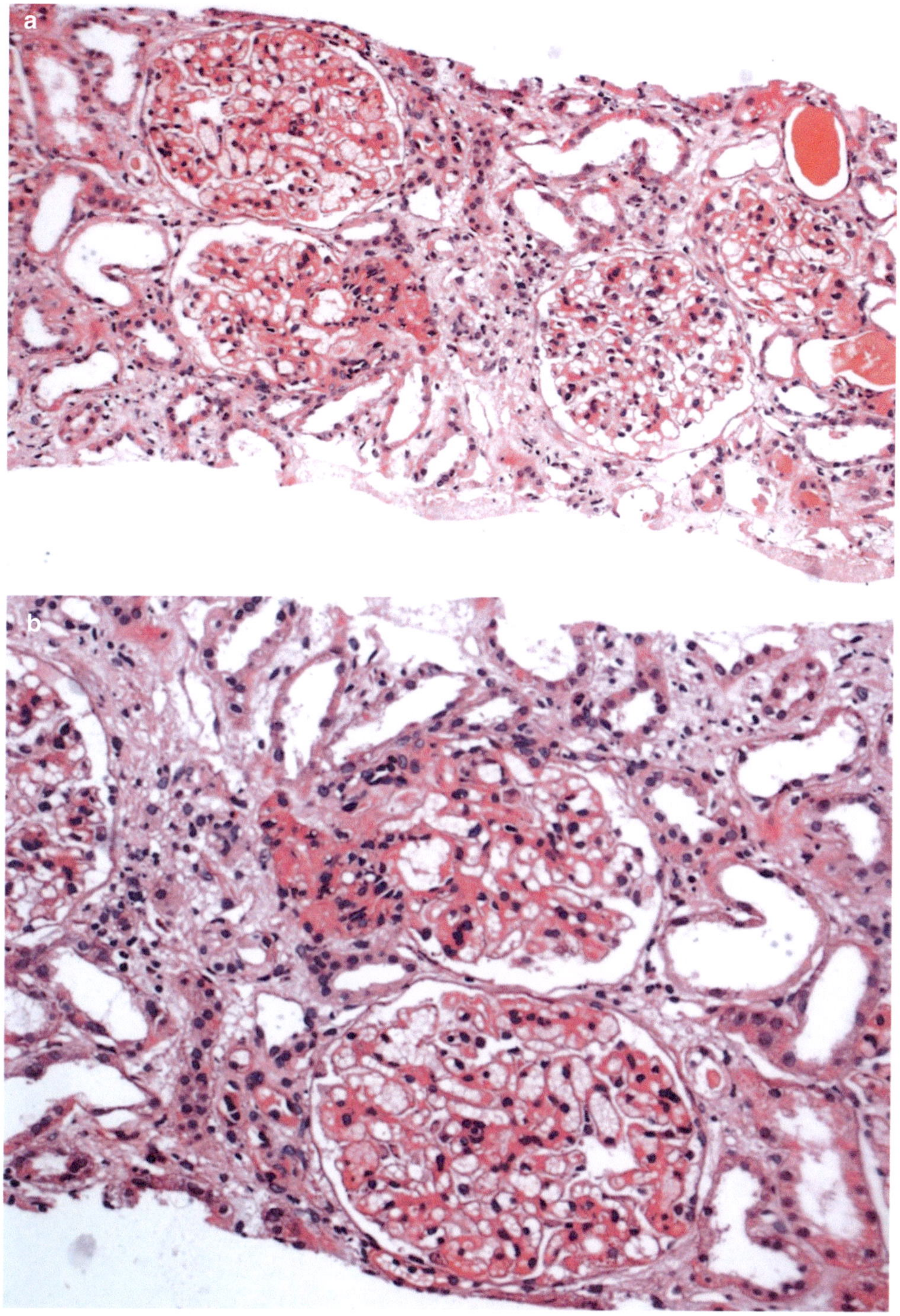

Fig. 3.2 **FSGS (Perihilar Variant)** A 62-years male patient presented with anasarca and facial puffiness. He had no h/o diabetes or hypertension. Urine analysis revealed protein 2+ with almost bland sediment; urinary 24 h protein was 11.9 g. Serum total protein/albumin being 5.0/1.7 g/dL. Serum creatinine was 4.38 mg/dL. Serum total cholesterol was 345 mg/dL with TG of 490 mg/dL. ANA, dsDNA, and ANCA were negative; serum complements C3 and C4 were wnl. One core renal biopsy was obtained which had 12 glomeruli, 10 were unremarkable and 2 showed perihilar sclerosis. Focal tubular atrophy with minimal interstitial lymphocytic infiltration and minimal fibrosis was present; renal blood vessels were unremarkable. IF revealed segmental mesangial IgM deposits. (**a**) HE ×100, (**b**) HE ×200, (**c**) HE ×400 and (**d**) MT ×400 (Contributor—Dr Megha Uppin, Associate Professor, Department of Pathology, Nizam's Institute of Medical Sciences, Hyderabad, India)

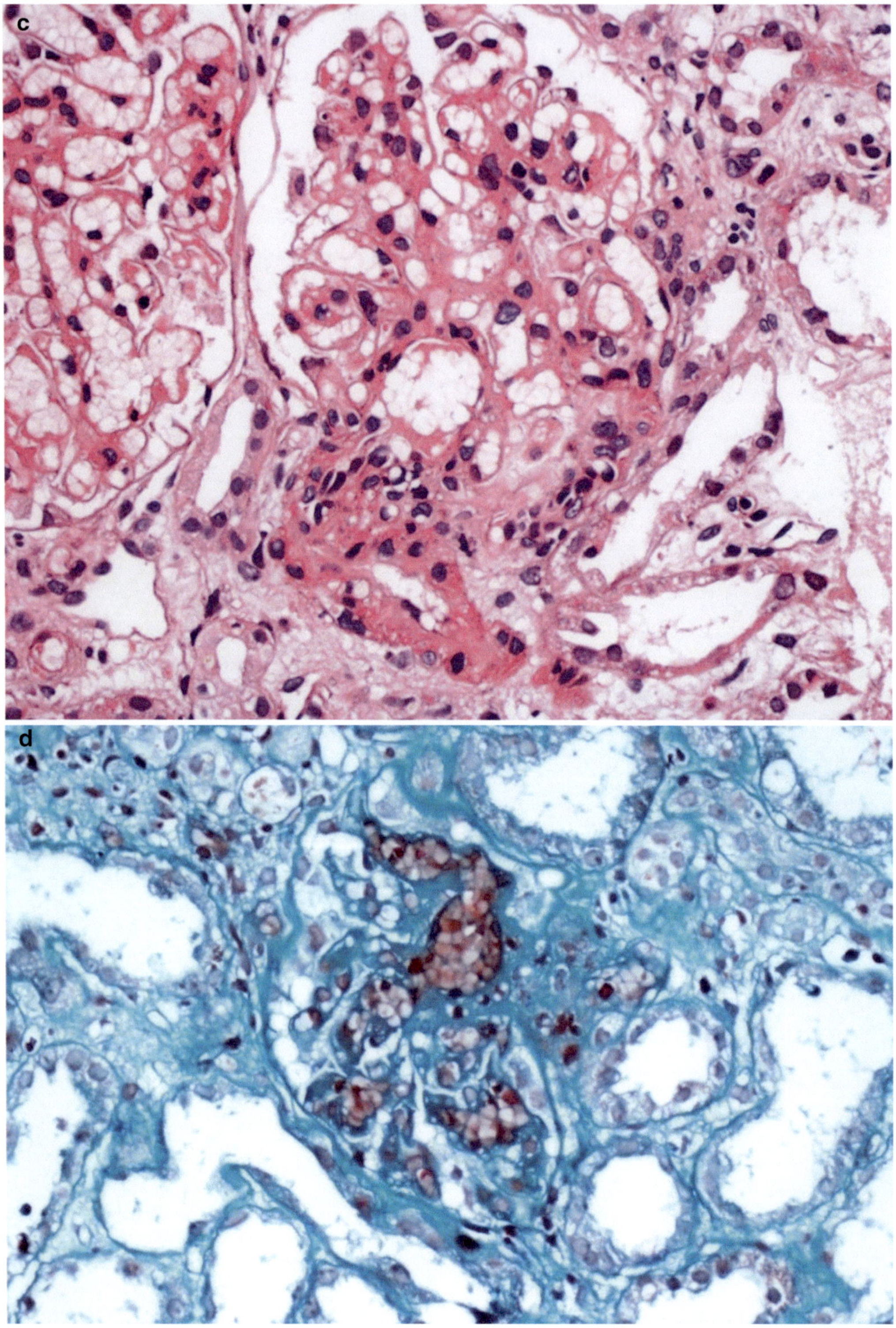

Fig. 3.2 (continued)

3.3 FSGS (Cellular Variant)

In this morphologic type >25% of glomerular capillary tuft of at least one glomerulus shows endocapillary hypercellularity. Hypercellularity could be due to endothelial cell proliferation, infiltrating leukocytes, or macrophages. Hyaline material, karyorrhexis, and fibrin deposition may be seen. Often there is accompanying hyperplasia of podocytes; pseudo-crescent formation can be seen. These patients have severe proteinuria and more frequently have nephrotic syndrome at presentation.

3.4 FSGS (Tip Variant)

In this morphologic type, peripheral 25% of the glomerular capillary tuft at the origin of the proximal tubule (tubular pole) will show either adhesion of glomerular capillary tuft with Bowman's capsule or confluence of podocytes with tubular or parietal epithelial cells. Endocapillary hypercellularity, foam cells, and hyalinosis can be seen. Collapsing variant should be excluded before making this diagnosis. This variant shows better steroid responsiveness (Fig. 3.3).

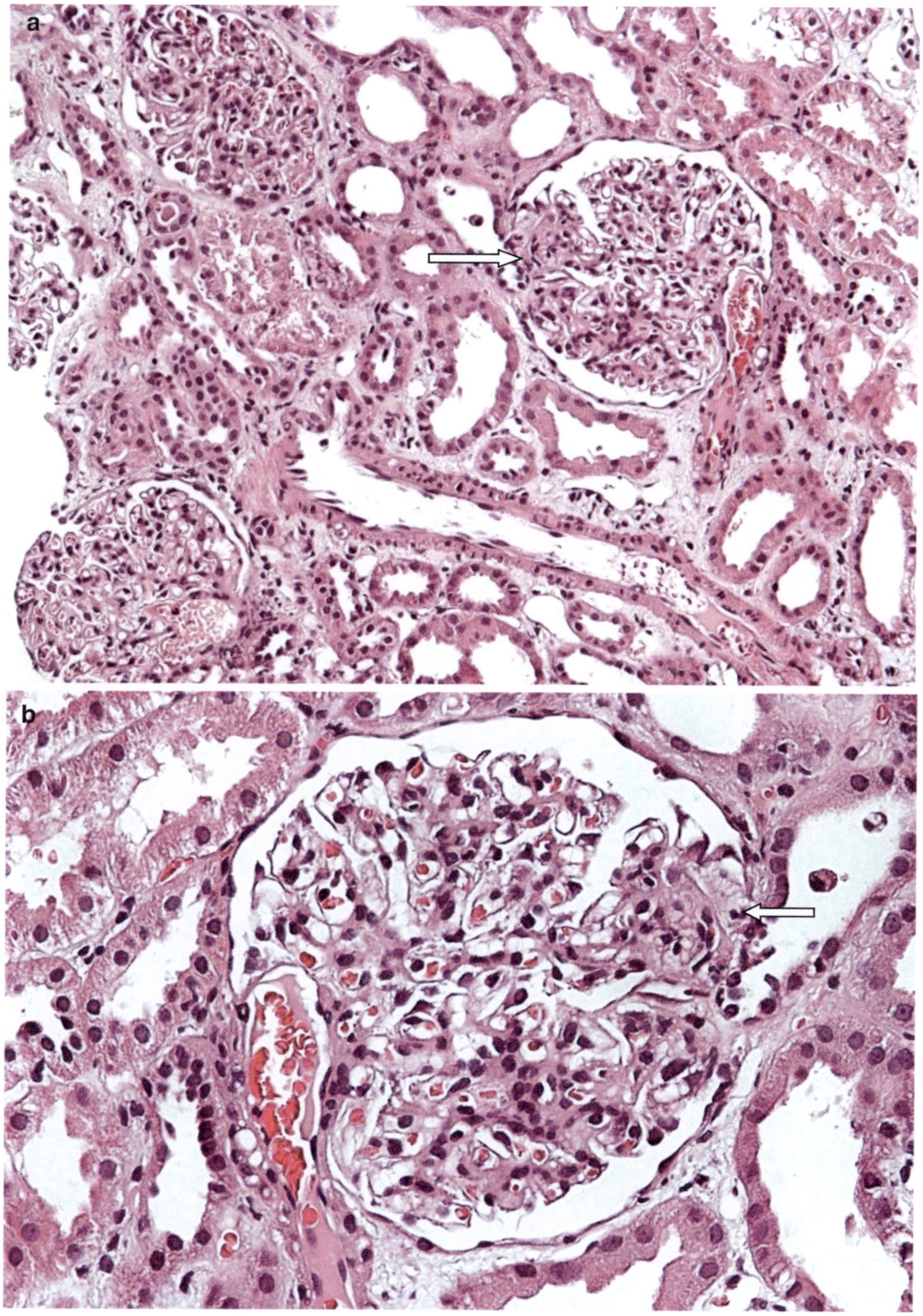

Fig. 3.3 **FSGS (Tip Variant)** A 41-years male patient known to be hypertensive for the past 2 years, presented with pedal edema. Urine analysis revealed proteinuria 3+ and the urinary sediment was bland. Urinary P:C ratio at admission was 3.84 which subsequently increased to 6.18. His serum creatinine was 1.1 mg/dL. Renal biopsy revealed 12 glomeruli, 3 of them showed sclerosis at antihilar pole (tubular pole) with synechia formation (white arrow) and prolapse into the tubular pole (black arrow). Focal tubular atrophy was present. (**a**) HE ×200, (**b**) and (**c**) HE ×400, and (**d**) PAS ×400

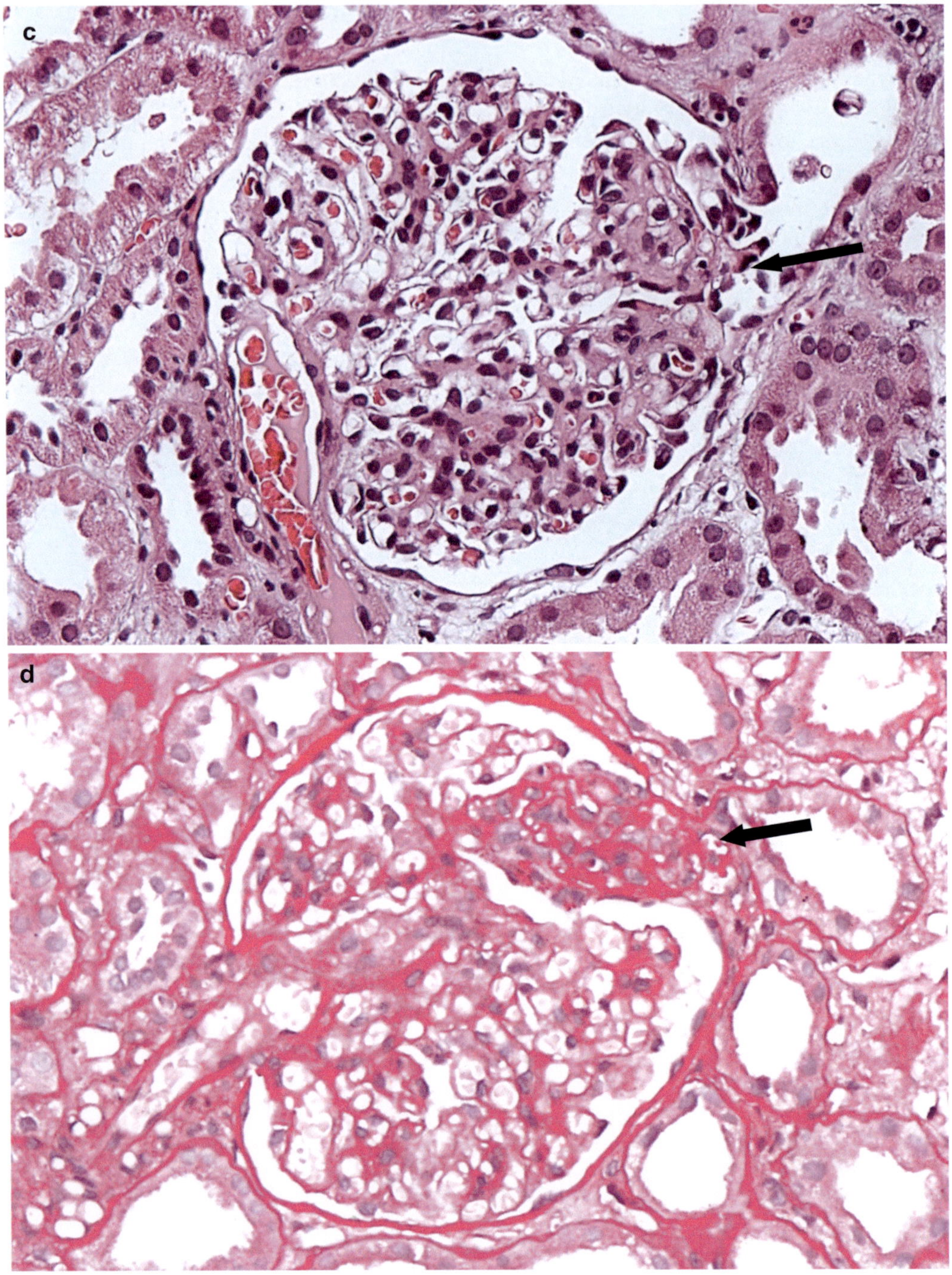

Fig. 3.3 (continued)

3.5 FSGS (Collapsing Variant)

In this morphologic variant, there is wrinkling and collapse of the glomerular capillary tuft involving at least one glomerulus. Segmental or global obliteration of glomerular capillaries can be seen. There is accompanying podocyte hypertrophy and hyperplasia. Ki-67 stain highlights the proliferative activity of podocytes. Pseudo-crescent formation can be seen. Podocytes will show a loss of mature podocyte phenotype characterized by the absence of WT-1, CALLA, synaptopodin, and GLEEP-1. These patients frequently have nephrotic syndrome and rapidly progressive renal failure (Fig. 3.4).

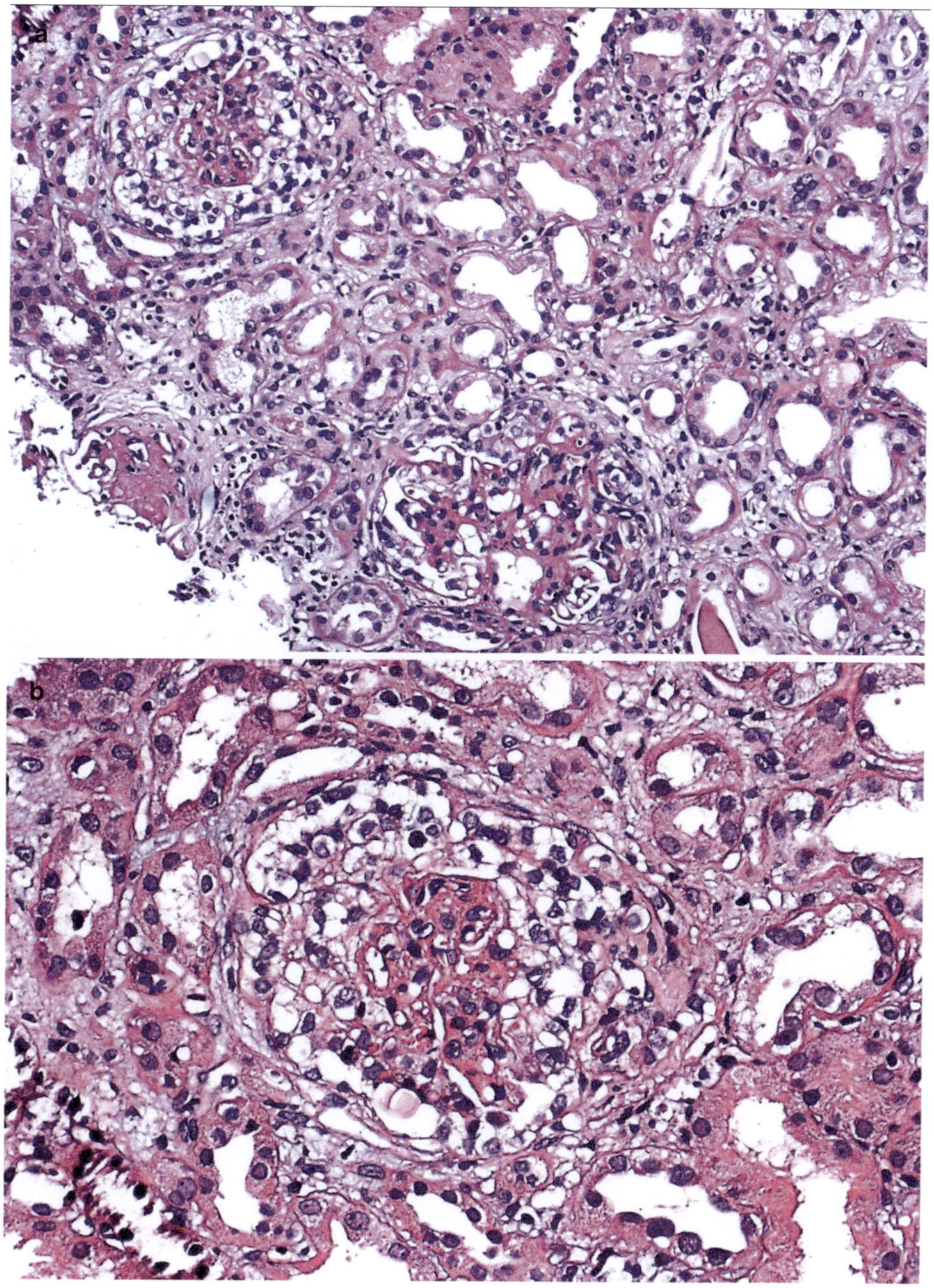

Fig. 3.4 **FSGS (Collapsing variant)** A 9-years male child, a known case of nephrotic syndrome for the last 5 years was on immunosuppressive drugs (Tab wysolone and Tab MMF). He presented with anasarca. During the last 2 years, he had 5–6 relapses of nephrotic syndrome. Laboratory workup revealed urinary protein 2+; M/E showed 0–5 pus cells/hpf and 6–10 rbc/hpf. Twenty-four-hour urinary protein was 5.4 g. Urinary protein creatinine ratio was 4.73 and the serum creatinine was 2.3 mg/dL. Serum total protein/albumin was 5.1/3.1 g/dL. Serum lipid profile revealed total serum cholesterol of 215 mg/dL with triglyceride being 490 mg/dL. ANA, DsDNA, and ANCA were negative. Serum C3 and C4 were low being 88 mg/L and 46 mg/L, respectively. Two core renal biopsy was obtained which contained 18 glomeruli, 8 of them showed podocyte hyperplasia and hypertrophy resembling pseudocrescents with the collapse of glomerular tuft of capillaries; 3 glomeruli showed mesangial matrix expansion and hypercellularity while other glomeruli were obsolescent. Tubulointerstitial compartment showed moderate tubular atrophy with thickening of tubular basement membrane with moderate lymphomononuclear interstitial infiltrate and fibrosis. IF showed segmental mesangial IgM deposits. (**a**) HE ×100, (**b**) HE ×200, (**c**) HE ×400, (**d**) Jones ×400, (**e**) PAS ×100 and (**f**) MT ×100. (**g**) The podocytes are highlighted by WT1 stain (WT1, HRP Polymer) ×400 (Contributor—Dr. Megha Uppin, Associate Professor, Department of Pathology, Nizam's Institute of Medical Sciences, Hyderabad, India)

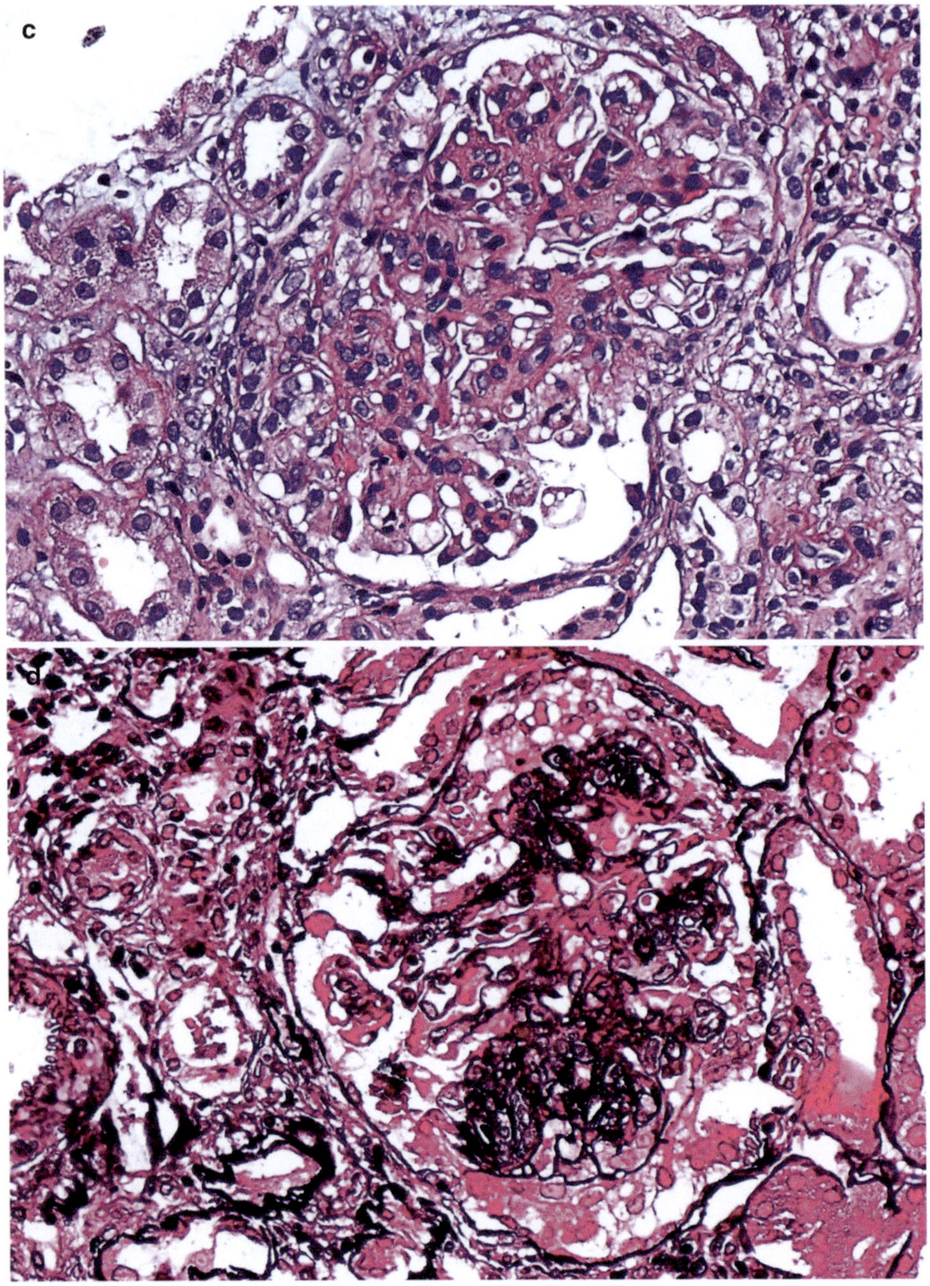

Fig. 3.4 (continued)

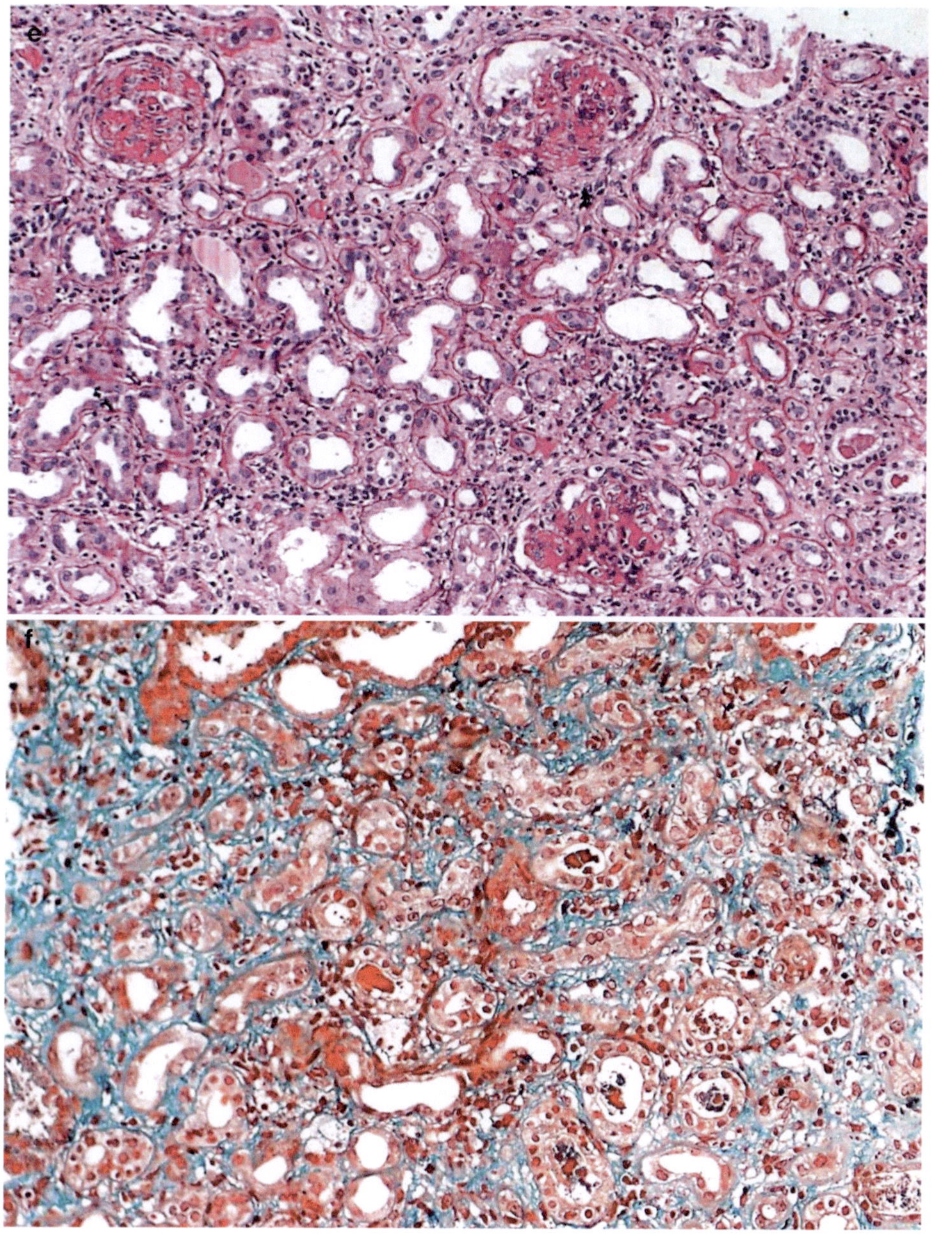

Fig. 3.4 (continued)

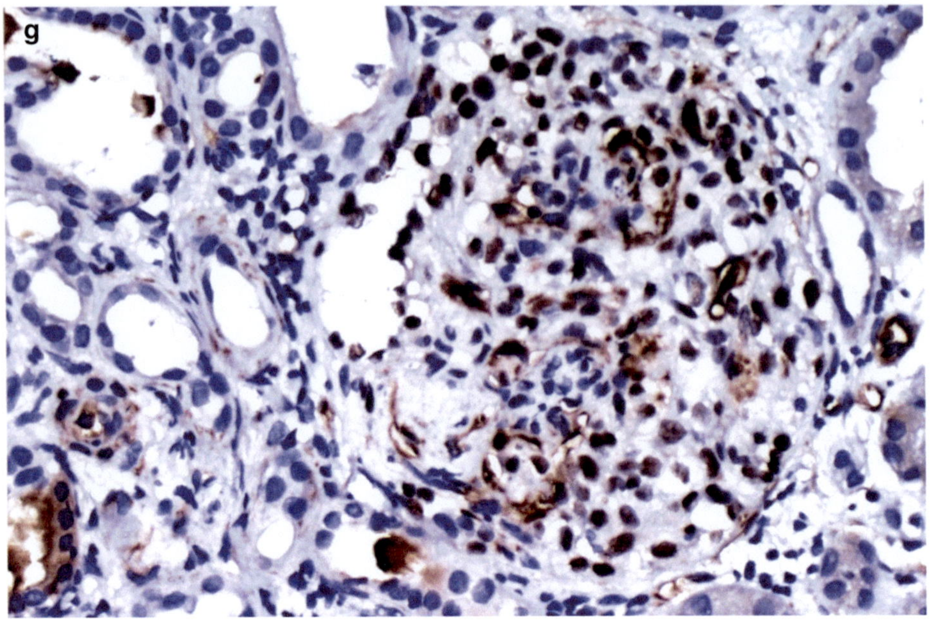

Fig. 3.4 (continued)

3.6 Secondary FSGS (Fig. 3.5)

a

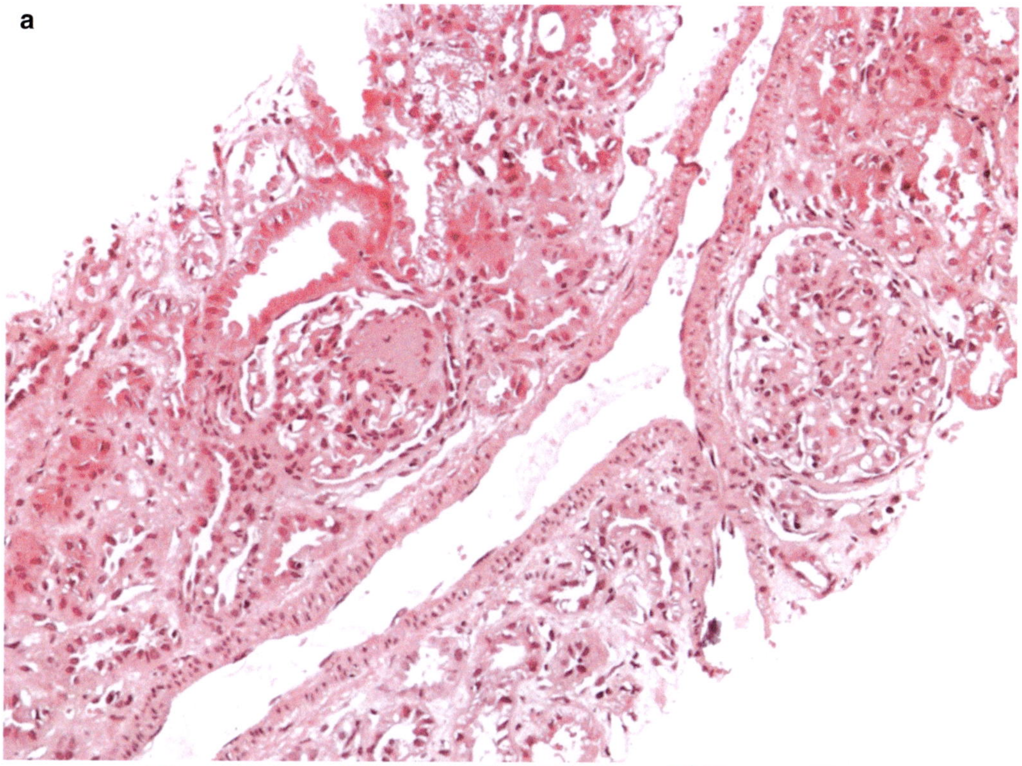

b

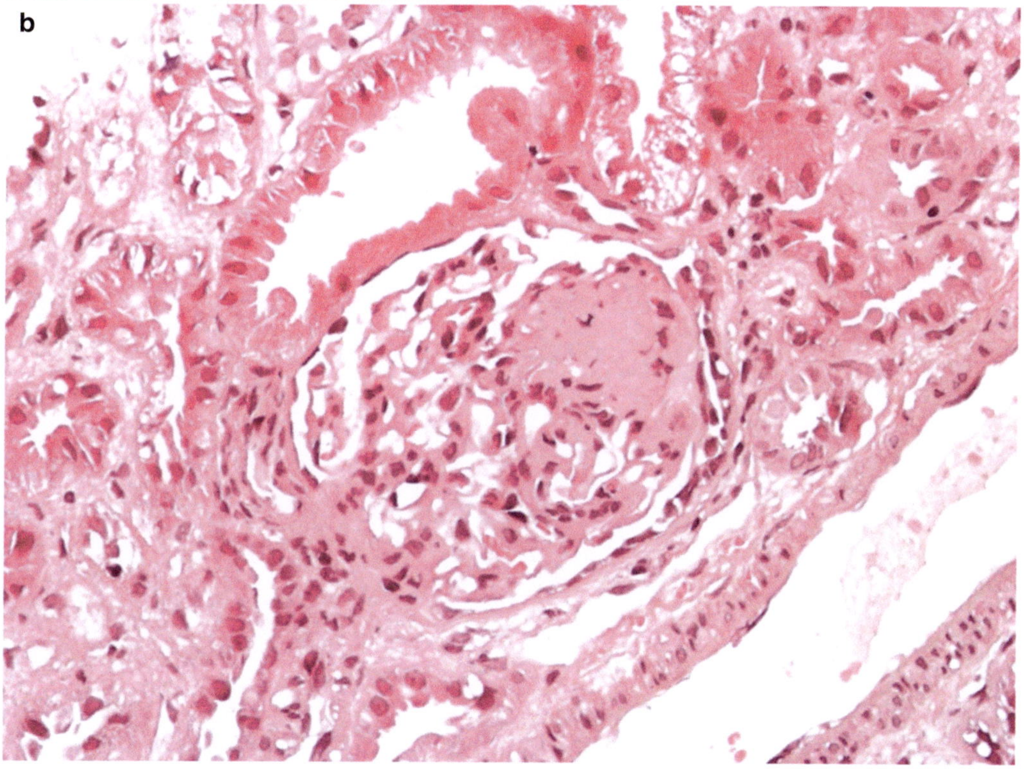

Fig. 3.5 **Secondary FSGS** A 38-years nondiabetic nonhypertensive male patient presented with bilateral pedal edema. On laboratory evaluation, he was found to have subnephrotic range proteinuria (24 h urine protein 2.4 g). Urine analysis showed 2+ protein and no active sediments. Serum creatinine was 1 mg/dL. Serum cholesterol was wnl. Renal biopsy showed 16 glomeruli, 4 showed segmental sclerosis. Of these one had sclerosis in perihilar area. There was mild focal tubular atrophy and interstitial fibrosis. Blood vessels were unremarkable. On immunofluorescence IgM segmental mesangial deposits were seen. No other immunoglobulin, complement, or light chain deposits were seen. On electron microscopy, focal effacement of foot processes of podocytes was seen without any immune complex deposits. (**a**) HE ×200, (**b**) and (**c**) HE ×400, (**d**) PAS ×400, (**e**) PSM ×400 and (**f**) EM ×2500

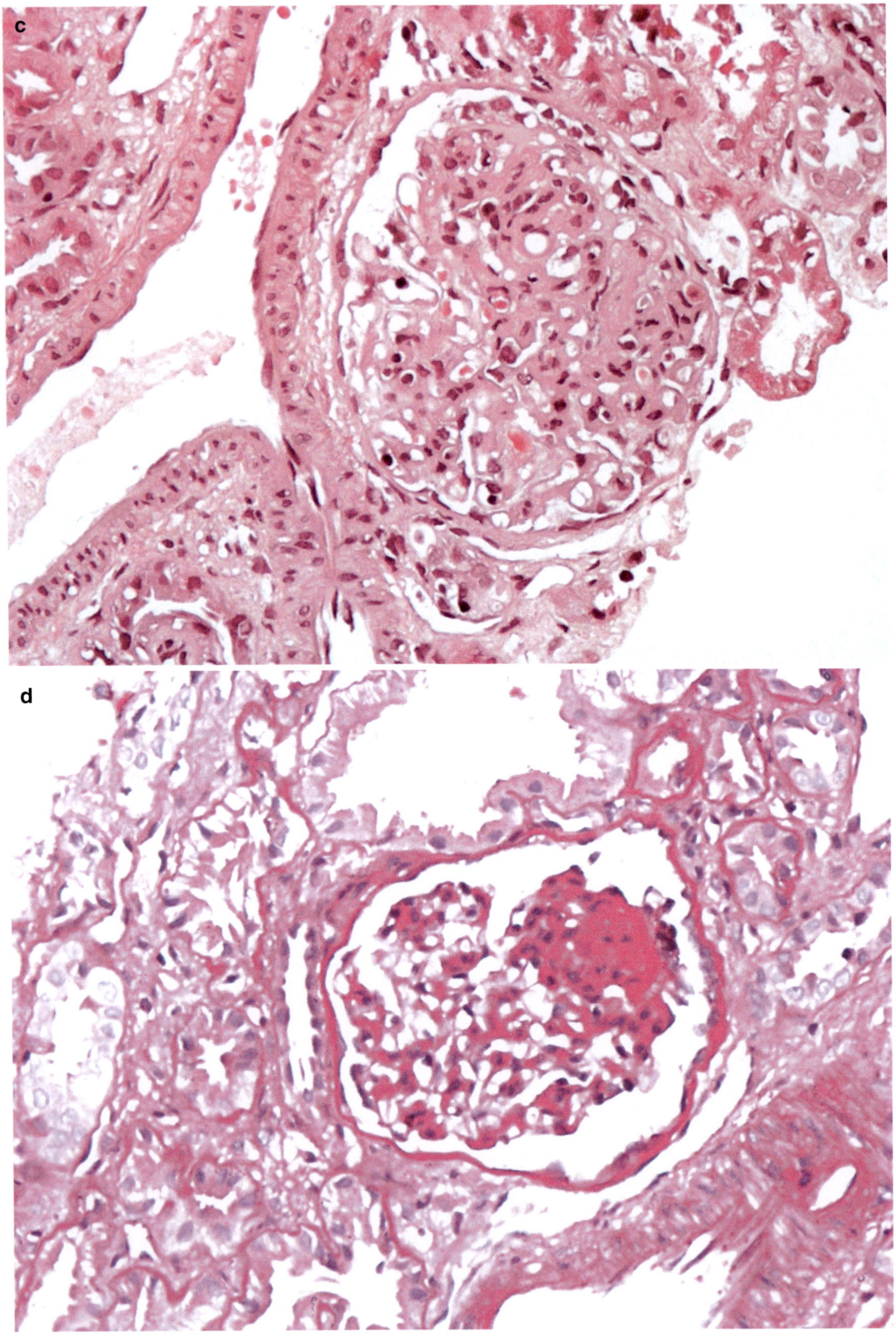

Fig. 3.5 (continued)

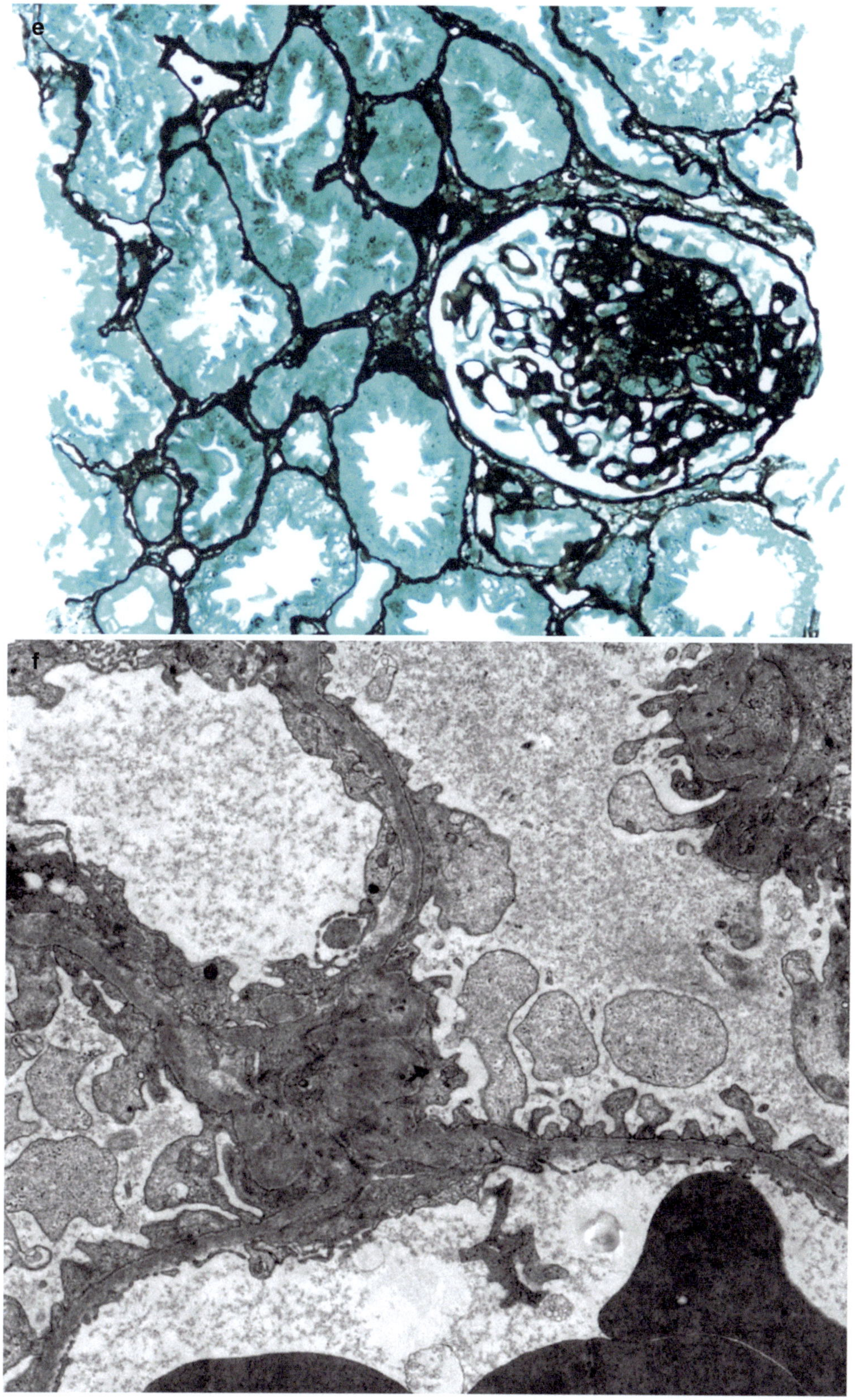

Fig. 3.5 (continued)

Further Reading

Allard L, Kwon T, Krid S, Bacchetta J, Garnier A, Novo R, Deschenes G, Salomon R, Roussey G, Allain-Launay E. Treatment by immunoadsorption for recurrent focal segmental glomerulosclerosis after paediatric kidney transplantation: a multicentre French cohort. Nephrol Dial Transplant. 2018;33:954–63.

D'Agati VD, Fogo AB, Bruijn JA, Jennette JC. Pathologic classification of focal segmental glomerulosclerosis: a working proposal. Am J Kidney Dis. 2004;43:368–82.

D'Agati VD, Alster JM, Jennette JC, Thomas DB, Pullman J, Savino DA, Cohen AH, Gipson DS, Gassman JJ, Radeva MK, Moxey-Mims MM, Friedman AL, Kaskel FJ, Trachtman H, Alpers CE, Fogo AB, Greene TH, Nast CC. Association of histologic variants in FSGS clinical trial with presenting features and outcomes. Clin J Am Soc Nephrol. 2013;8:399–406.

De Vriese AS, Sethi S, Nath KA, Glassock RJ, Fervenza FC. Differentiating primary, genetic, and secondary FSGS in adults: a clinicopathologic approach. J Am Soc Nephrol. 2018;29:759–74.

Gulati A, Sharma A, Hari P, Dinda AK, Bagga A. Idiopathic collapsing glomerulopathy in children. Clin Exp Nephrol. 2008;12:348–53.

Kachurina N, Chung CF, Benderoff E, Babayeva S, Bitzan M, Goodyer P, Kitzler T, Matar D, Cybulsky AV, Alachkar N, Torban E. Novel unbiased assay for circulating podocyte-toxic factors associated with recurrent focal segmental glomerulosclerosis. Am J Physiol Renal Physiol. 2016;310:F1148–56.

Raja R, Nada R, Yadav AK, Kumar A, Goyal A, Kumar V, Rathi M, Kohli HS, Gupta KL, Sakhuja V, Jha V. A prospective study of collapsing focal segmental glomerulosclerosis. Ren Fail. 2016;38:894–8.

Rosenberg AZ, Kopp JB. Focal segmental glomerulosclerosis. Clin J Am Soc Nephrol. 2017;12:502–17.

4 Membranous Glomerulopathy (MGN)

Membranous glomerulopathy (MGN) accounts for majority of cases of adult onset nephrotic syndrome and nephrotic range proteinuria in adults. On light microscopy, the glomeruli are often enlarged. Its characteristic morphological feature is the diffuse thickening of the glomerular capillary basement membrane with or without epimembranous argyrophylic spikes or glomerular capillary basement membrane vacoulations. On Immunofluorescence granular subepithelial deposits of IgG often accompanied by C3 are seen. Electron microscopy shows subepithelial electron-dense to pale deposits on the outer aspect of glomerular capillary basement membrane. A variable degree of foot process effacement can be seen.

Membranous glomerulopathy can be primary or secondary. Primary membranous glomerulopathy is an autoimmune disorder caused by antibodies against M-type phospholipase receptor (anti-PLA2r) in up to 85% of patients. It can also be caused by antibodies against thrombospondin type I domain (THSD7A) in 3–5% of cases. Recent studies have described anti-Nell-1 antibody as the second most common antibody associated with primary membranous nephropathy (positive in 16% of PLA2r negative membranous nephropathy). Many other autoantibodies are now implicated and are a matter of ongoing research. Secondary causes of membranous glomerulopathy include infections such as hepatitis B and C, malignancy, drugs, toxins and autoimmune diseases such as SLE. Patients having positive serum anti-PLA2r/THSD7A antibodies and proteinuria >3.5 g/day are treated with immunosuppressive regimen. Patients with negative serum anti-PLA2r/THSD7A antibodies and negative staining for PLA2r and THSD7A on renal biopsies are considered to have secondary membranous glomerulopathy. They are given supportive care with treatment of the underlying cause. Cases with negative serum Anti-PLA2r/THSD7A but positive staining on renal biopsies are considered to have inactive primary membranous glomerulopathy and are given supportive care. A case each of PLA2r positive membranous nephropathy (Fig. 4.1), Nell-1 associated membranous nephropathy (Fig. 4.2), and Thrombospondin associated membranous nephropathy (Fig. 4.3) are illustrated below.

P. Gupta, R. K. Gupta, *Pathology of Glomerular Diseases*, https://doi.org/10.1007/978-981-19-1430-0_4

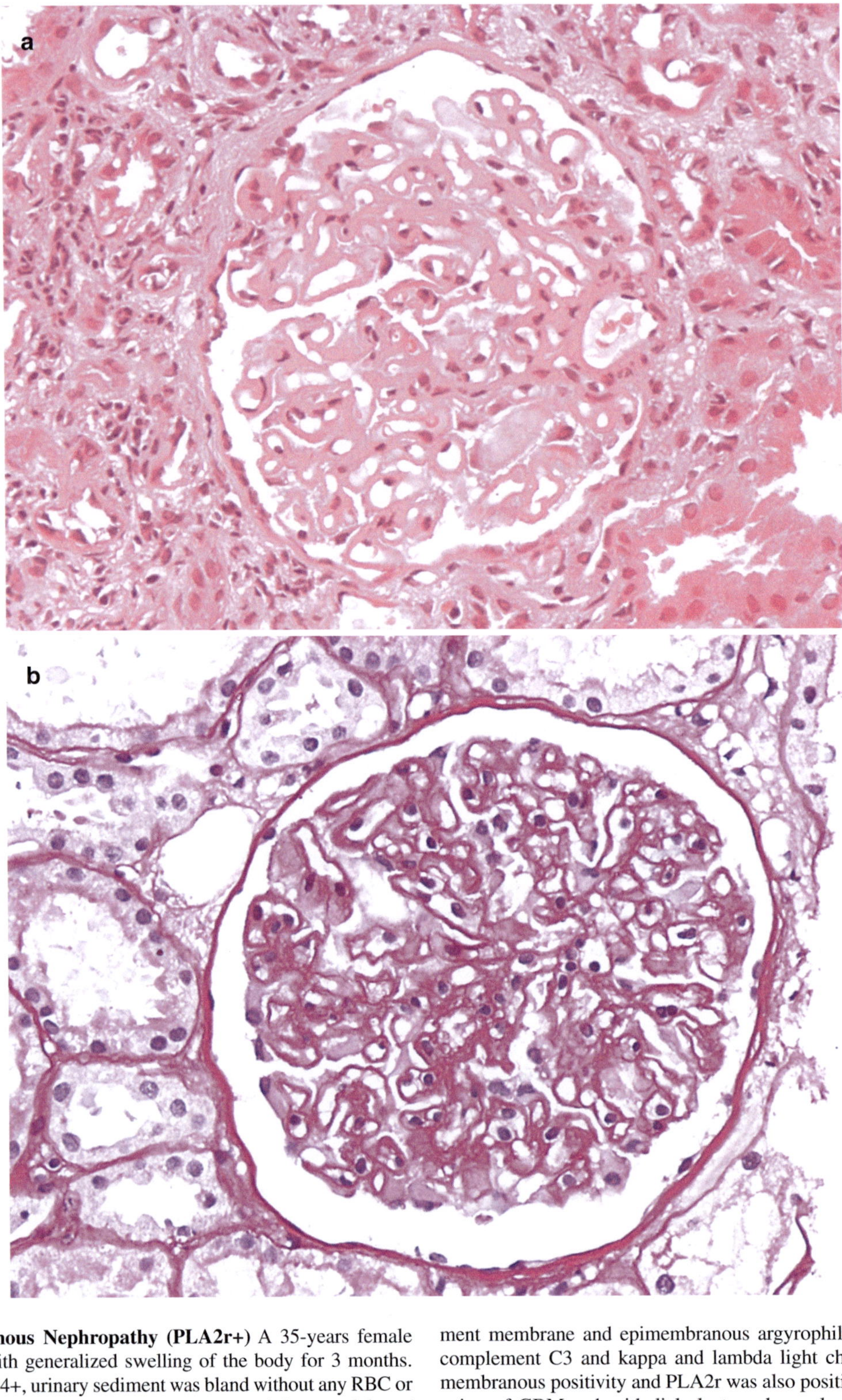

Fig. 4.1 **Membranous Nephropathy (PLA2r+)** A 35-years female patient presented with generalized swelling of the body for 3 months. Urinary protein was 4+, urinary sediment was bland without any RBC or pus cells. Urinary P:C ratio was 4.8. Her serum creatinine was 0.9 mg/dL and serum cholesterol was 250 mg/dL. Her serum PLA2r was positive and ANA was negative by IIF. Renal biopsy showed nine glomeruli, all of them were enlarged with thickening of glomerular capillary basement membrane and epimembranous argyrophilic spikes. IF for IgG, complement C3 and kappa and lambda light chains showed granular membranous positivity and PLA2r was also positive. EM showed thickening of GBM, subepithelial electron-dense deposits, and intervening connective tissue spikes with effacement of visceral epithelial cell foot processes. (**a**) HE ×400, (**b**) PAS ×400, (**c**) PSM ×400, (**d**) PSM ×1000, (**e–i**) IF ×400 and (**j**) EM (identity of the patient has been concealed)

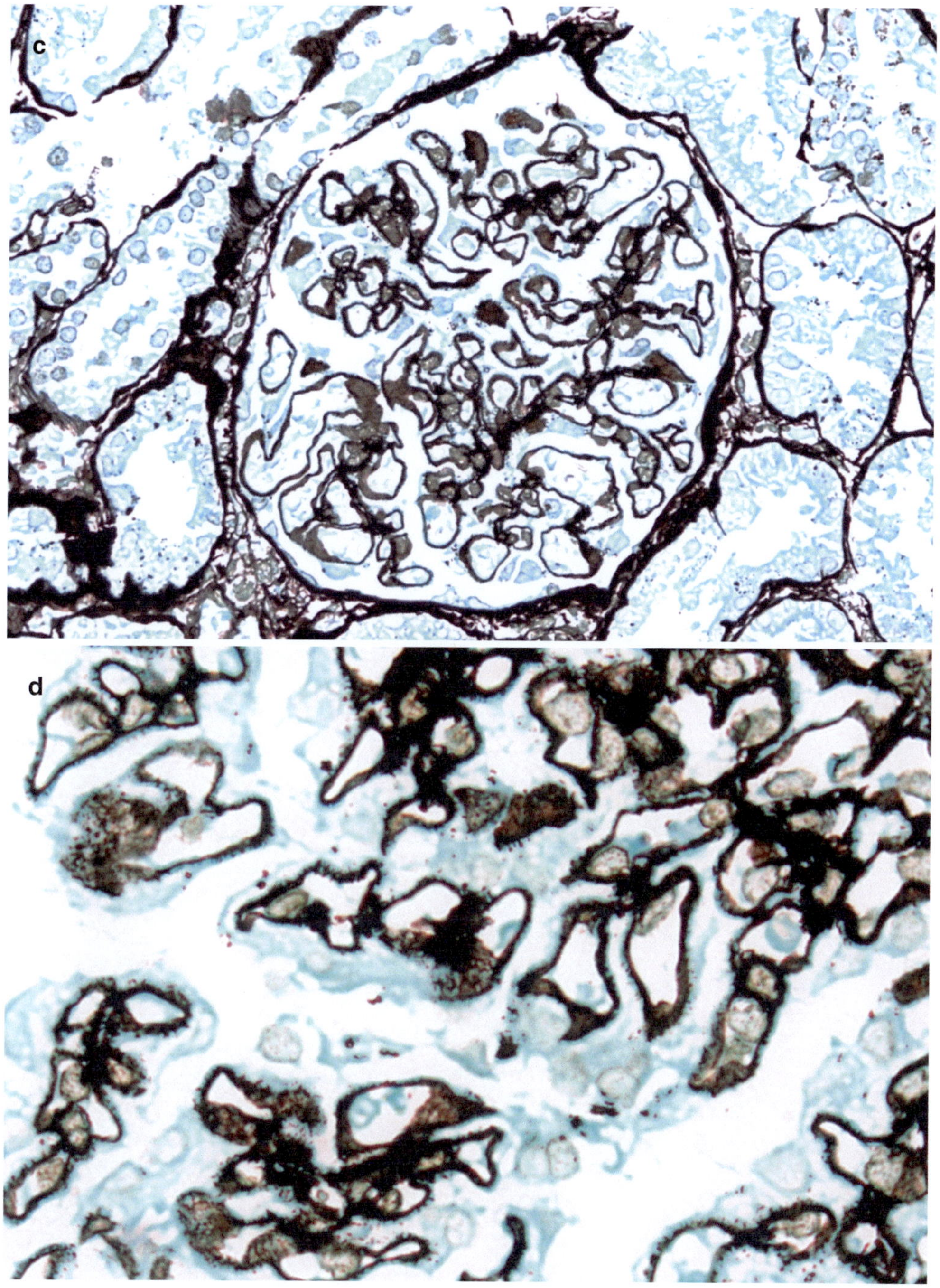

Fig. 4.1 (continued)

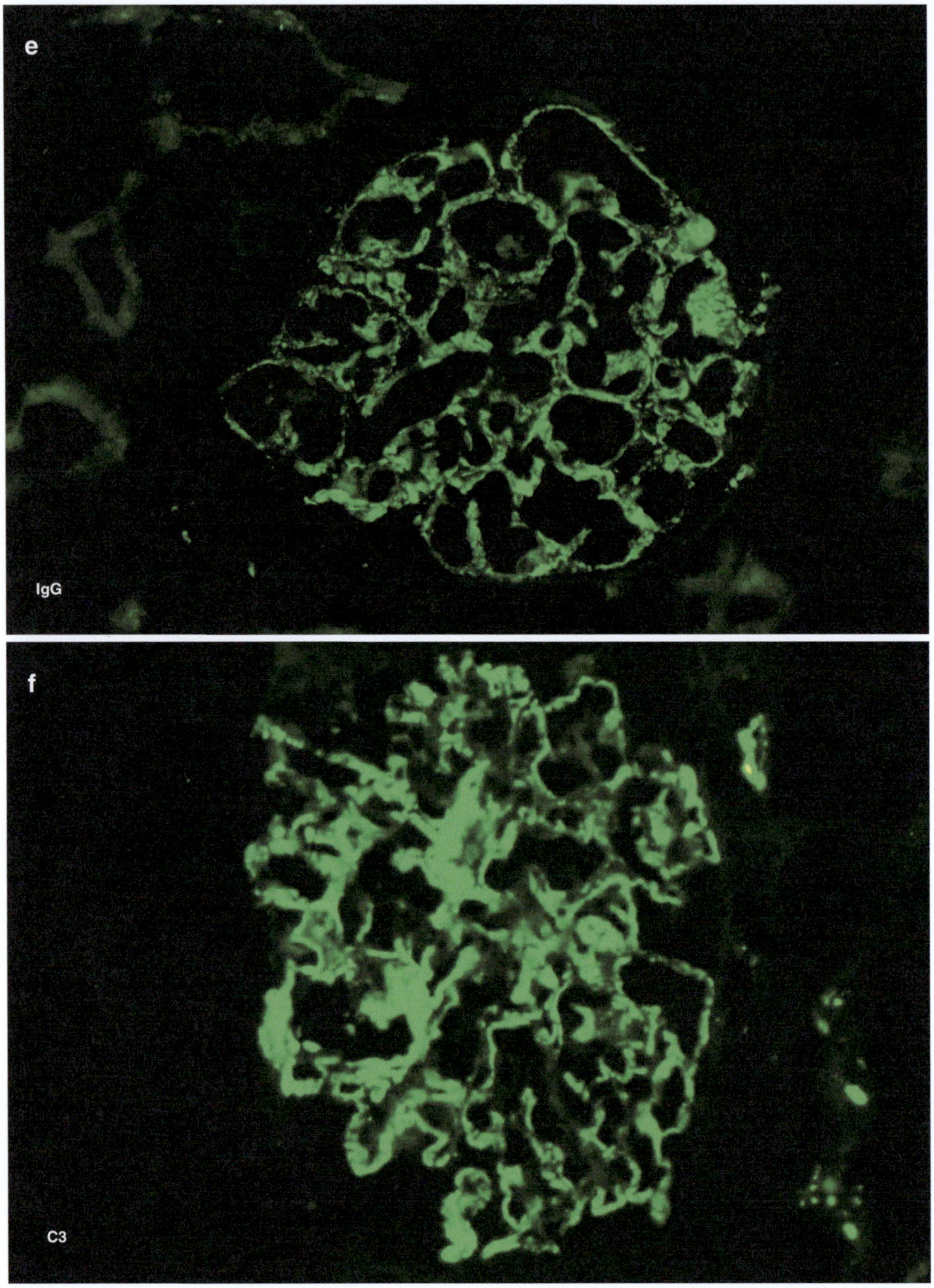

Fig. 4.1 (continued)

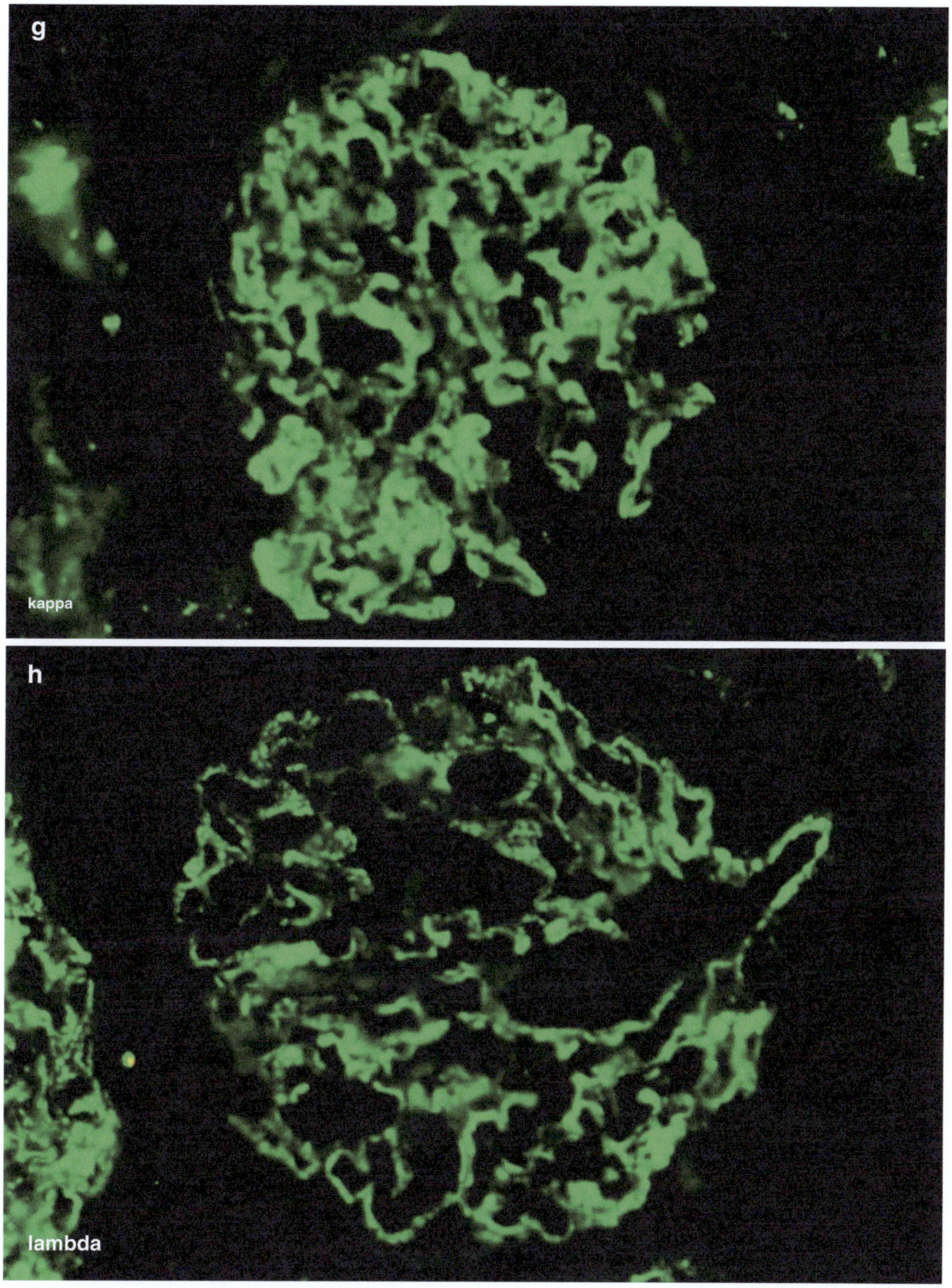

Fig. 4.1 (continued)

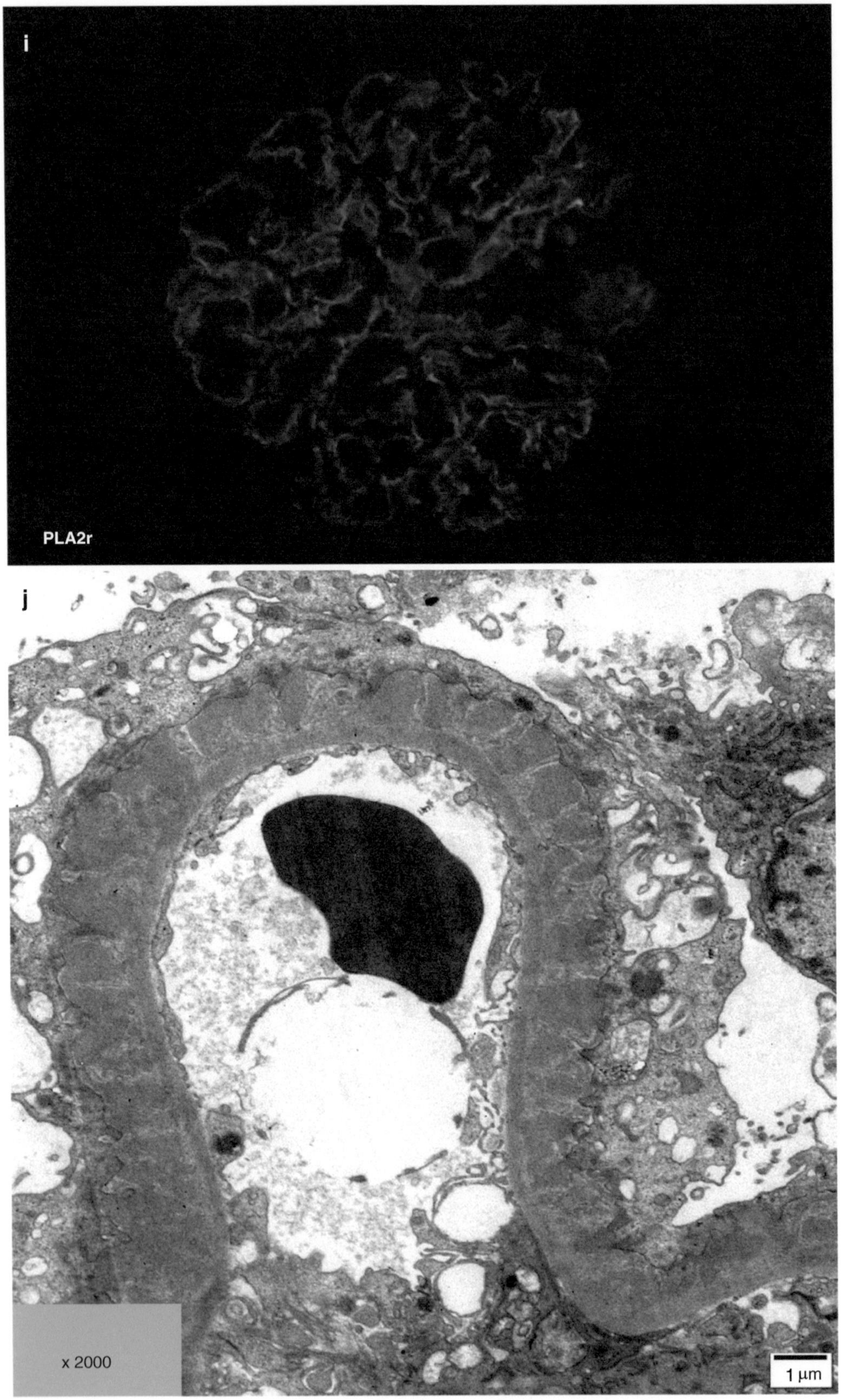

Fig. 4.1 (continued)

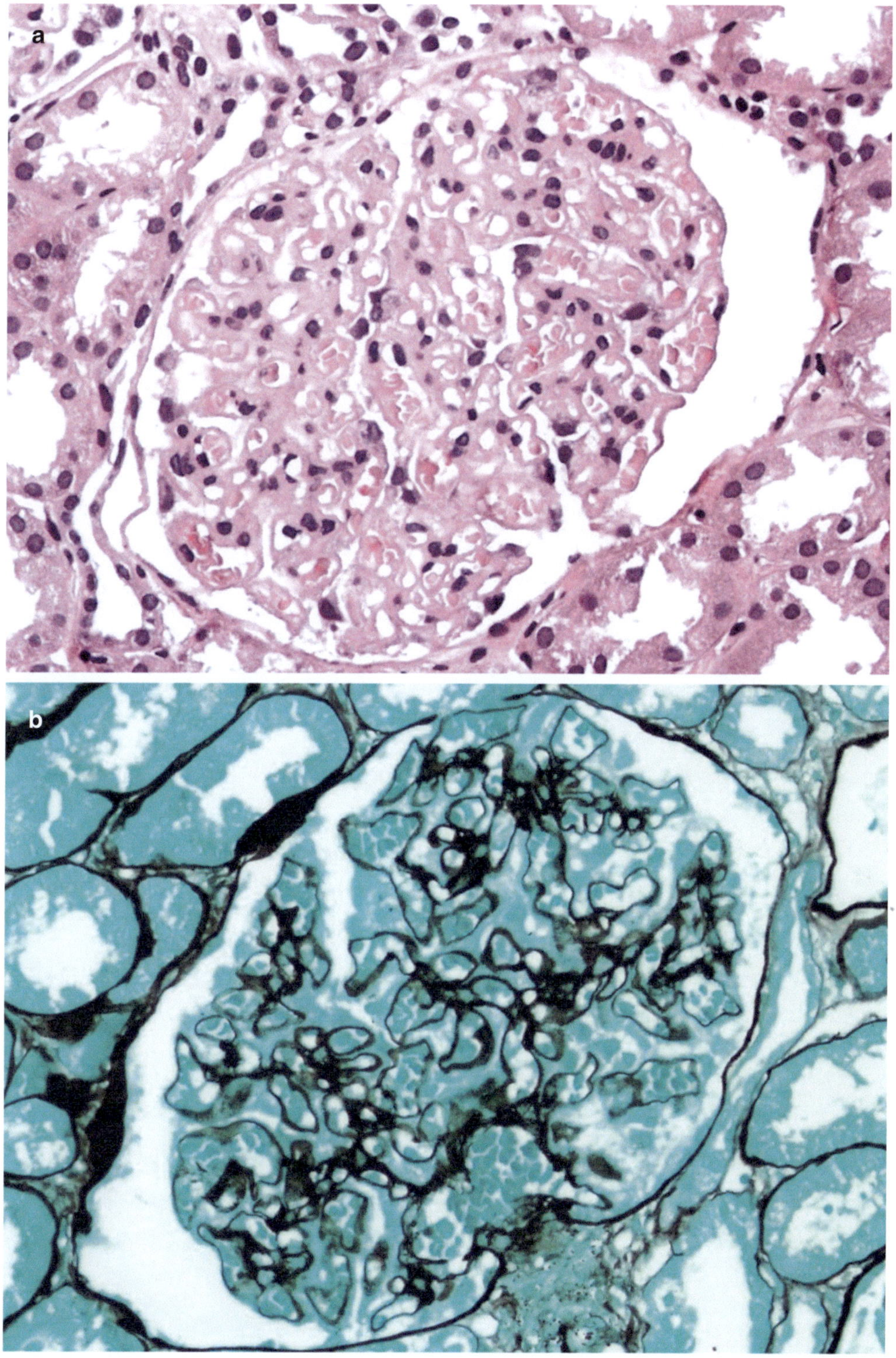

Fig. 4.2 **Membranous Nephropathy (NELL-1 +)** A 53-years male patient presented with generalized swelling of body for 2 months. Urinary protein was 3+, urinary sediment was bland without any RBC or pus cells. Urinary P:C ratio was 3.6. His serum creatinine was 1.2 mg/dL. Serum PLA2r was negative and ANA was negative by IIF. Renal biopsy showed seven glomeruli, all of them showing thickening of glomerular capillary basement membrane and epimembranous argyrophilic spikes. IF for IgG, complement C3 and kappa and lambda light chains showed granular membranous positivity. PLA2r and THSD7A were negative on biopsy. IHC for anti-NELL-1 antibody showed granular positivity along glomerular capillary basement membrane similar to IgG positivity. (**a**) HE ×400, (**b**) PSM ×400, (**c**) IgG (DIF) ×400, and (**d**) anti-NELL-1 (IHC) ×400

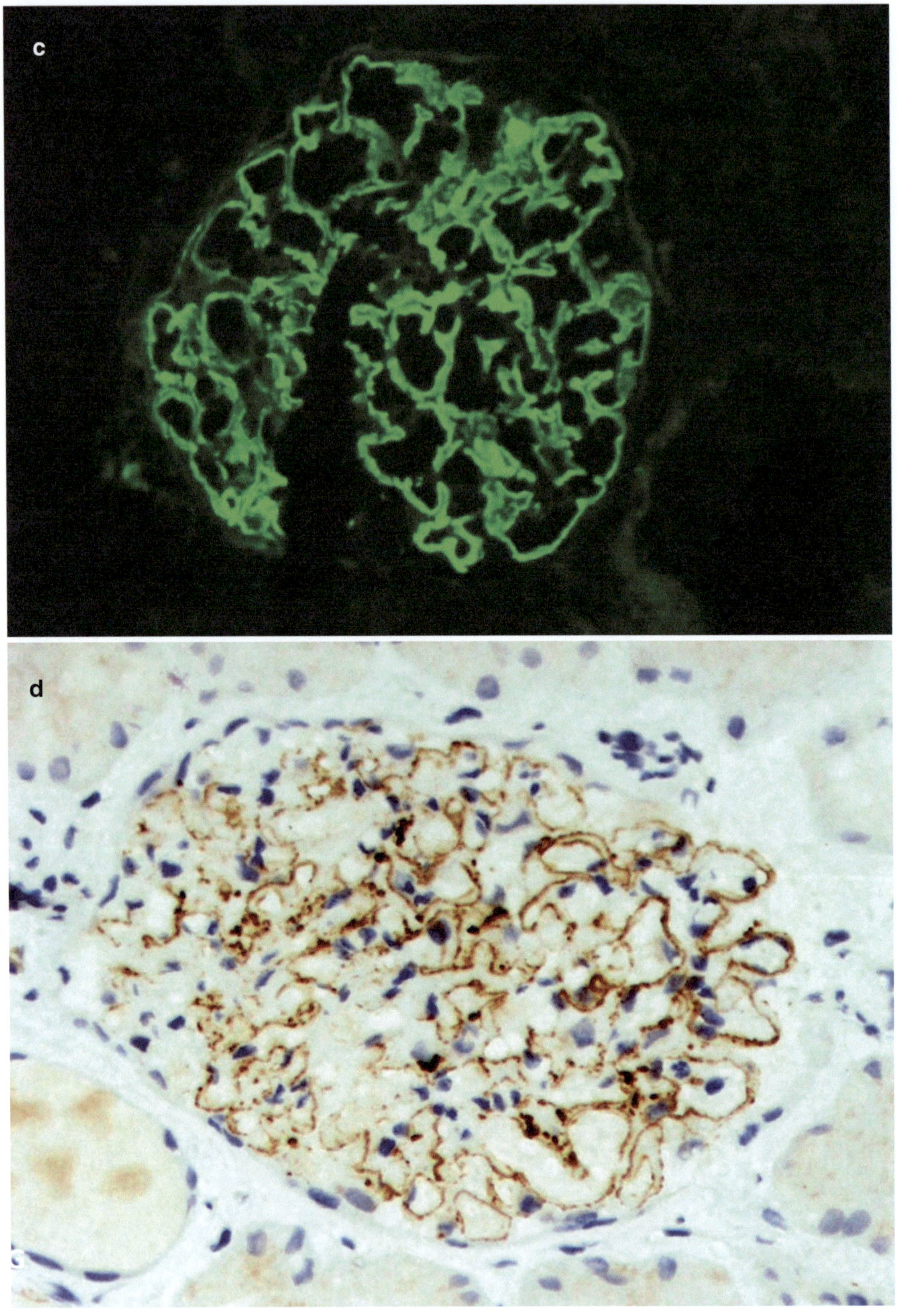

Fig. 4.2 (continued)

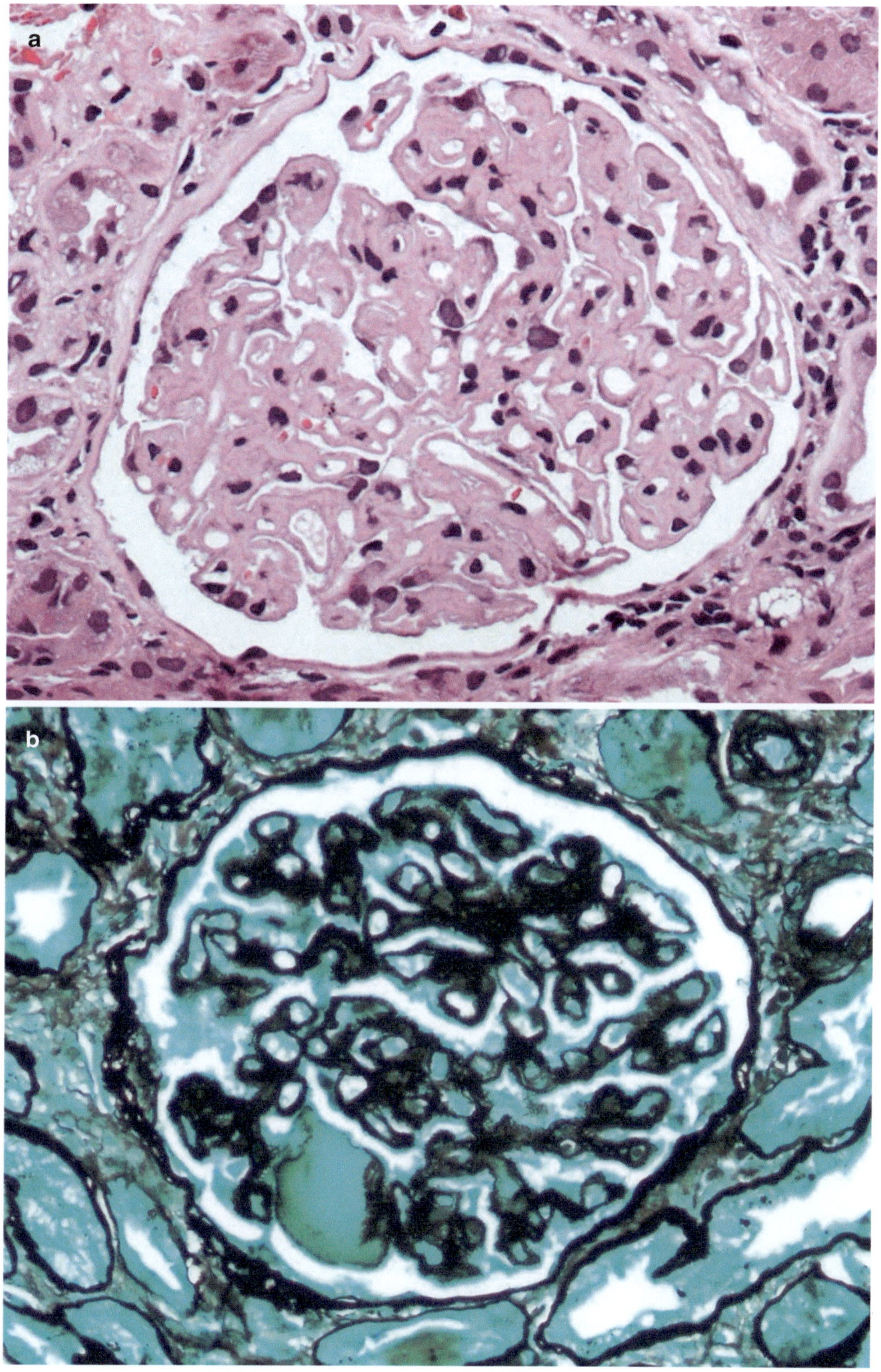

Fig. 4.3 **Membranous Nephropathy (THSD7A +)** A 34-years male patient presented with pedal edema. Urinary protein was 3+, urinary sediment was bland without any RBC or pus cells. Urinary P:C ratio was 4.1. His serum creatinine was 0.6 mg/dL. Serum PLA2r was negative and ANA was negative by IIF. Renal biopsy showed nine glomeruli, one was globally sclerosed, remaining glomeruli showed thickening of glomerular capillary basement membrane and epimembranous argyrophilic spikes. IF for IgG, complement C3 and kappa and lambda light chains showed granular membranous positivity. PLA2r was negative on the biopsy. IHC for THSD7A antibody showed granular positivity along glomerular capillary basement membrane similar to IgG positivity. (**a**) HE ×400, (**b**) PSM ×400, (**c**) IgG (DIF) ×400, (**d**) anti-THSD7A (IHC) ×400

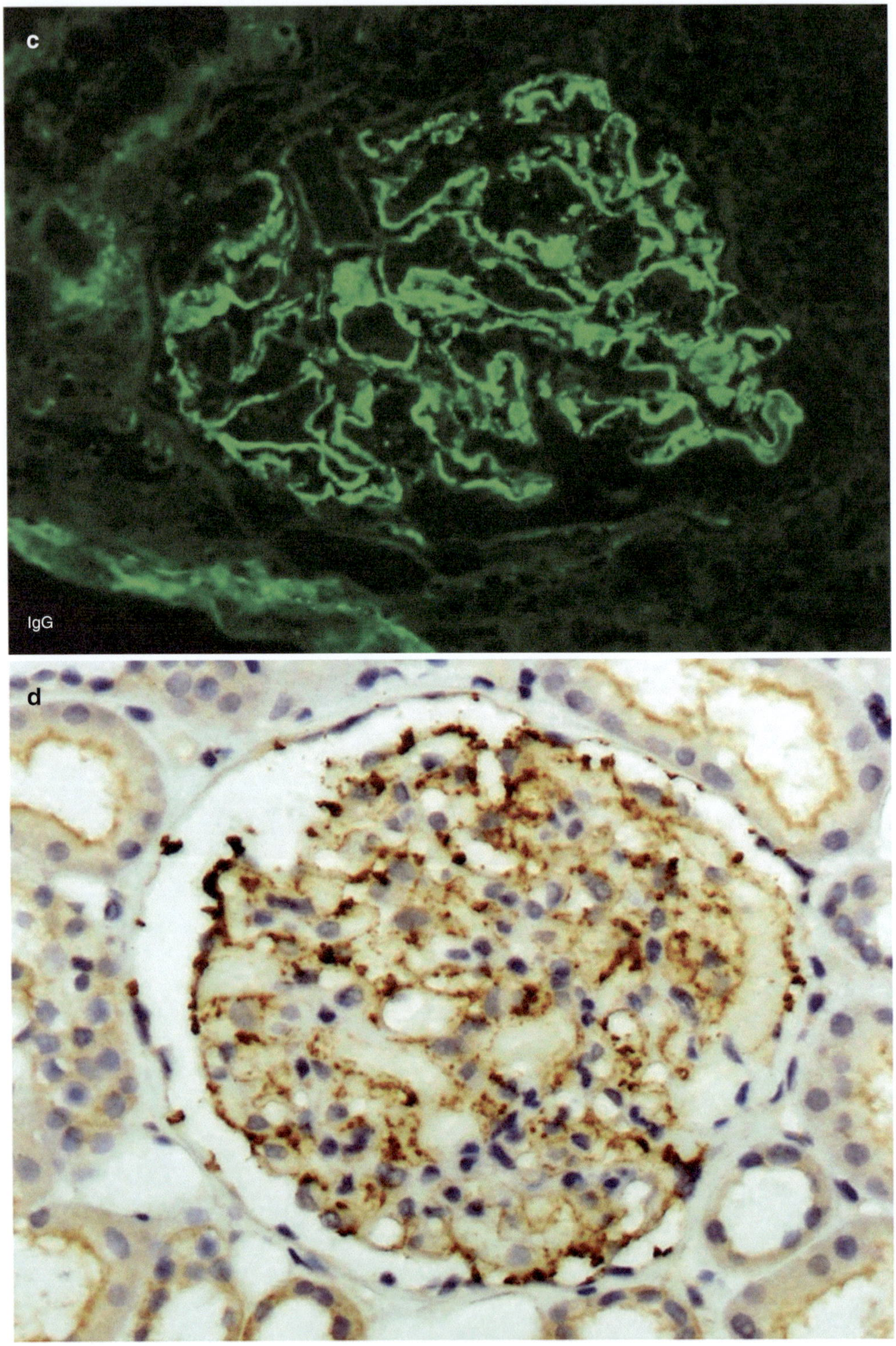

Fig. 4.3 (continued)

Further Reading

Alsharhan L, Beck LH Jr. Membranous nephropathy: core curriculum 2021. Am J Kidney Dis. 2021;77:440–53.

Cattran DC, Brenchley PE. Membranous nephropathy: integrating basic science into improved clinical management. Kidney Int. 2017;91:566–74.

Sethi S, Debiec H, Madden B, Charlesworth MC, Morelle J, Gross L, Ravindran A, Buob D, Jadoul M, Fervenza FC, Ronco P. Neural epidermal growth factor-like 1 protein (NELL-1) associated membranous nephropathy. Kidney Int. 2020;97:163–74.

Couser WG. Primary membranous nephropathy. Clin J Am Soc Nephrol. 2017;12:983–97.

De Vriese AS, Glassock RJ, Nath KA, Sethi S, Fervenza FC. A proposal for a serology-based approach to membranous nephropathy. J Am Soc Nephrol. 2016;28:421–30.

Debiec H, Ronco P. Immune response against autoantigen PLA2R is not gambling: implications for pathophysiology, prognosis and therapy. J Am Soc Nephrol. 2016;27:1275–7.

Salant DJ, CattranDC. Chapter 20: Membranous nephropathy. In: Floege J, Johnson RJ, Feehally J, editors. Comprehensive clinical nephrology. 5th ed. St. Louis, MI: Saunders, an imprint of Elsevier Inc.; 2015. p. 239–51.

5 Immune Complex-Mediated MPGN (Previously MPGN Type I)

Immune complex-mediated MPGN is a disease of young adults and children who frequently present with hematuria, proteinuria, nephrotic or nephritic syndrome. Progression to end-stage renal disease can be seen in 40% of patients over a period of 10 years. The renal biopsy would reveal that the glomeruli are enlarged with accentuated lobular pattern and look pale with a global increase of glomerular cellularity caused by endocapillary hyperplasia and mesangial cells proliferation as well as infiltration of polymorphonuclear inflammatory cells in some cases. The glomerular capillary basement membrane shows reduplication (tram track/double contour). On immunofluorescence immunoglobulins along with complement deposits are seen in subendothelial and mesangial compartments. On electron microscopy, patients have subendothelial and mesangial electron-dense deposits with variable subepithelial and intramembranous deposits. Thickening and double contours of glomerular capillary basement membrane are seen. It is one of the common causes of recurrent glomerulonephritis (27–65%) after renal transplantation.

Membranoproliferative glomerulonephritis (MPGN) has been reclassified into immune complex-mediated MPGN and complement-mediated disease which comprises C3 glomerulonephritis and dense deposit disease.

Immune complex-mediated MPGN is caused secondary to infections like hepatitis B, C, autoimmune disorders like SLE, Sjogren's syndrome, cryoglobulinemia, etc. or due to monoclonal gammopathies including monoclonal gammopathy of renal significance. It is caused by activation of the classical complement pathway. A case of immune complex mediated MPGN is illustrated (Fig. 5.1).

P. Gupta, R. K. Gupta, *Pathology of Glomerular Diseases*, https://doi.org/10.1007/978-981-19-1430-0_5

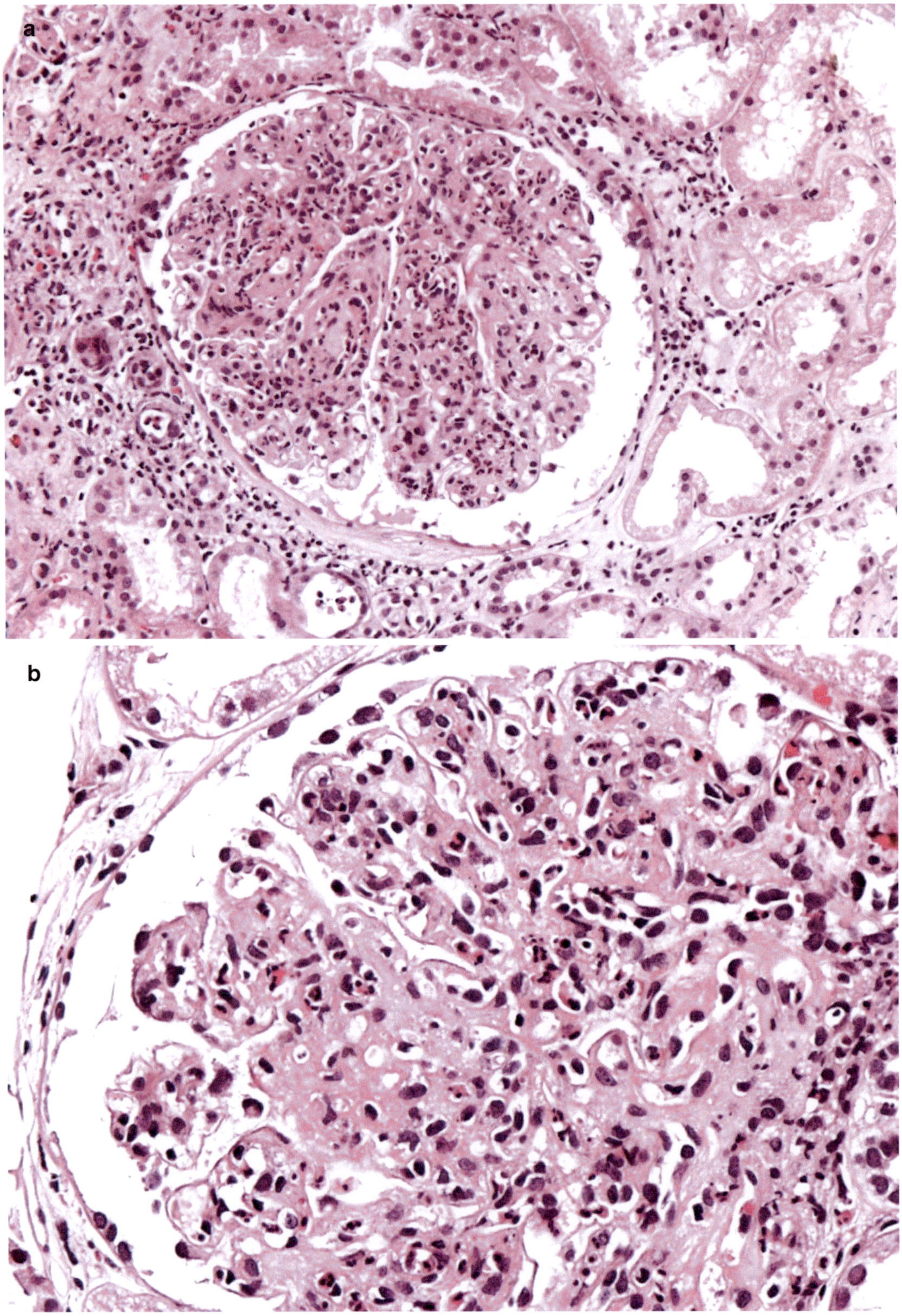

Fig. 5.1 Immune Complex Mediated MPGN A 32-years male patient, known to be hypertensive for the past 3 years and suffering from hypothyroidism for the past 18 months, presented with pedal edema. Urine analysis revealed proteinuria (2+) with 10–15 RBC/hpf; P/C ratio was 4.2. The patient was anemic with a hemoglobin of 9.4 g/dL. Serum creatinine was 1.74 mg/dL. Serum C3 was 542 mg/L and C4 was 143 mg/L. ENA profile and serology for HBsAg and HCV were negative. Renal biopsy had 11 glomeruli which showed endocapillary hyperplasia with increased mesangial cellularity, few polymorphs along with thickening and reduplication of capillary basement membrane. Occasional foci of tubular atrophy with mild lymphocytic interstitial infiltration were present. Blood vessels were unremarkable. IF showed IgG (3+), C3 (3+), IgM (2+), and C1q (1+) granular deposits along the GBM and mesangium; IgA was negative. EM showed thickened basement membrane with subendothelial, mesangial, few subepithelial and intramembranous electron-dense deposits. GBM double contour and widespread effacement of foot processes of visceral epithelial cells were also seen, (**a**) HE ×200, (**b**) HE ×400, (**c** and **d**) PAS ×400, (**e**) PSM ×200, (**f**) PSM ×400, (**g** and **h**) IF ×400, (**i** and **j**) EM (identity of the patient has been concealed)

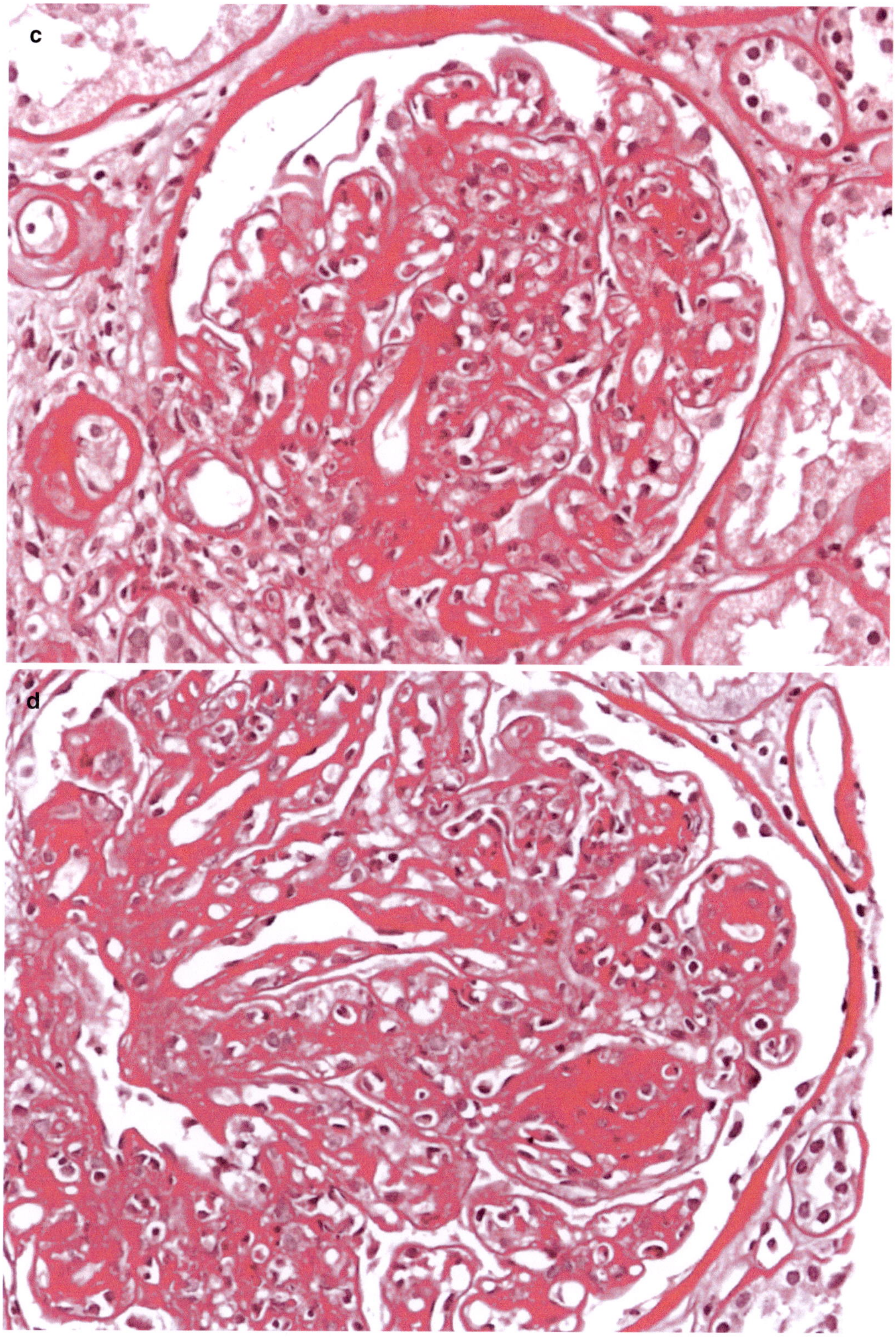

Fig. 5.1 (continued)

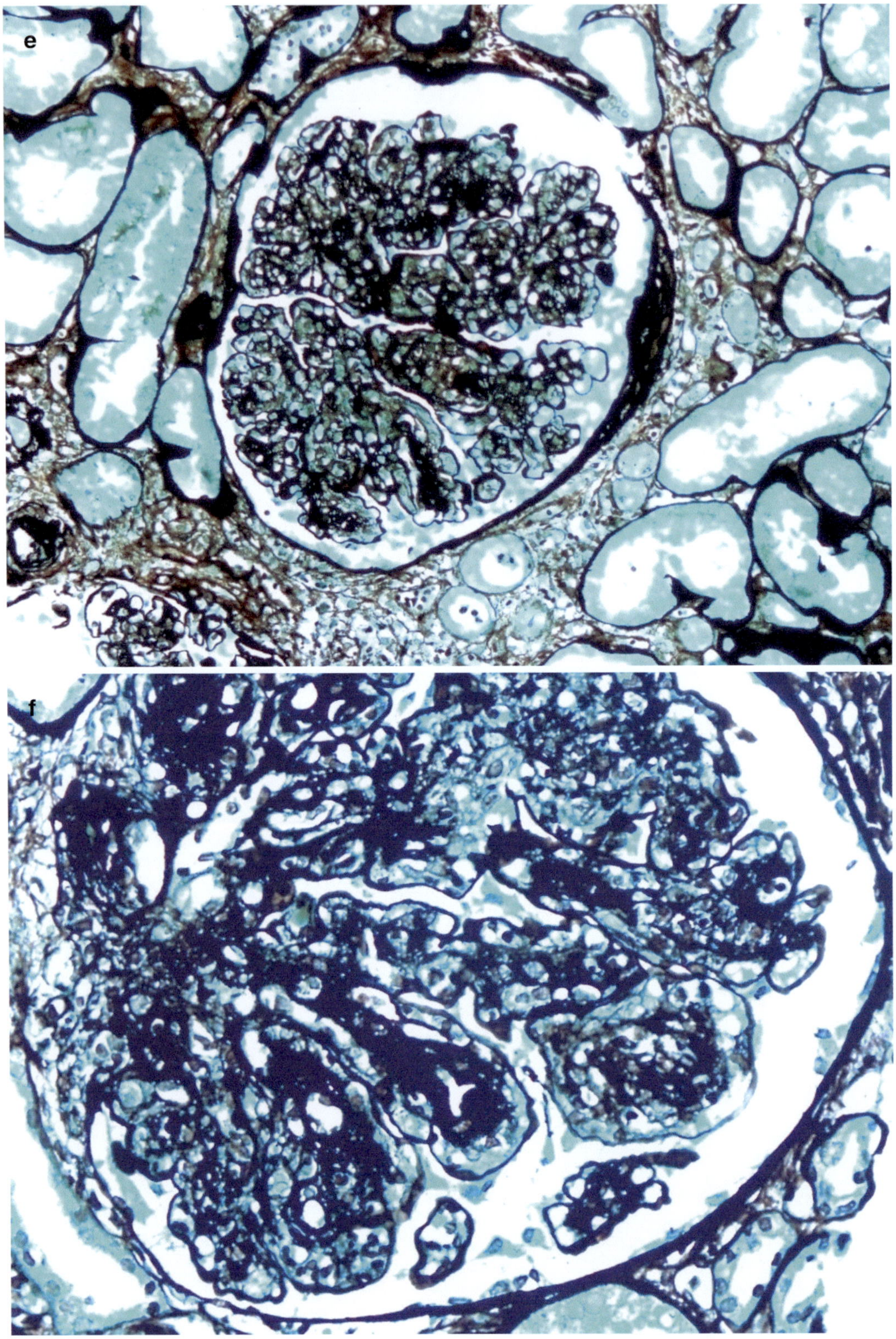

Fig. 5.1 (continued)

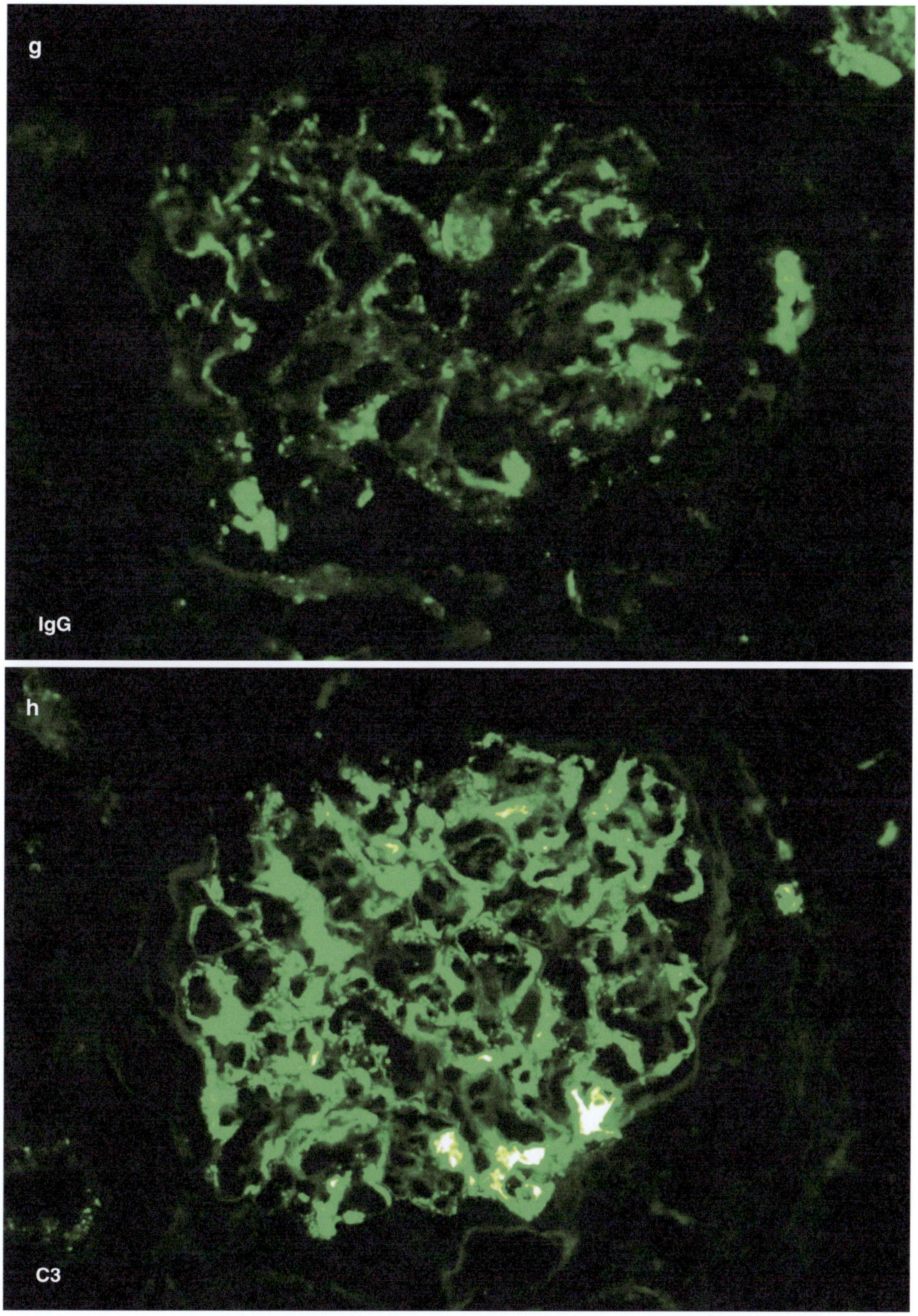

Fig. 5.1 (continued)

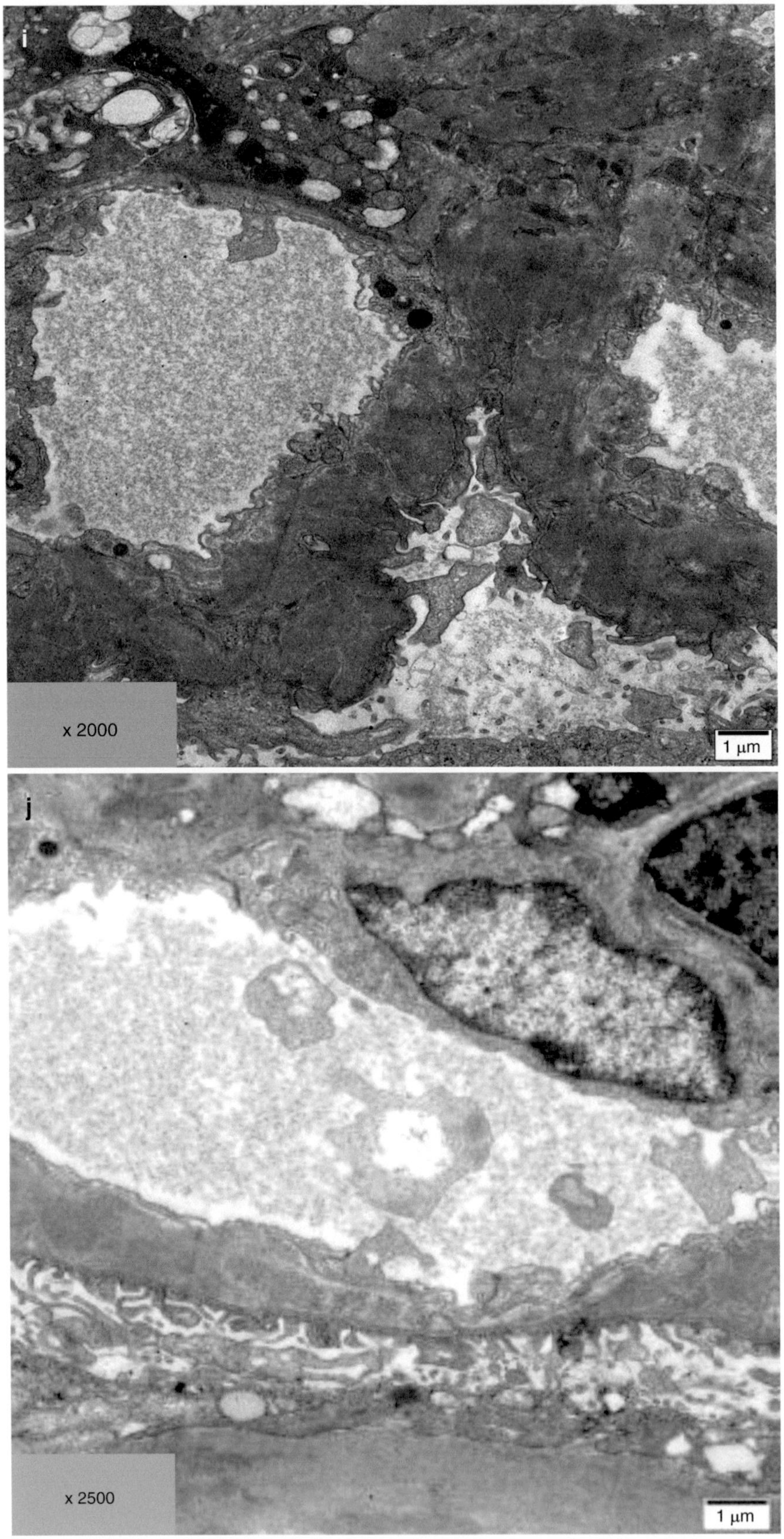

Fig. 5.1 (continued)

Further Reading

Bomback AS, Appel GB. Pathogenesis of the C3 glomerulopathies and reclassification of MPGN. Nat Rev Nephrol. 2012;8:634–42.

Cook HT, Pickering MC. Histopathology of MPGN and C3 glomerulopathies. Nat Rev Nephrol. 2015;11:14–22.

Salvadori M, Rosso G. Reclassification of membranoproliferative glomerulonephritis: identification of a new GN: C3GN. World J Nephrol. 2016;5:308–20.

Sethi S, Fervenza FC. Membranoproliferative glomerulonephritis–a new look at an old entity. N Engl J Med. 2012;366:1119–31.

Sethi S, Fervenza FC. Membranoproliferative glomerulonephritis: pathogenetic heterogeneity and proposal for a new classification. Semin Nephrol. 2011;31:341–8.

6 C3 Glomerulopathy

C3 glomerulopathy is a rare group of glomerular disorders comprising of C3 glomerulonephritis and dense deposit disease (DDD). It is caused by dysfunction in the alternate complement pathway due to antibodies targeted against C3 or C5 convertases or due to genetic variation in complement-related genes including complement factor H(CFH), complement factor B(CFB), CFHR1-5, and C3. Clinically patients present with hematuria, proteinuria and may have hypertension. Anti-factor H antibodies in association with C3 nephritic factor have also been seen in these patients. Serum C3 levels are low in the majority of patients at presentation. Light microscopic appearance can be commonly membranoproliferative, however mesangioproliferative, endocapillary hyperplasia or even crescentic morphology can be seen. On immunofluorescence microscopy, only C3 deposits are seen. Sometimes they may be accompanied by minimal immunoglobulin deposits with a difference of two staining intensities between C3 and immunoglobulins. The site of C3 deposits can be intramembranous, mesangial or capillary wall and deposits can be granular to semilinear. Tubular basement membrane deposits can be seen in patients with dense deposit disease.

Electron microscopy is essential in differentiating between dense deposit disease and C3 glomerulonephritis. Dense deposit disease shows characteristic intramembranous highly osmiophilic electron-dense band-like or sausage-shaped deposits. Deposits can also be seen within mesangium, subendothelial locations, or as subepithelial humps. Electron-dense deposits can also be observed within Bowman's capsule and in the tubular basement membrane.

In C3 glomerulonephritis, deposits are amorphous, less electron-dense as compared to dense deposit disease and bland with the extracellular matrix. They can be located within mesangium, subendothelial or intramembranous locations, or as subepithelial humps.

Dense deposit disease is frequently seen in children in the first decade of life and young adults with majority of cases being between 5 and 15 years of age. C3 glomerulonephritis is usually seen in the second decade of life but can also be seen in children.

Both dense deposit disease and C3 glomerulonephritis have a high recurrence rate following renal transplantation.

P. Gupta, R. K. Gupta, *Pathology of Glomerular Diseases*, https://doi.org/10.1007/978-981-19-1430-0_6

6.1 C3 Glomerulonephritis (Fig. 6.1)

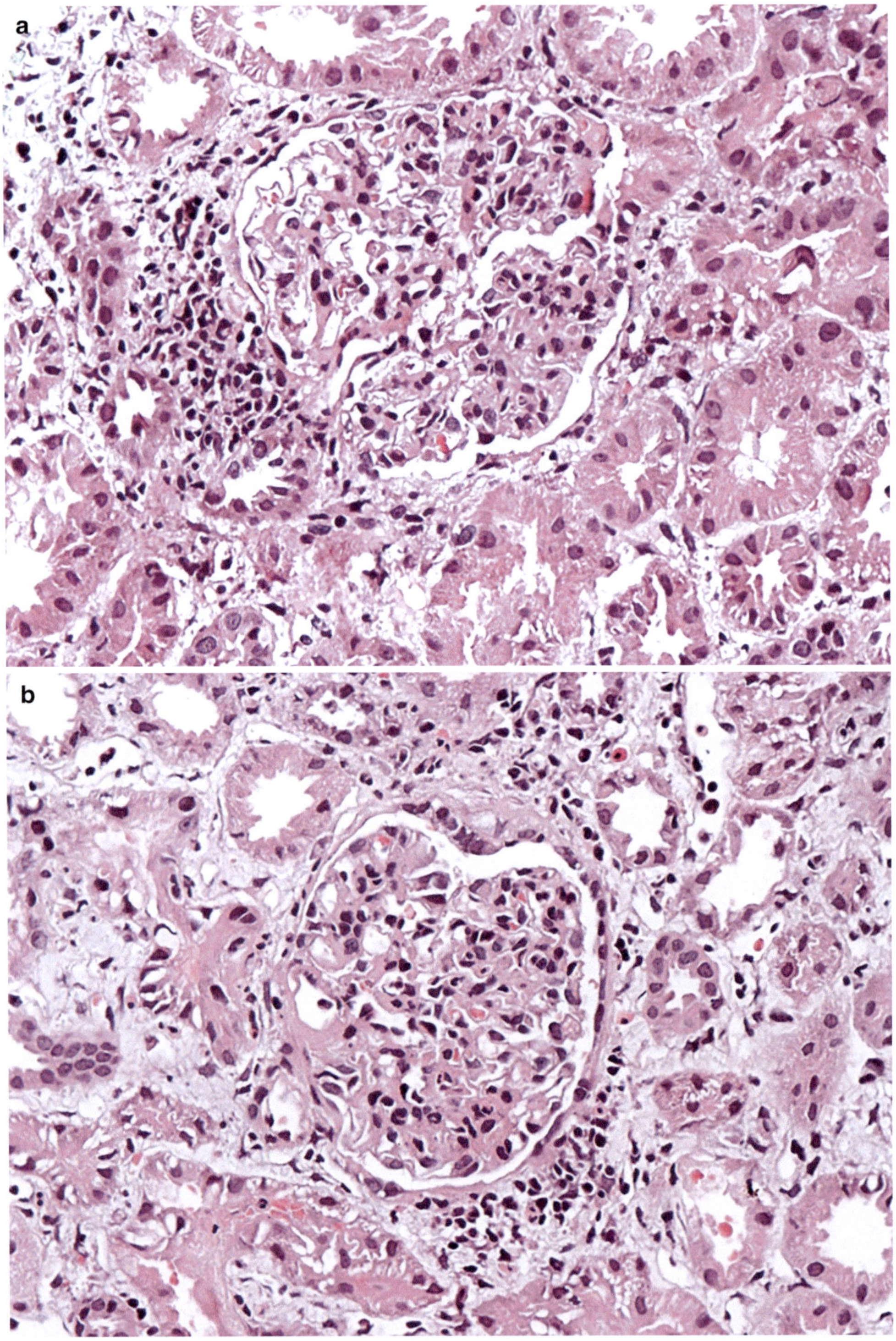

Fig. 6.1 **C3 Glomerulonephritis** A 6-years male child presented with gross hematuria with fever and skin rash for 3 weeks. He had no h/o joint pain, redness of eyes, or dysuria. Current episode was triggered by URI with intermittent hematuria. No family h/o renal disease was present. Urine analysis revealed 2+ proteinuria with 10–15 WBC and numerous RBC/hpf; there were no casts. CBC was wnl. Serum creatinine was 1.79 mg/dL. Serum total protein was 6.1 g/dL with serum albumin of 3.04 g/dL, serum globulin of 3.06 g/dL, and A/G ratio of 0.99. Serum total cholesterol was 139 mg/dL. ASO titer was <200 IU/L. C-ANCA, P-ANCA and ANA were negative. Serum complement C3 was low, 675 mg/L and C4 was 437 mg/L. Single-core renal biopsy was obtained which had 11 glomeruli, out of which 1 was globally sclerosed, 3 showed partial fibrocellular crescents; other glomeruli showed an increase in mesangial cellularity with mild neutrophilic infiltration and segmental endocapillary hyperplasia. IF revealed granular deposits of C3 along GBM and mesangium. IgG, IgM, IgA, C1q, kappa and lambda were negative. EM showed a glomerular capillary loop with subendothelial and few intramembranous electron-dense deposits along with a subepithelial hump. (**a** and **b**) HE ×200, (**c** and **d**) PAS ×200, (**e**) IF ×400, (**f** and **g**) EM (identity of the patient has been concealed)

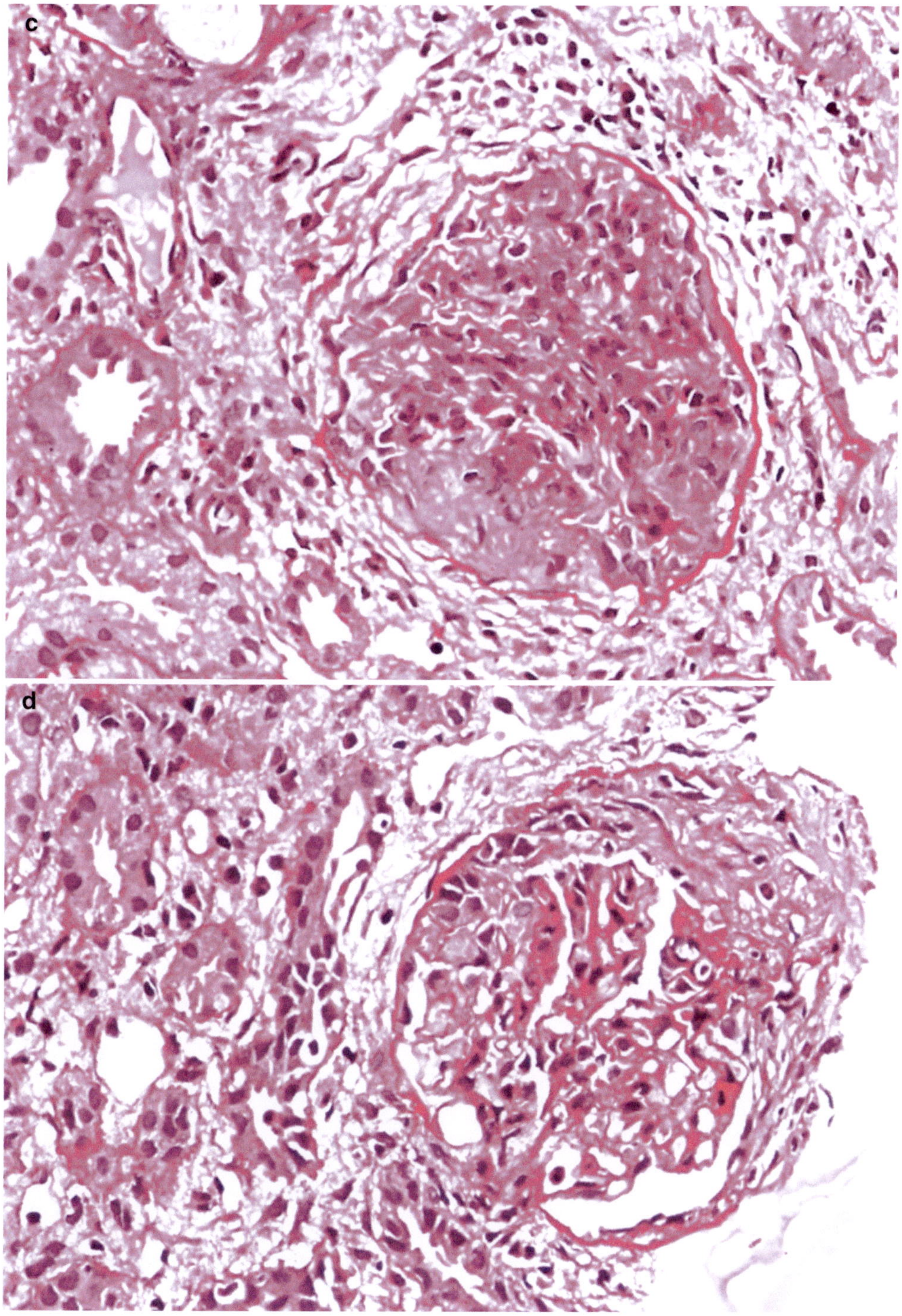

Fig. 6.1 (continued)

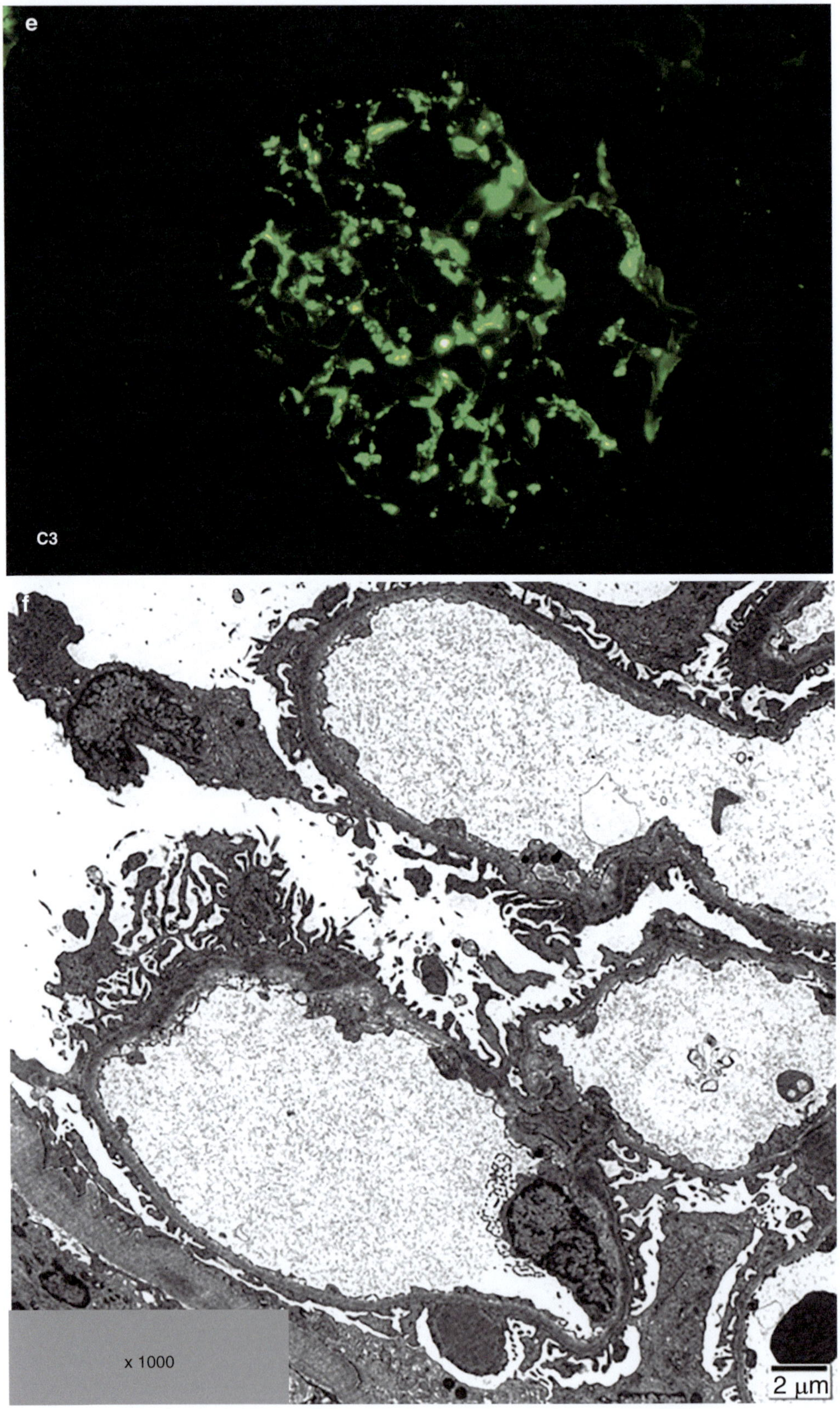

Fig. 6.1 (continued)

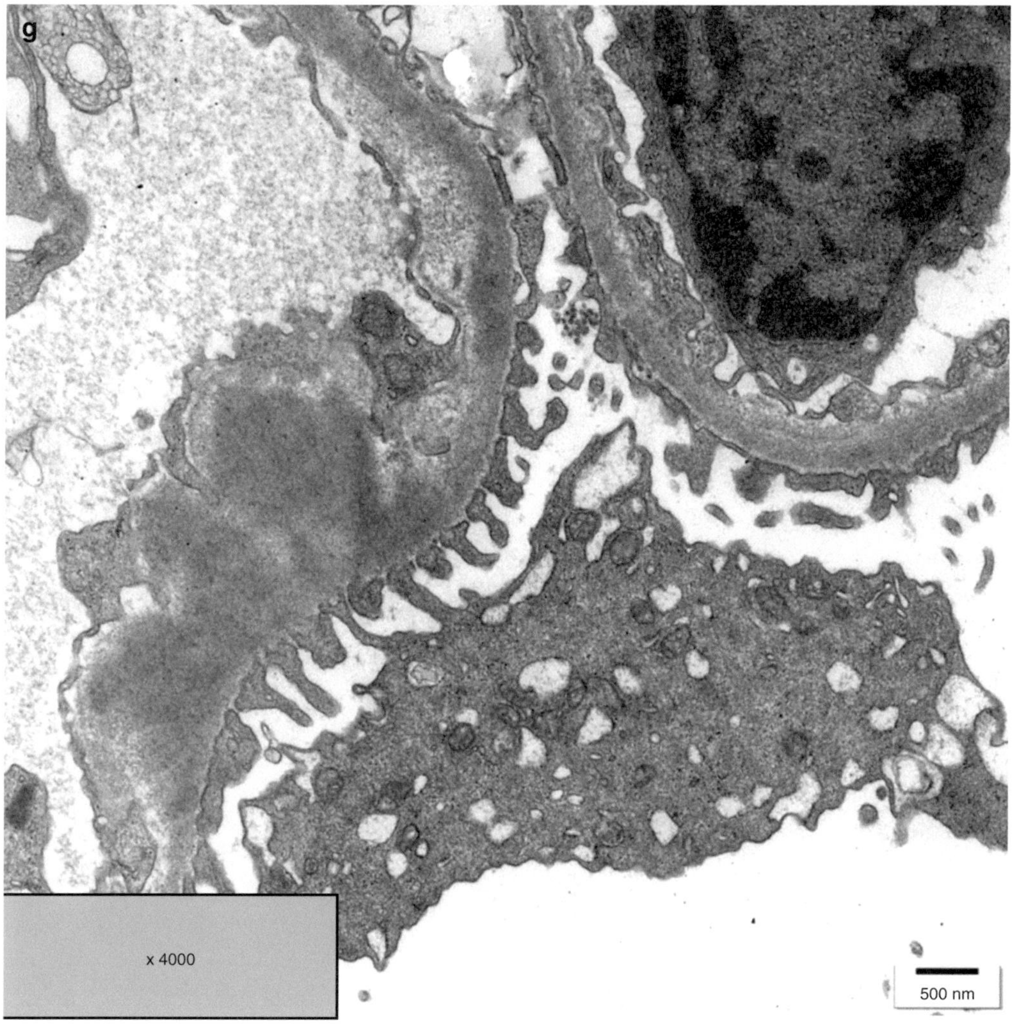

Fig. 6.1 (continued)

6.2 Dense Deposit Disease (DDD) (Fig. 6.2)

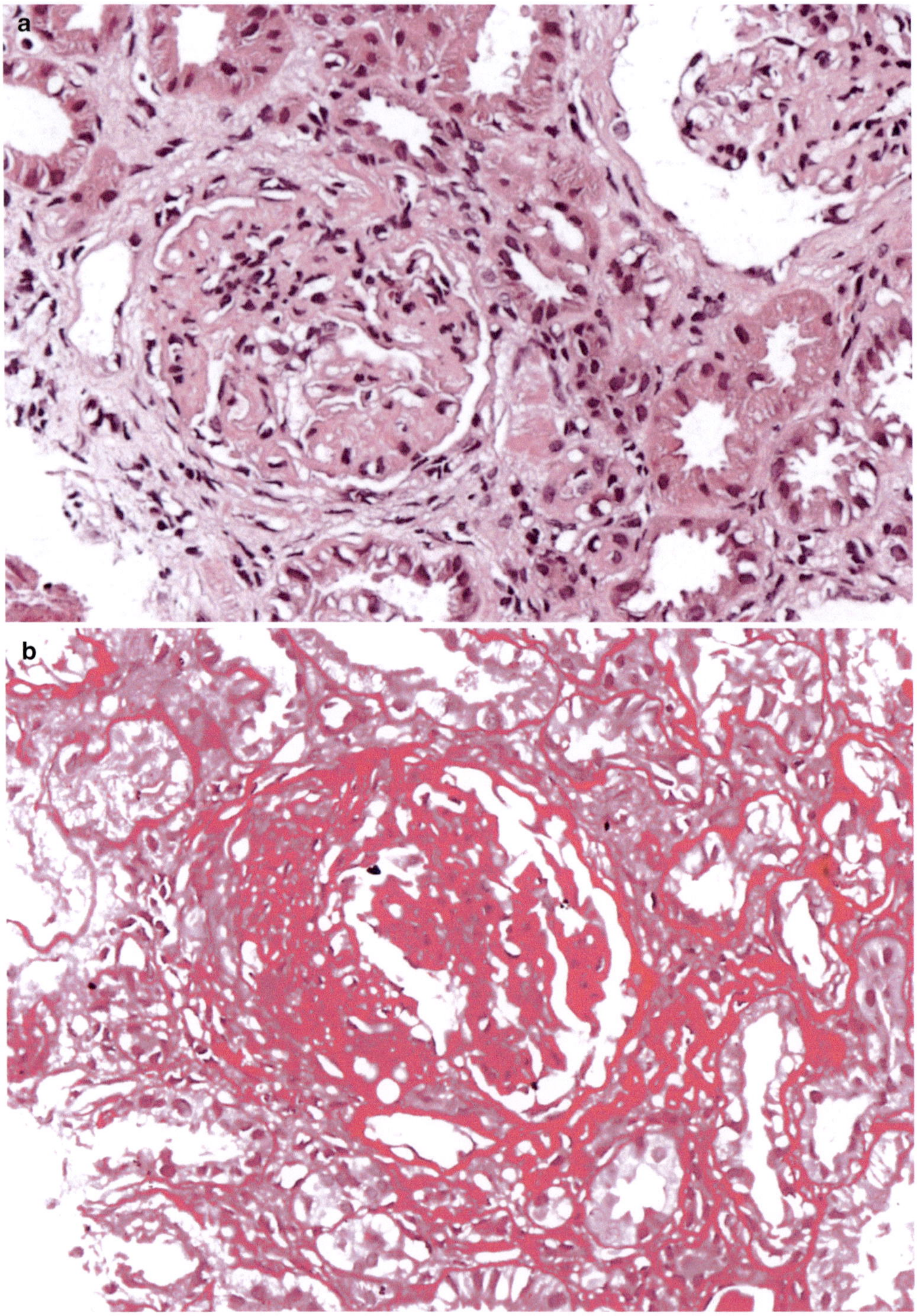

Fig. 6.2 **Dense Deposit Disease** A 13-years female patient presented with bilateral pedal edema and hypertension. On workup, she was found to have nephrotic range proteinuria. Urine analysis revealed proteinuria (+++) with no RBC; urinary P:C ratio was 5.8. Her serum creatinine was 1.7 mg/dL. Serum C3 was reduced being 763 mg/L and serum C4 was wnl being 289 mg/L. Renal biopsy had eight glomeruli, two of them were globally sclerosed and one showed segmental sclerosis. The remaining glomeruli showed mild increase in mesangial matrix and cellularity along with thickening and segmental reduplication of GBM. Endocapillary hyperplasia and crescents were seen in two glomeruli each; one of the crescent was fibrous and the other was fibrocellular. Patchy tubular atrophy was evident. Interstitium showed a moderate amount of lymphocytic infiltrate. Blood vessels were unremarkable. IF showed complement C3 granular to smudgy deposits (+++) along GBM and mesangium. IF for IgG, IgM, IgA and complement C1q were negative. EM showed intramembranous ribbon-like highly osmiophilic deposits within the glomerular capillaries and focally in mesangial areas. Occasional tubules also showed electron-dense deposits along the tubular basement membrane. (**a**) HE ×400, (**b**) PAS ×400, (**c**) PSM ×400, (**d**) IF ×400, (**e** and **f**) EM (identity of the patient has been concealed)

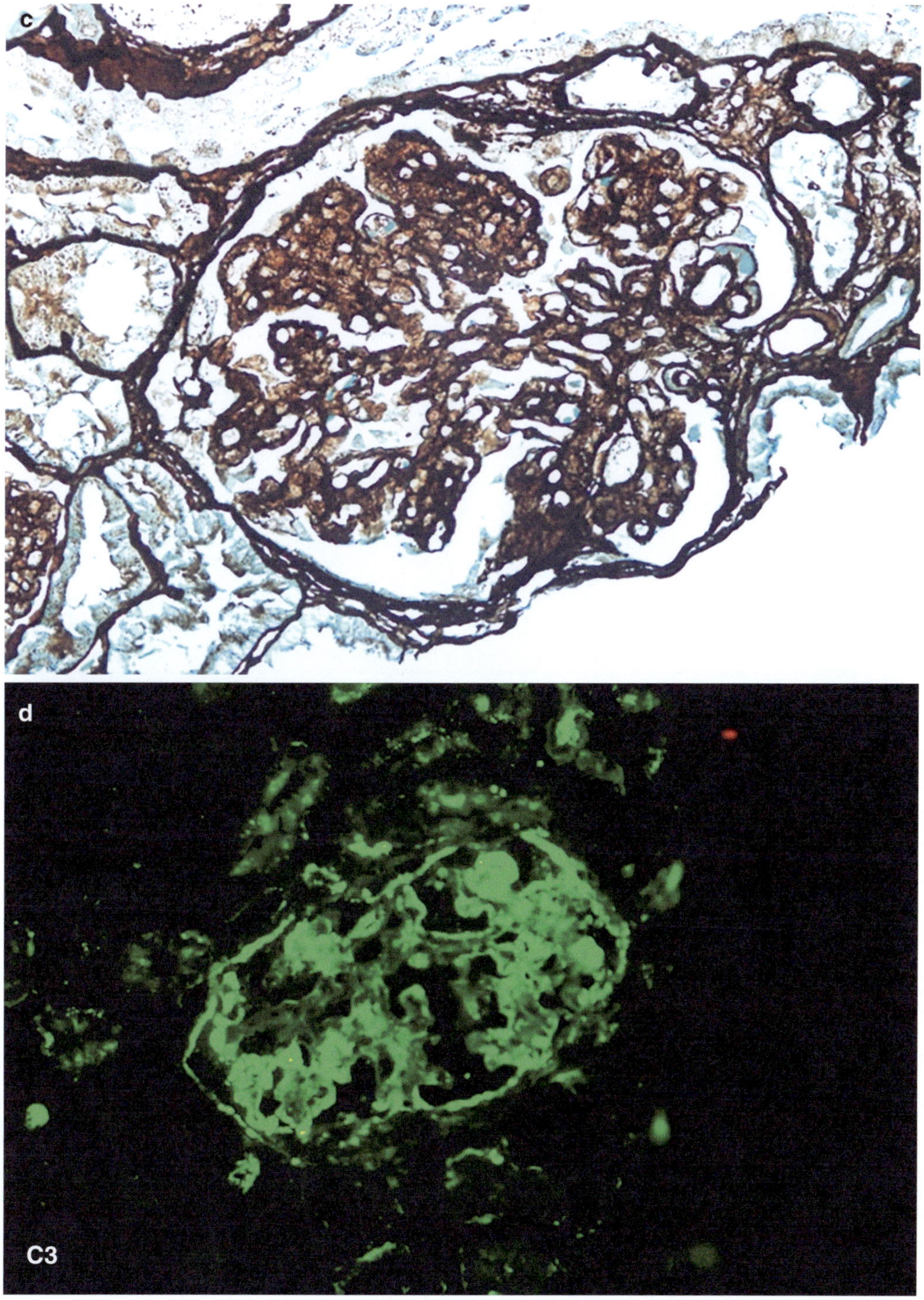

Fig. 6.2 (continued)

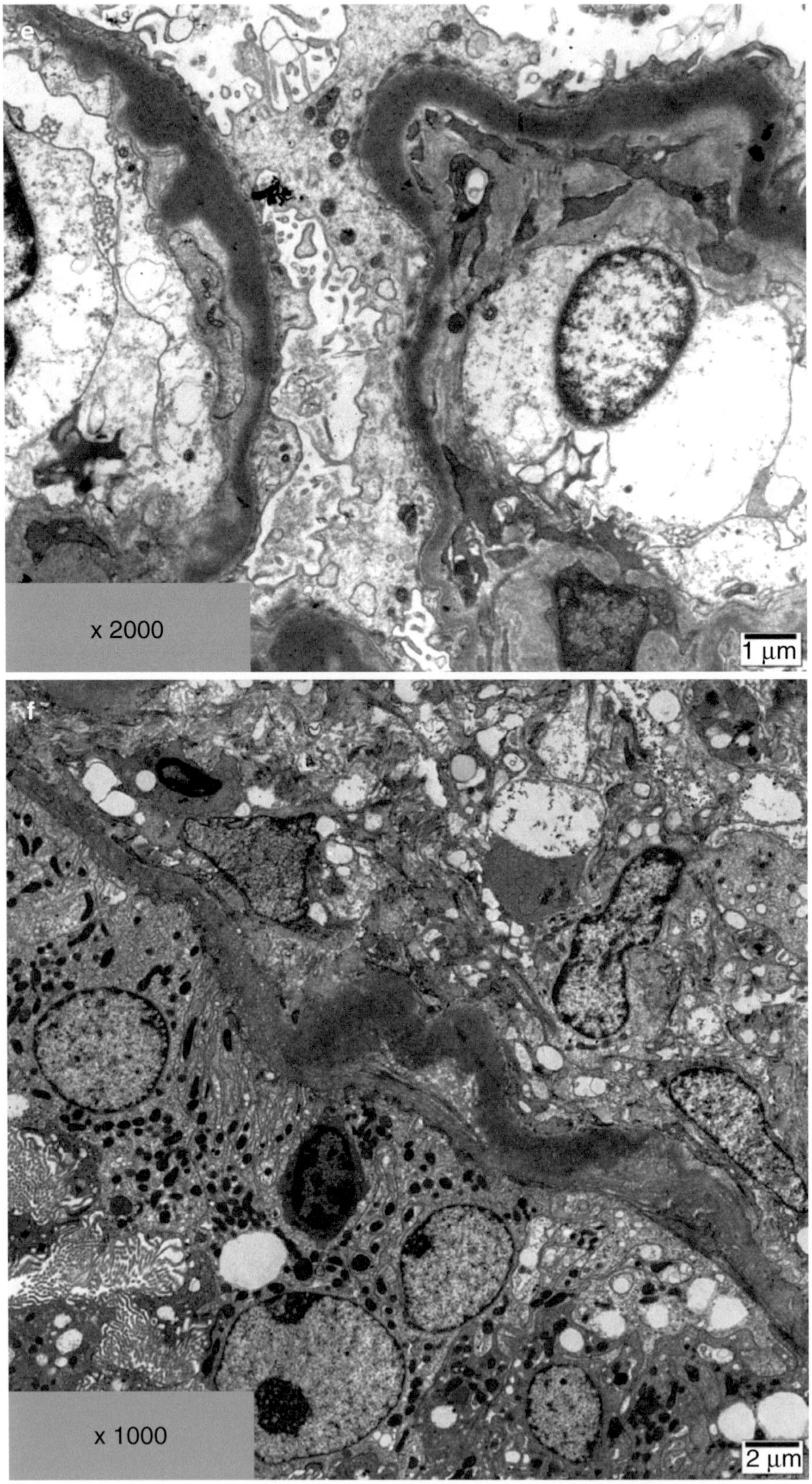

Fig. 6.2 (continued)

6.3 Post-transplant Recurrent DDD (Fig. 6.3)

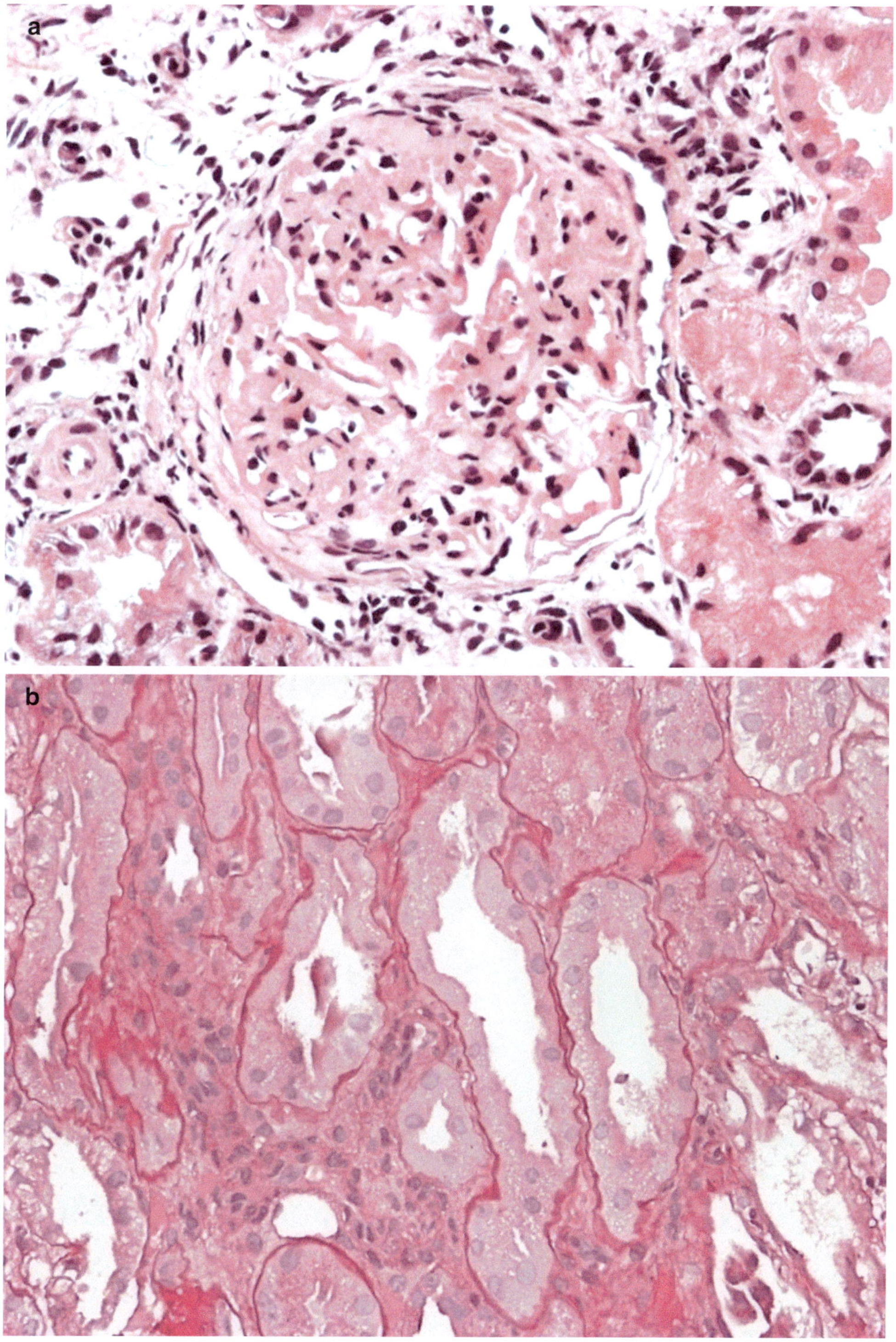

Fig. 6.3 Post Transplant Recurrent DDD A 22-years male patient diagnosed as MPGN 8 years ago, received live related renal allograft 18 months back. Now he presented with proteinuria 3+, urinary sediment had 10–15 RBC/hpf; urine spot P/C ratio was 6.0 and his serum creatinine was 0.69 mg/dL. Serum complement C3 was 820 mg/L and serum C4 was 210 mg/L. Renal biopsy had ten glomeruli, all of them showed marked thickening of GBM and a few showed increased mesangial cellularity. Thickening of tubular basement membrane was seen. Focal tubular atrophy with mild lymphocytic interstitial infiltration was evident. Blood vessels were unremarkable. IHC for C4d was negative in peritubular capillaries. IF revealed granular C3 (4+) deposits along GBM, mesangium, and TBM; IgM was (+) while IgG, IgA, C1q and kappa and lambda were negative. EM showed that the GBM was thickened, ribbon-like highly osmiophilic intramembranous electron-dense deposits were seen in the GBM and focally in the mesangial areas and also along TBM. (**a**) HE ×400, (**b**) PAS ×400, (**c**) PSM ×400, (**d**) IF ×400, and (**e**) EM (identity of the patient has been concealed)

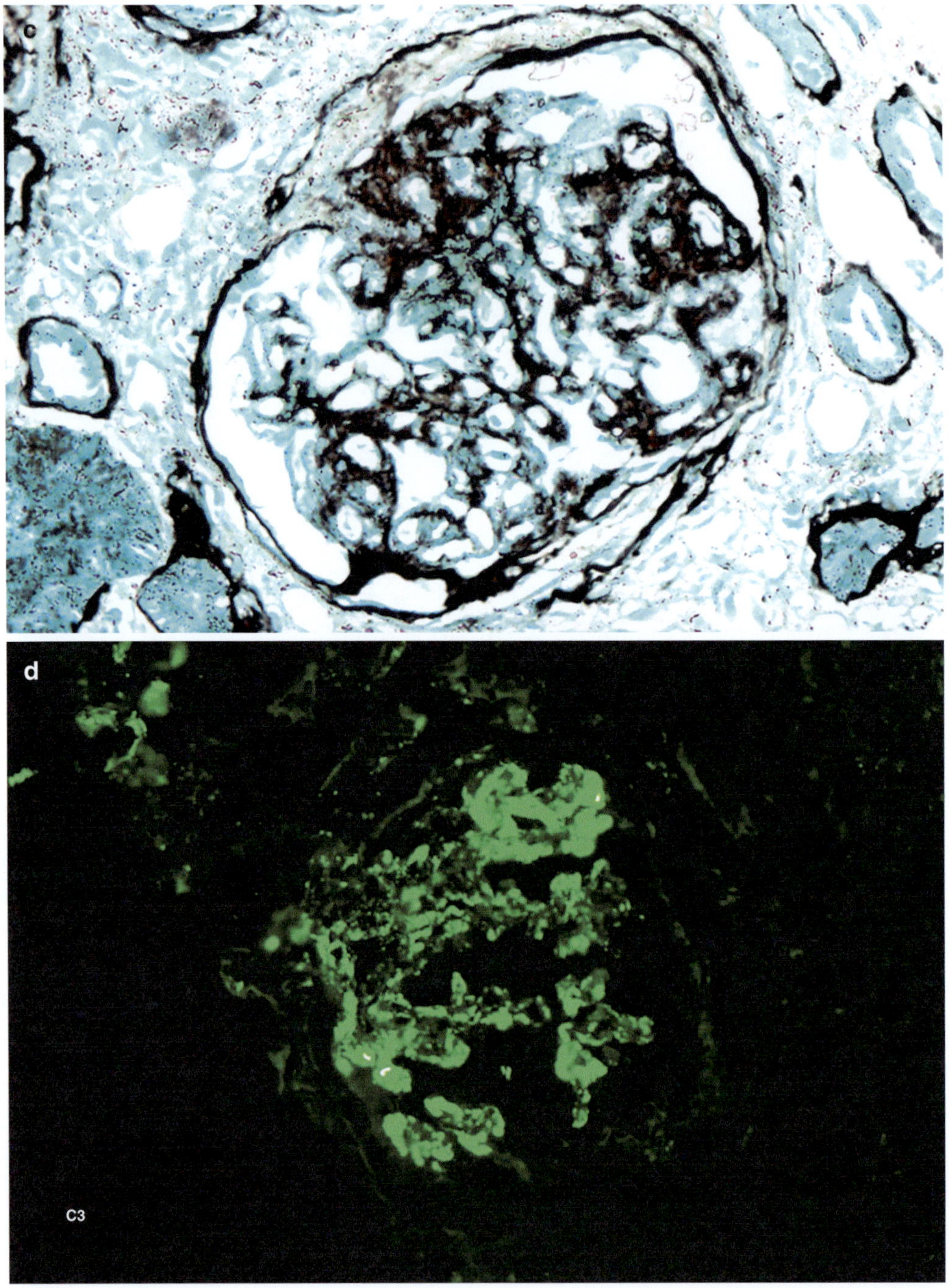

Fig. 6.3 (continued)

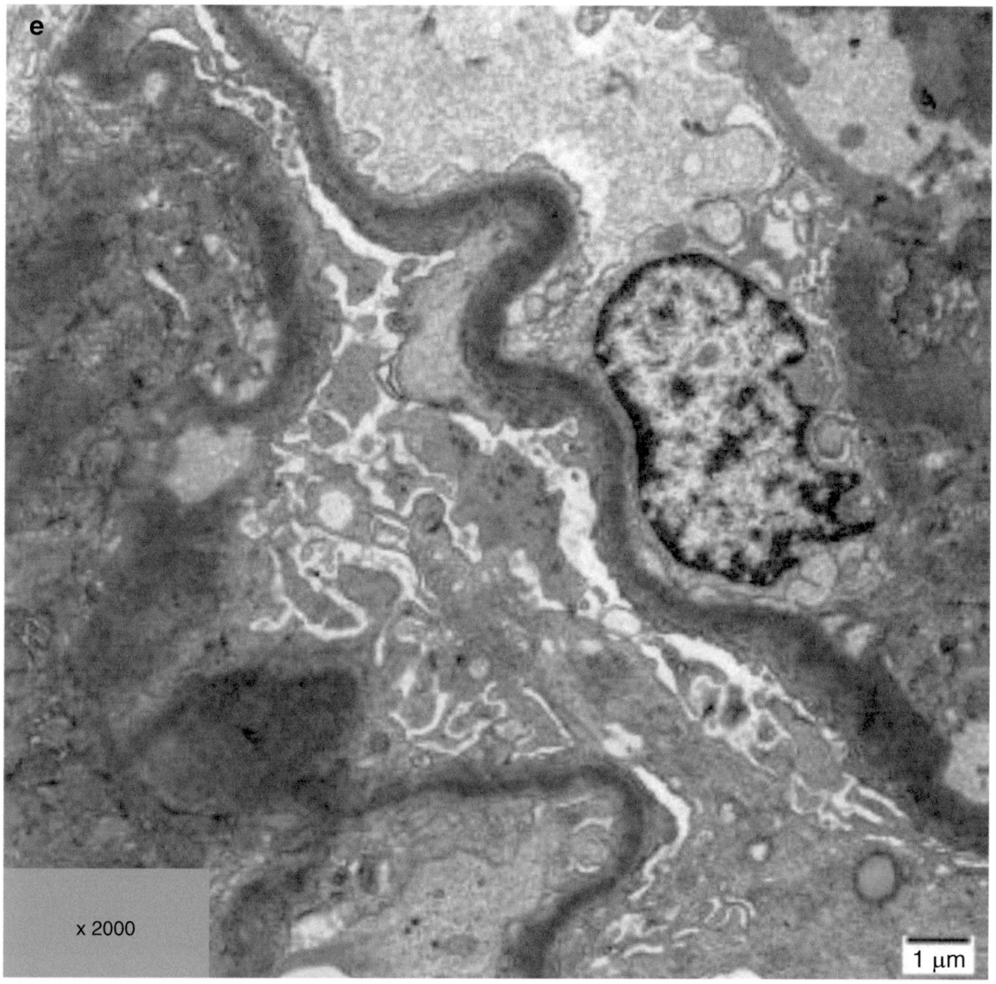

Fig. 6.3 (continued)

Further Reading

Ito N, Ohashi R, Nagata M. C3 glomerulopathy and current dilemmas. Clin Exp Nephrol. 2017;21:541–51.

Pickering MC, D'Agati VD, Nester CM, Smith RJ, Haas M, Appel GB, Alpers CE, Bajema IM, Bedrosian C, Braun M, Doyle M, Fakhouri F, Fervenza FC, Fogo AB, Frémeaux-Bacchi V, Gale DP, Goicoechea de Jorge E, Griffin G, Harris CL, Holers VM, Johnson S, Lavin PJ, Medjeral-Thomas N, Paul Morgan B, Nast CC, Noel LH, Peters DK, Rodríguez de Córdoba S, Servais A, Sethi S, Song WC, Tamburini P, Thurman JM, Zavros M, Cook HT. C3 glomerulopathy: consensus report. Kidney Int. 2013;84:1079–89.

Ravindran A, Fervenza FC, Smith RJH, De Vriese AS, Sethi S. C3 glomerulopathy: ten years' experience at Mayo Clinic. Mayo Clin Proc. 2018;93:991–1008.

Regunathan-Shenk R, Avasare RS, Ahn W, Canetta PA, Cohen DJ, Appel GB, Bomback AS. Kidney transplantation in C3 glomerulopathy: a case series. Am J Kidney Dis. 2019;73(3):316–23.

Smith RJH, Appel GB, Blom AM, Cook HT, D'Agati VD, Fakhouri F, Fremeaux-Bacchi V, Józsi M, Kavanagh D, Lambris JD, Noris M, Pickering MC, Remuzzi G, de Córdoba SR, Sethi S, Van der Vlag J, Zipfel PF, Nester CM. C3 glomerulopathy – understanding a rare complement-driven renal disease. Nat Rev Nephrol. 2019;15:129–43.

7 Infection Related Glomerulonephritis (IRGN)

Infection related glomerulonephritis include post-infectious (post-streptococcal) glomerulonephritis, IgA dominant post-infectious glomerulonephritis, endocarditis associated glomerulonephritis etc. Post-infectious (post-streptococcal) glomerulonephritis (PIGN) is the leading cause of acute nephritic syndrome/acute glomerulonephritis in children. It is less often seen in adults. It is usually caused secondary to upper respiratory tract streptococcal infection with a latent period of 1–2 weeks. Streptococcal pyrogenic exotoxin B and nephritis-associated plasmin receptor are two common antigens that cause activation of the alternate complement pathway and are involved in the pathogenesis of PIGN. In adults, it is usually seen in association with risk factors such as diabetes, alcohol abuse, malignancies, etc. It can also be caused by other bacteria such as staphylococci and pneumococcal infection. Gram-negative bacteria and certain viral and parasitic infections associated PIGN have also been described. The most common presentation is nephritic syndrome, but nephrotic syndrome and rapidly progressive glomerulonephritis can also be seen. Light microscopic appearances show enlarged glomeruli with lobular accentuation and diffuse proliferative glomerulonephritis with endocapillary hyperplasia along with neutrophilic infiltration. Crescents can also be seen. In the resolving phase of the disease, glomeruli are less cellular with only mesangial proliferation. Subepithelial humps can be observed in some cases under oil immersion in Masson's trichrome-stained sections. On immunofluorescence, typical cases show coarse granular deposits of IgG and complement C3 along glomerular capillary wall. In the resolving phase mesangial granular IgG and C3 deposits are seen or sometimes only C3 deposits can be evident. On electron microscopy, characteristic finding is the presence of electron-dense deposits in the form of subepithelial humps. Endothelial cell swelling, mesangial cell swelling, and polymorphs are also visualized.

In majority of these patients, the disease has a self-resolving clinical course. Some of the patients may succumb to acute illness due to renal or cardiac causes. A small percentage of cases can have persistence of hematuria, hypertension, proteinuria, and hypocomplementemia.

P. Gupta, R. K. Gupta, *Pathology of Glomerular Diseases*, https://doi.org/10.1007/978-981-19-1430-0_7

7.1 Post-infectious Glomerulonephritis (PIGN) (Fig. 7.1)

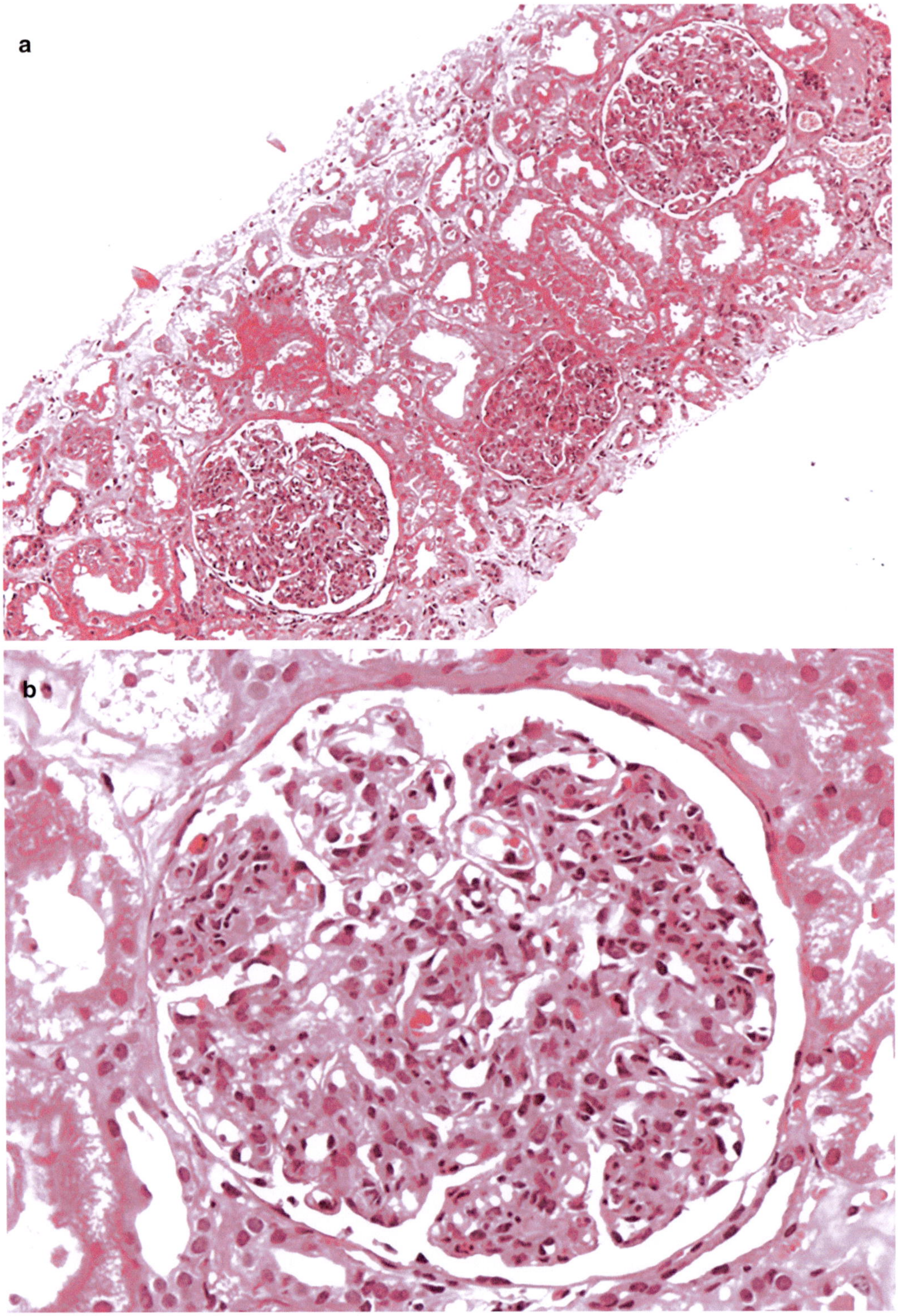

Fig. 7.1 **PIGN** A 12-years male patient presented with fever and h/o sore throat for 2 weeks. There was no h/o hemoptysis or vomiting. For the past 2 days, he had been passing dark (cola-colored) urine. He did not have any pedal edema. Urine analysis revealed albumin 3+ with 30–40 RBC/hpf. Serum creatinine was 3.5 mg/dl, ASO titre was >800 IU. Serum procalcitonin was 36.84 and serum C3 was low (640 mg/L); C4 was wnl. c-ANCA, p-ANCA, ANA, and DsDNA were negative. Single-core renal biopsy had 16 glomeruli, all were enlarged and showed lobular accentuation. Endocapillary proliferation with neutrophilic infiltration in glomeruli was observed. There was no splitting or thickening of GBM, nor there were any areas of segmental or global sclerosis. Focal tubular atrophy was observed. The interstitium had focal lymphocytic infiltrate; blood vessels were unremarkable. IF showed 3+ granular deposits of IgG, C3, C1q, kappa and lambda along GBM; IgM and IgA were negative. EM showed several subepithelial humps. (**a**) HE ×100, (**b**) HE ×400, (**c**) PAS ×400, (**d**) PSM ×400, (**e** and **f**) IF ×400, (**g**) EM (identity of the patient has been concealed)

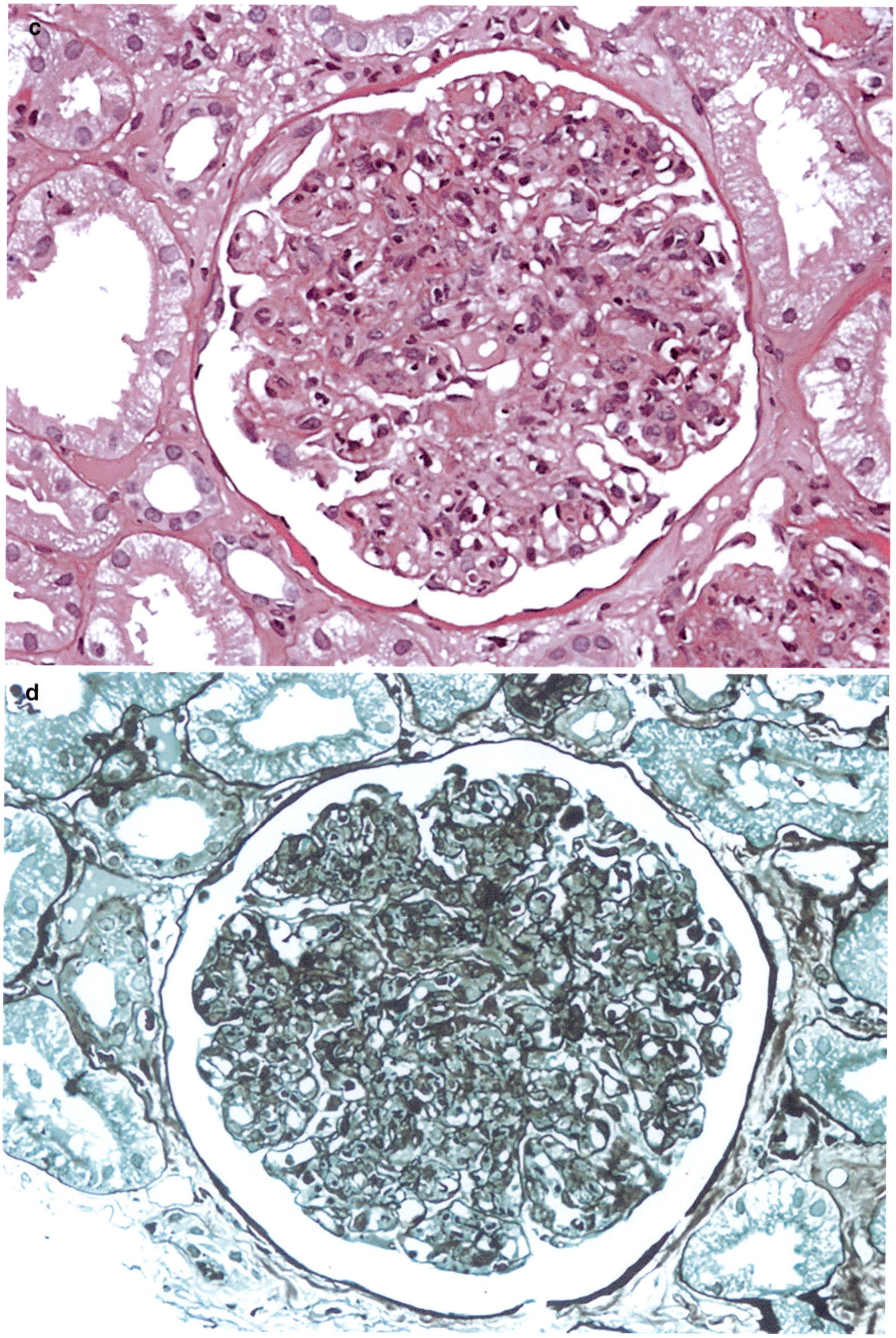

Fig. 7.1 (continued)

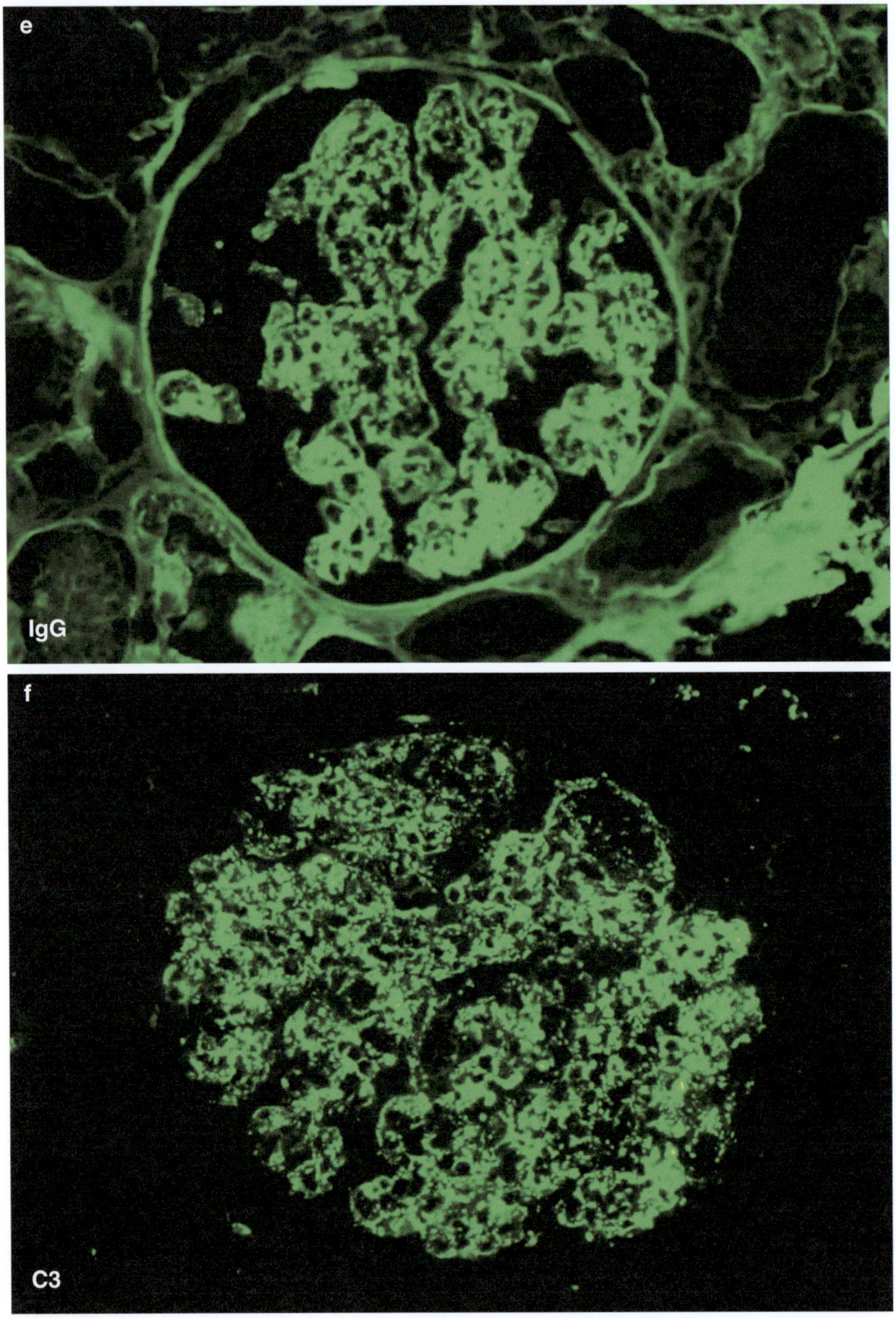

Fig. 7.1 (continued)

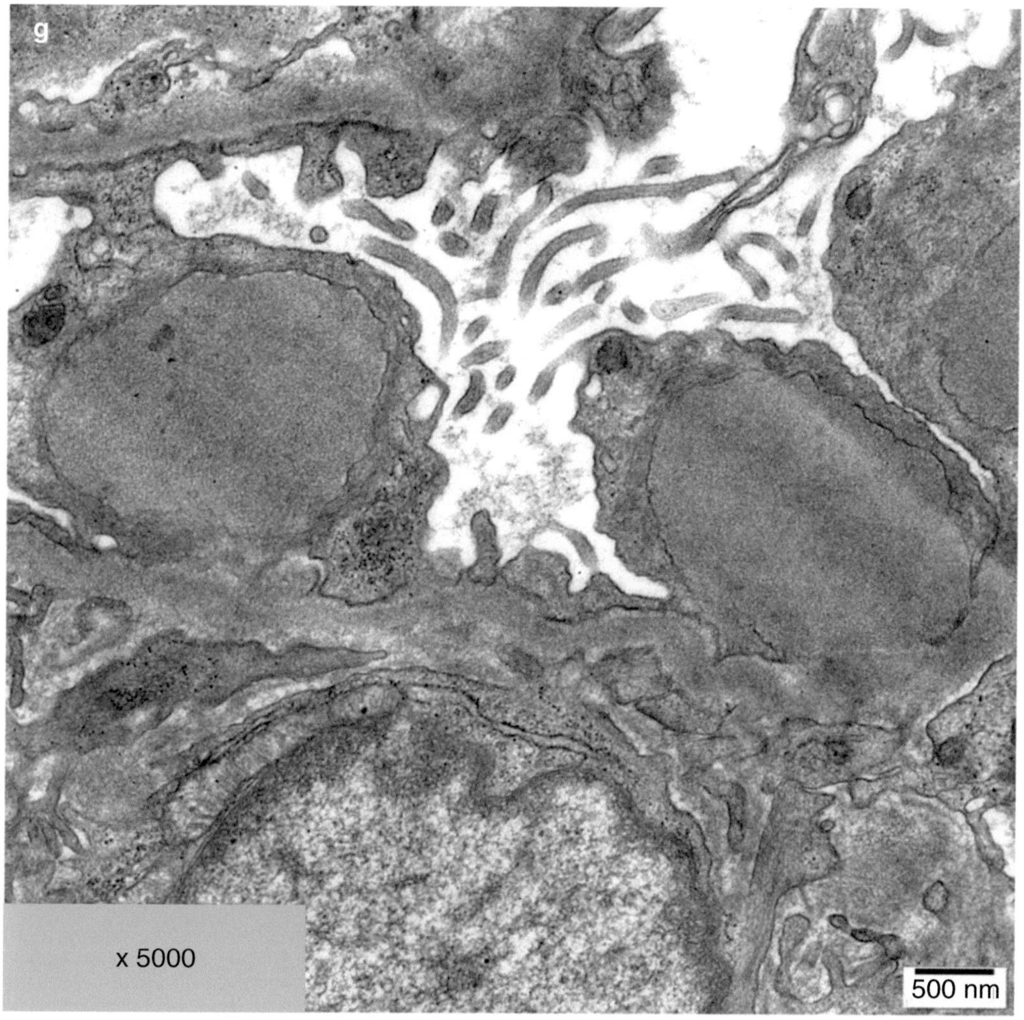

Fig. 7.1 (continued)

7.2 IgA Dominant PIGN (Fig. 7.2)

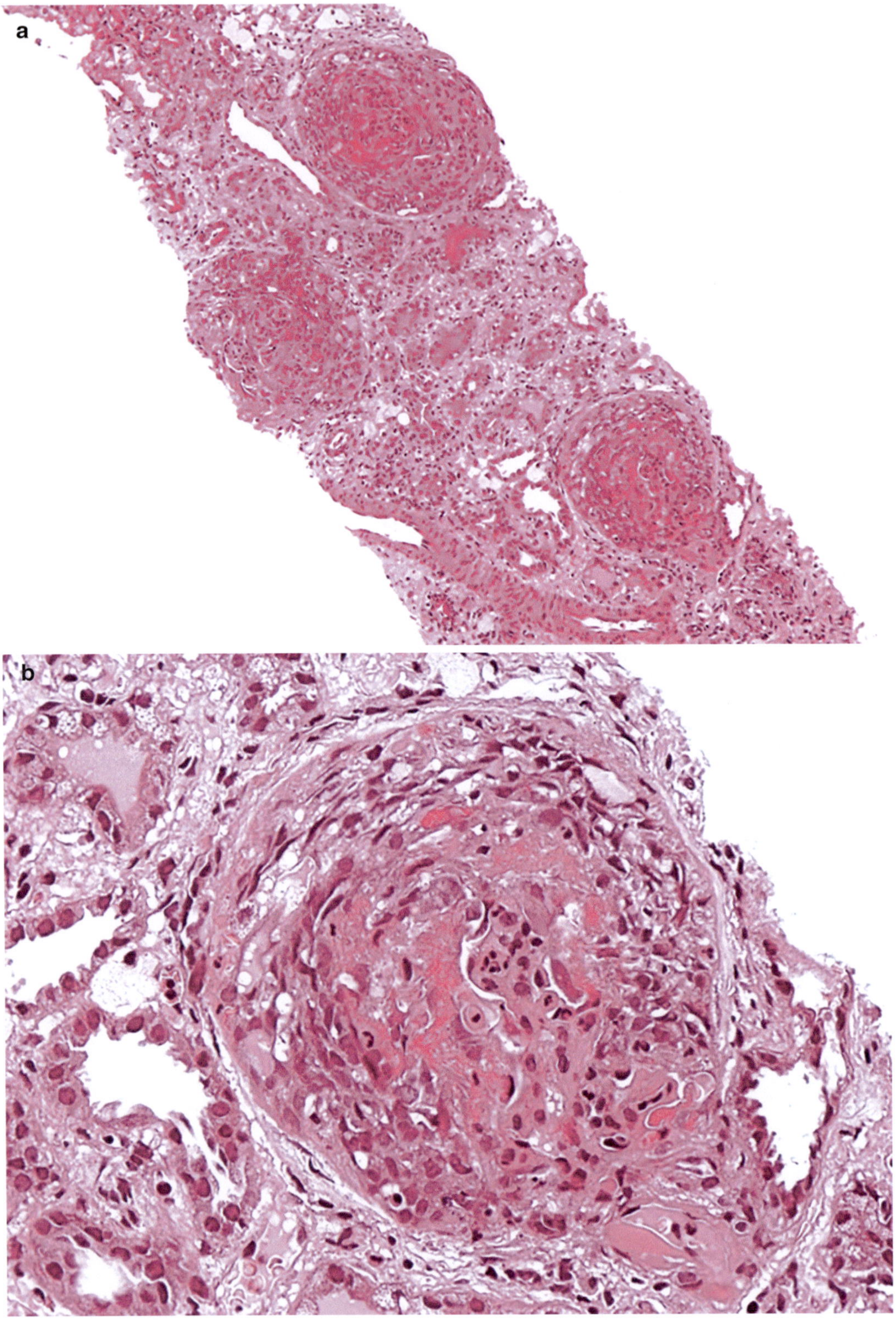

Fig. 7.2 **IgA dominant PIGN** A 20-years male patient presented with oliguria, pedal edema along with hematuria and nephrotic range proteinuria for 10 days. He had h/o upper respiratory tract Infection 1 week ago prior to the onset of symptoms. Serum creatinine was 4.8 mg/dL, urinary protein was 3+; urinary sediment had 20–30 RBC/hpf. Serum C3 was low (710 mg/L) and ASO titer was >200; serum ANA was negative. Renal biopsy had 14 glomeruli, 13 of them showed circumferential cellular crescents with neutrophilic infiltration and collapsed glomerular tuft. Mild tubulointerstitial mononuclear cell infiltration with the presence of interstitial foam cells was noted. Blood vessels were unremarkable. IF showed granular deposits of IgA ++, C3 ++++, kappa ++ and lambda ++ along the GBM; IgG and IgM were negative. EM revealed many subepithelial humps with effacement of visceral epithelial foot processes over the humps and few subendothelial deposits. (**a**) HE ×100, (**b**) HE ×400, (**c**) PAS ×400, (**d**) PSM ×400, (**e** and **f**) IF × 400, (**g**) EM ×5000 (identity of the patient has been concealed)

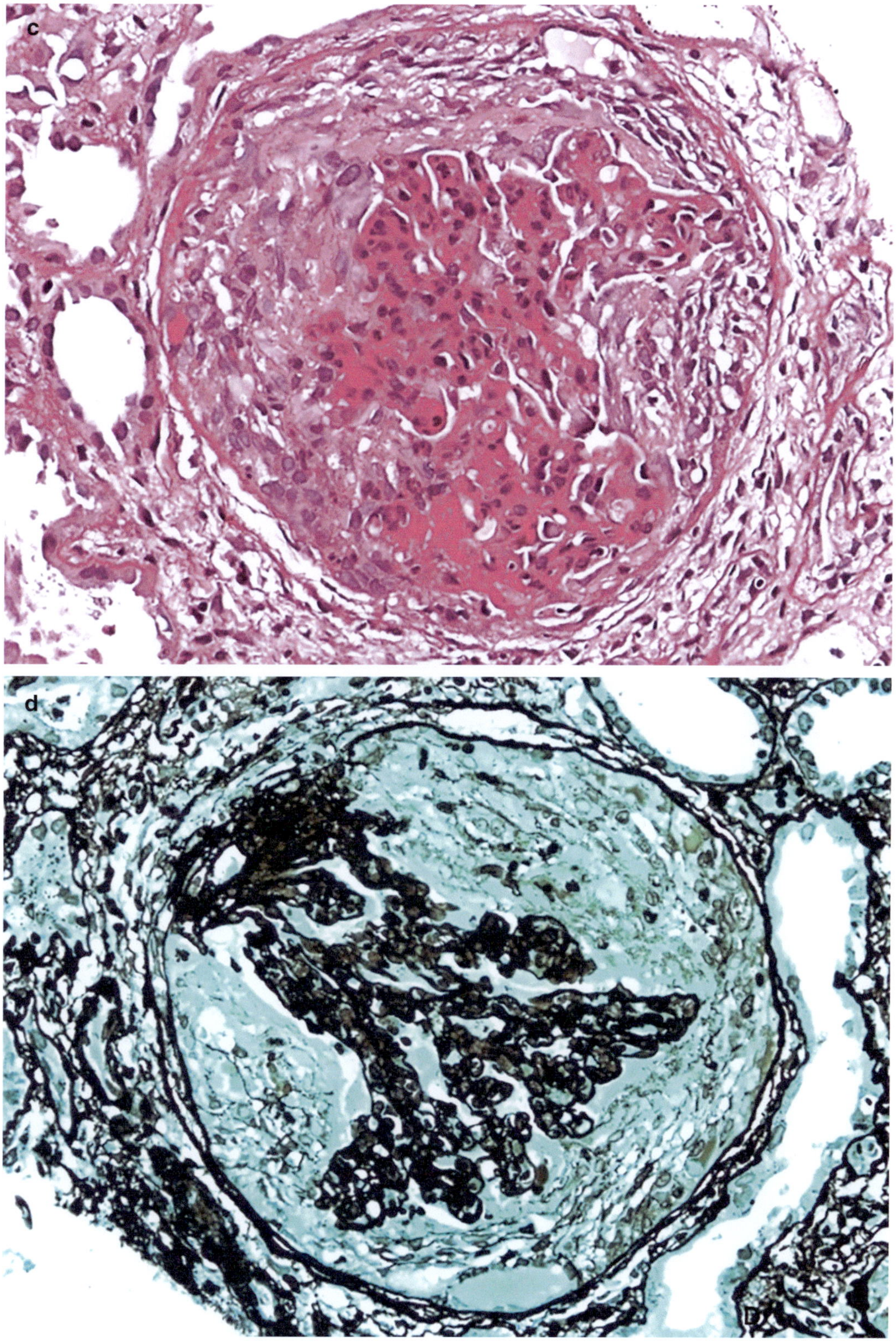

Fig. 7.2 (continued)

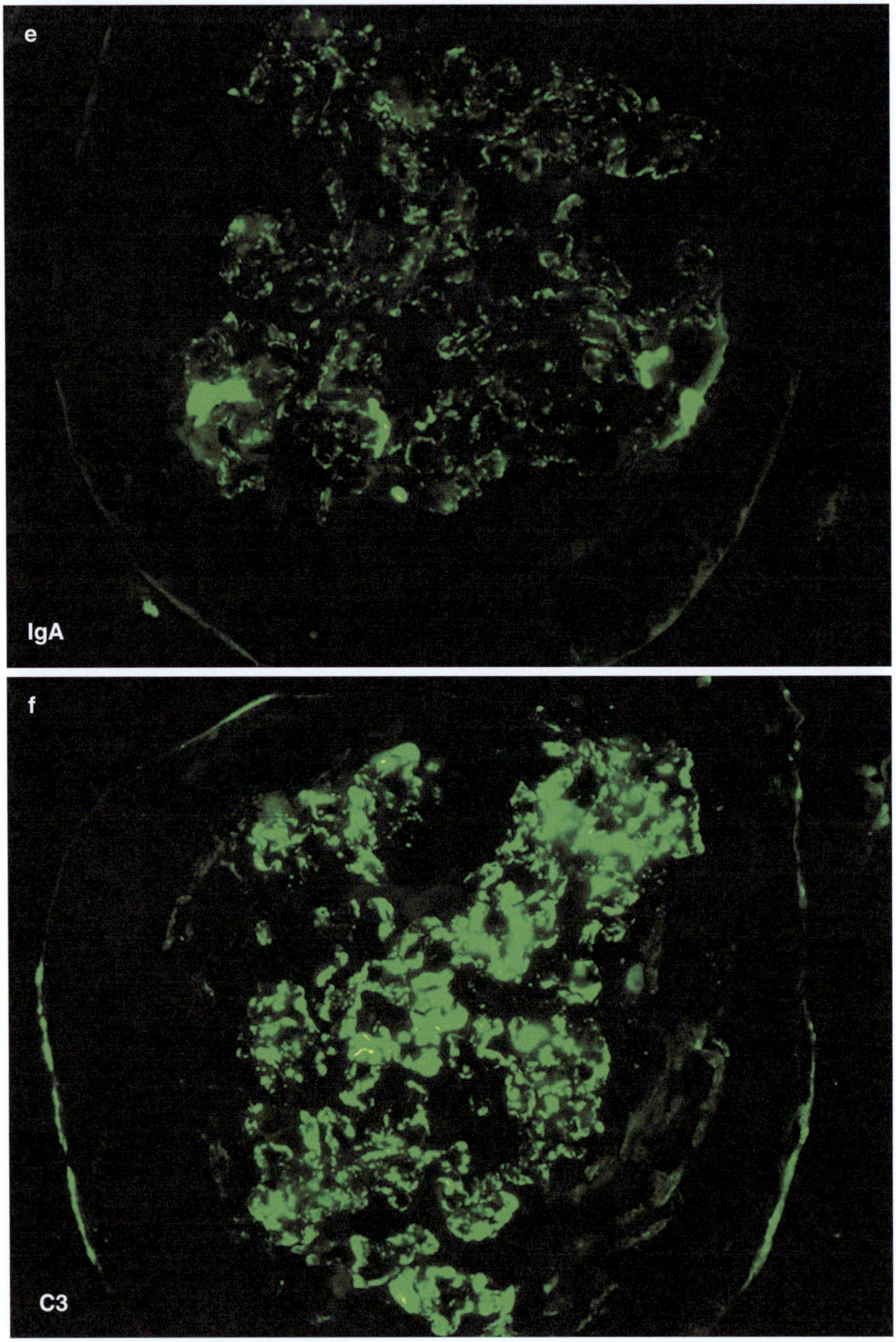

Fig. 7.2 (continued)

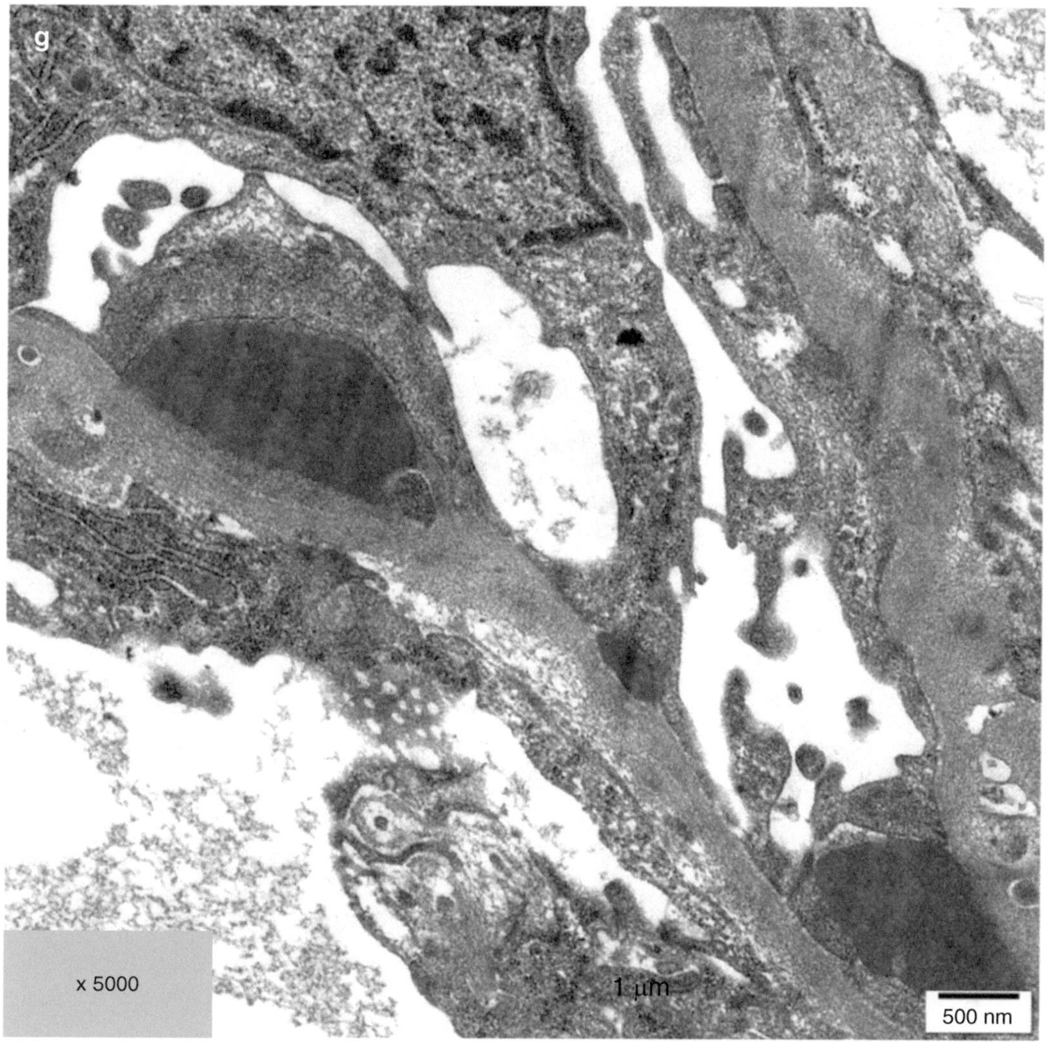

Fig. 7.2 (continued)

Further Reading

Balasubramanian R, Marks SD. Post-infectious glomerulonephritis. Paediatr Int Child Health. 2017;37:240–7.

D'Agati VD, Jennette JC, Olson JL. Heptinstall's pathology of the kidney. 7th ed. Wolters Kluwer; 2014.

Glassock RJ, Alvarado A, Prosek J, Hebert C, Parikh S, Satoskar A, Nadasdy T, Forman J, Rovin B, Hebert LA. Staphylococcus-related glomerulonephritis and poststreptococcal glomerulonephritis: why defining "post" is important in understanding and treating infection-related glomerulonephritis. Am J Kidney Dis. 2015;65:826–32.

Khalighi MA, Wang S, Henriksen KJ, Bock M, Keswani M, Meehan SM, Chang A. Revisiting post-infectious glomerulonephritis in the emerging era of C3 glomerulopathy. Clin Kidney J. 2016;9:397–402.

8 IgA Nephropathy and IgA Vasculitis (Henoch–Schonlein Purpura)

8.1 IgA Nephropathy

IgA nephropathy is the most common glomerular disease worldwide. Clinical features can range from microscopic hematuria, nephrotic syndrome to even rapidly progressive renal failure. It is characterized by dominant or co-dominant glomerular IgA deposits on immunofluorescence. On light microscopy, it can have mesangioproliferative, endocapillary proliferative, crescentic or focal segmental glomerulosclerosis like glomerular morphology. The histological changes including tubulointerstitial changes are scored by MEST-C scoring (Oxford classification). Patients having endocapillary proliferative changes and crescentic morphology often respond to immunosuppressive therapy. For other patients, supportive treatment is given including renin–angiotensin system blockade. On immunofluorescence, mesangial IgA deposits are more common although capillary wall deposits can be seen. It is often accompanied by complement C3 deposition and sometimes accompanying IgG deposits may also be seen. On electron microscopy, mesangial and paramesangial deposits are seen without any substructure. Subendothelial capillary wall deposits may accompany mesangial deposits. Capillary wall IgA deposits have more active histological changes and carry an unfavorable prognosis. Recurrent IgA nephropathy can be seen in about 30% of cases after renal transplantation. A case of IgA nephropathy is illustrated (Fig. 8.1).

P. Gupta, R. K. Gupta, *Pathology of Glomerular Diseases*, https://doi.org/10.1007/978-981-19-1430-0_8

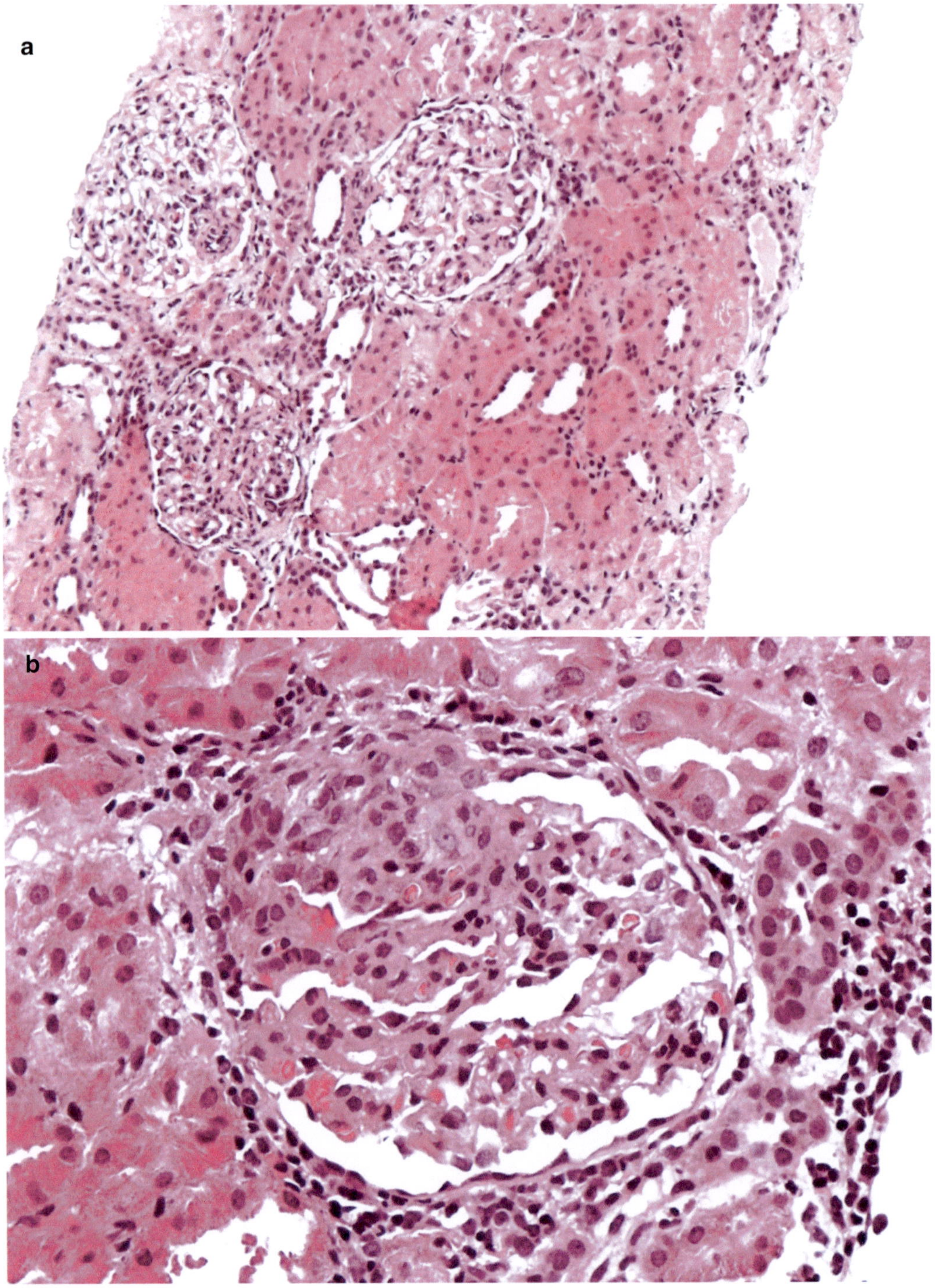

Fig. 8.1 **IgA Nephropathy** A 9-years male child presented with recurrent episodes of gross hematuria synchronic with URTI. He was normotensive. His urinary protein was 2+ with fields full of RBC. Serum creatinine was 0.47 mg/dL. Serum C3 was wnl. Anti DNAse, ANA, c-ANCA and p-ANCA were all negative. Renal biopsy revealed 20 glomeruli, all had mesangial proliferation which was not associated with endocapillary hyperplasia. Two glomeruli had partial cellular crescents. There was no segmental or global glomerulosclerosis. Few tubules showed red blood cells; focal tubular atrophy with patchy interstitial lymphocytic infiltration was present. Blood vessels were unremarkable. IF showed granular mesangial and focal capillary wall deposits of IgA (3+), C3 (2+), lambda (3+) and kappa (2+); IgG, IgM, and C1q were negative. EM showed electron-dense deposits (conventional) in mesangial and paramesangial regions along with expanded mesangium and occasional subendothelial deposits. (**a**) HE ×200, (**b** and **c**) HE ×400, (**d**) PAS ×400, (**e**) PSM ×200, (**f–i**) IF ×400, (**j** and **k**) EM (identity of the patient has been concealed)

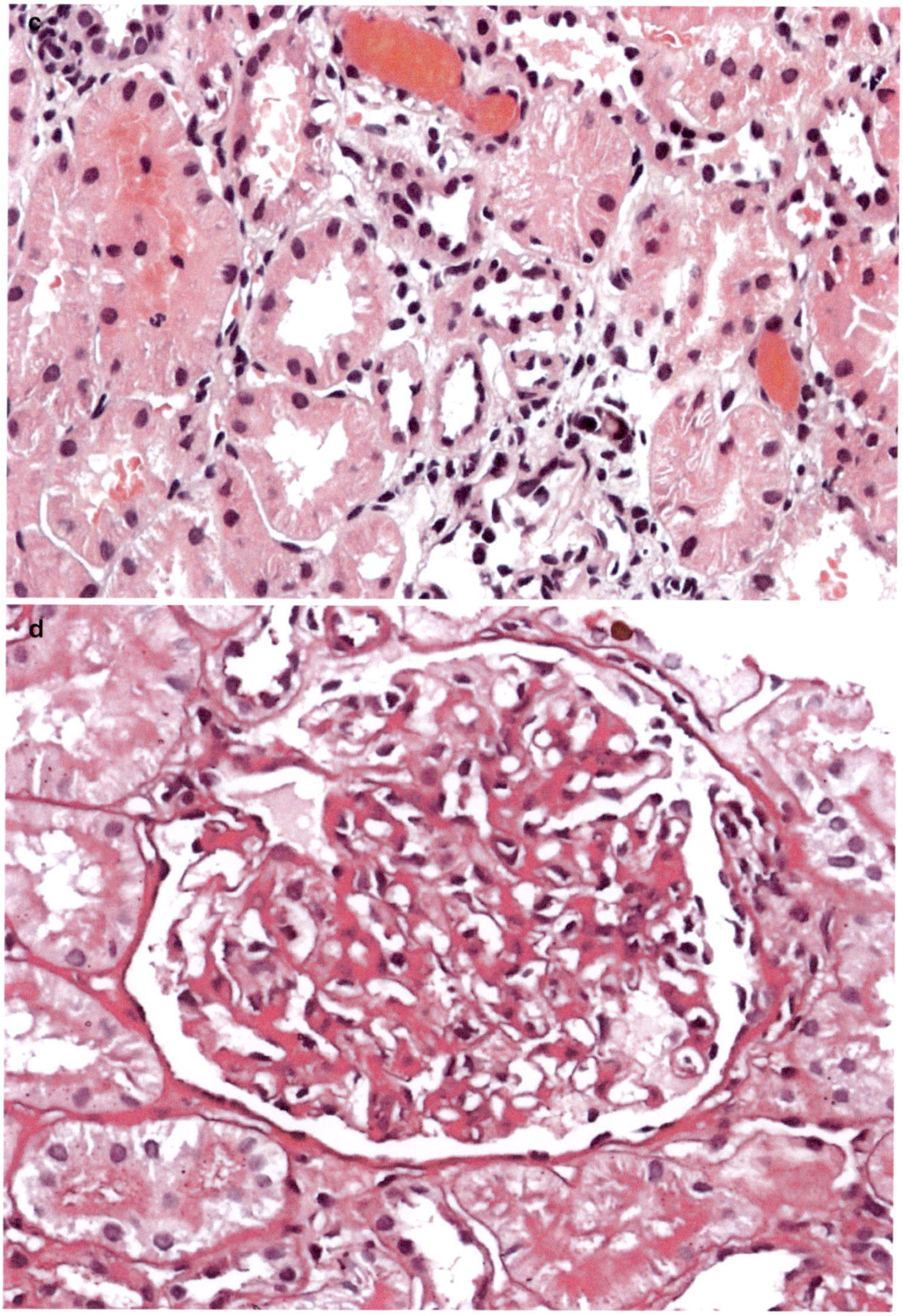

Fig. 8.1 (continued)

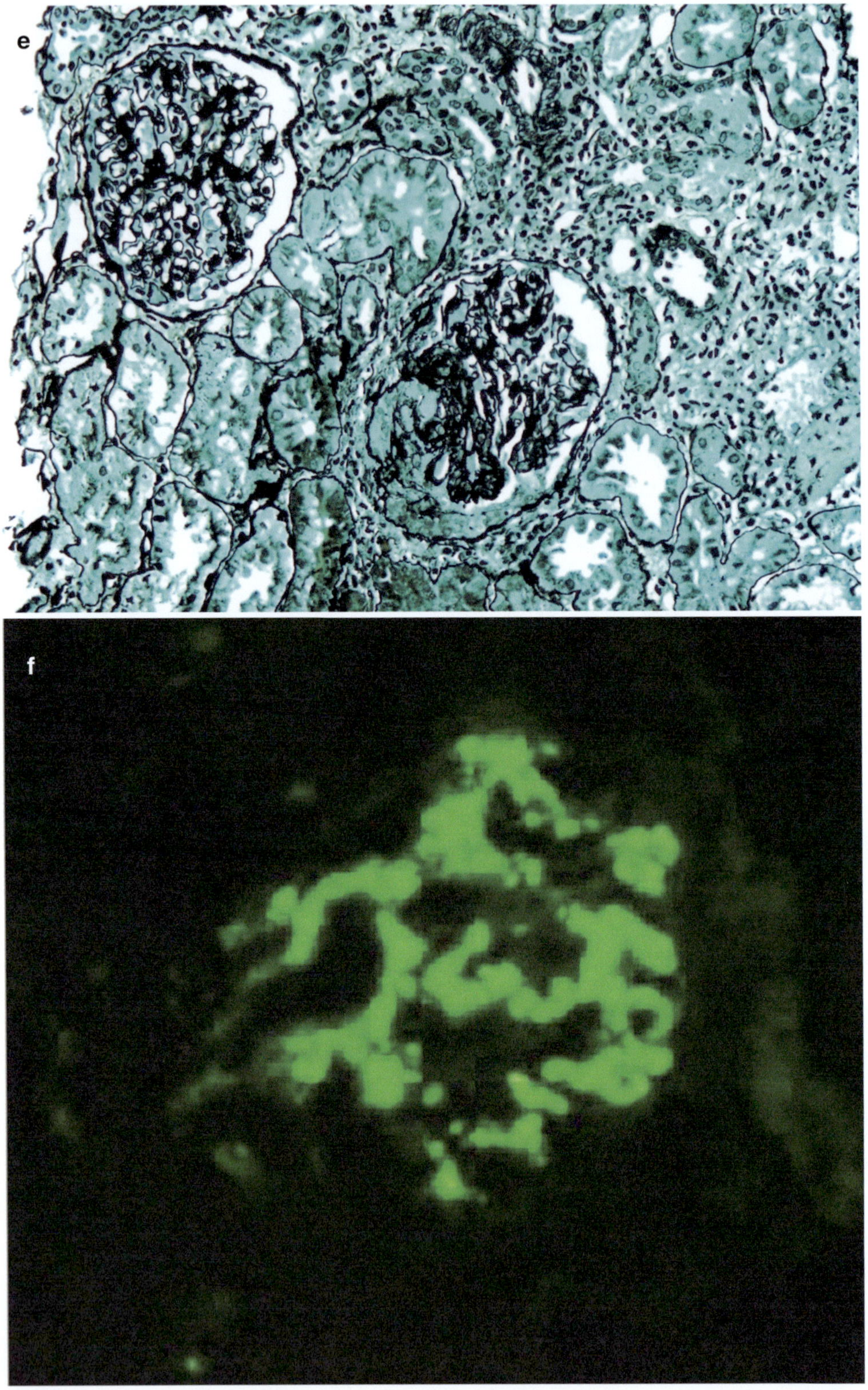

Fig. 8.1 (continued)

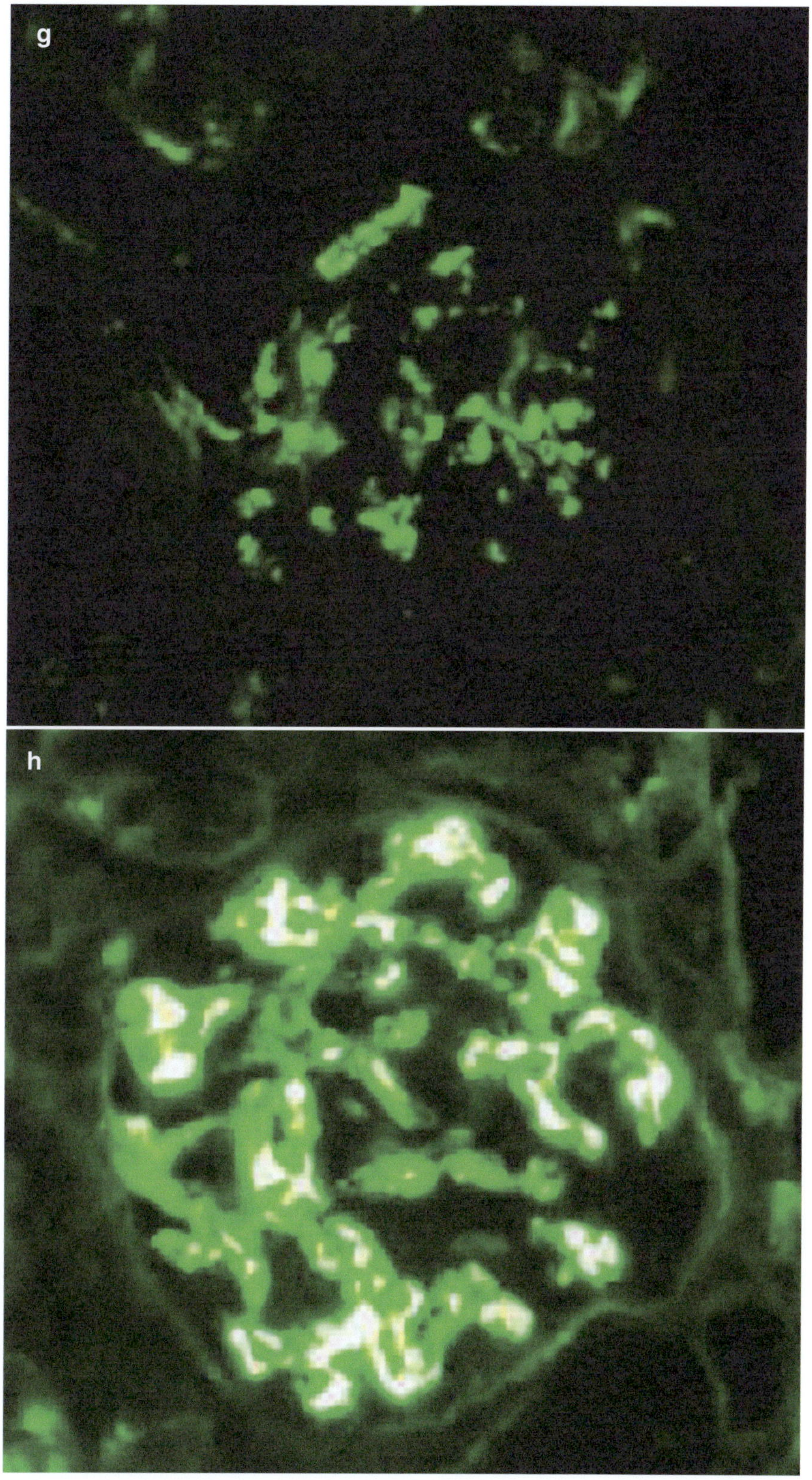

Fig. 8.1 (continued)

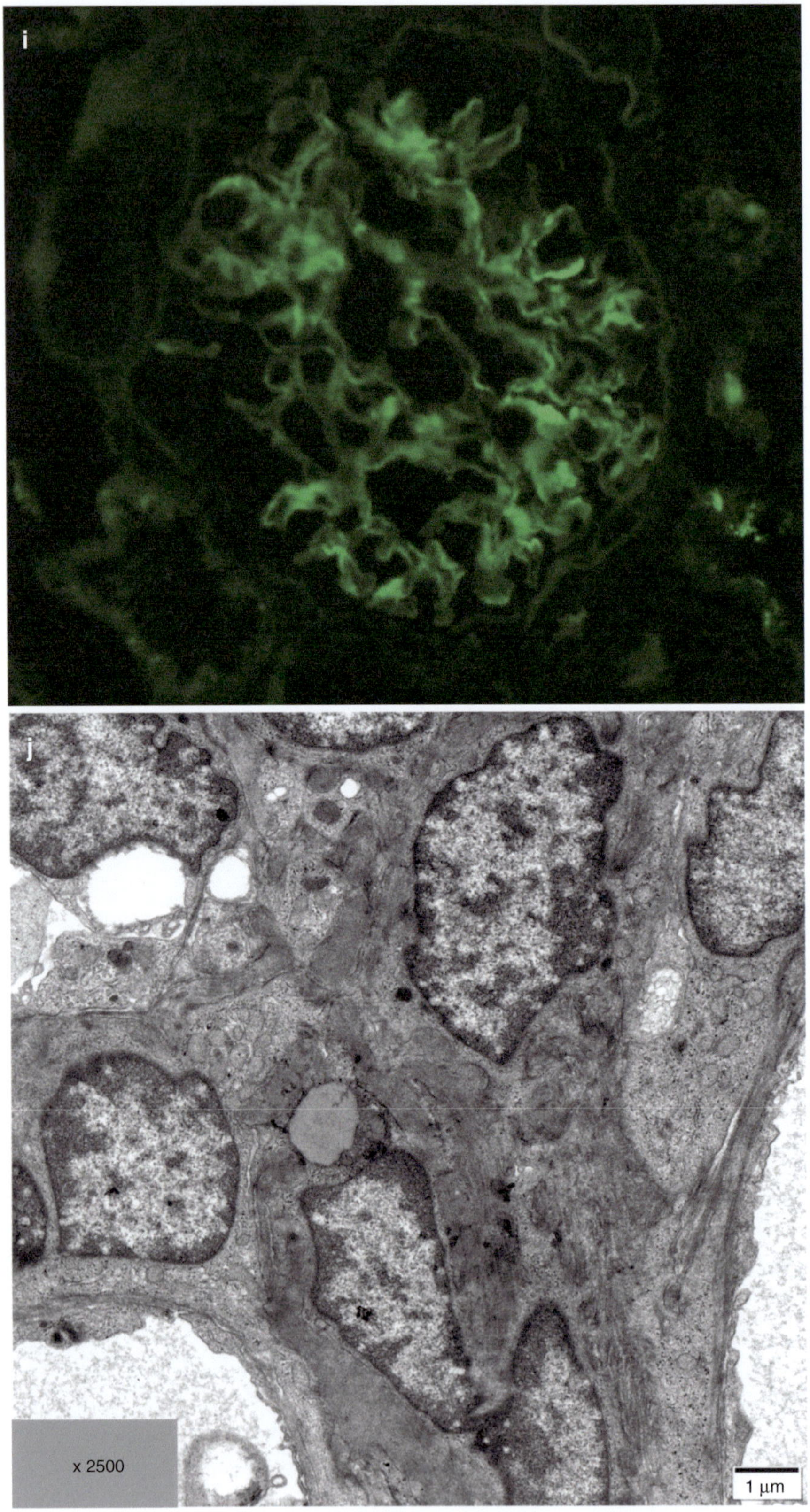

Fig. 8.1 (continued)

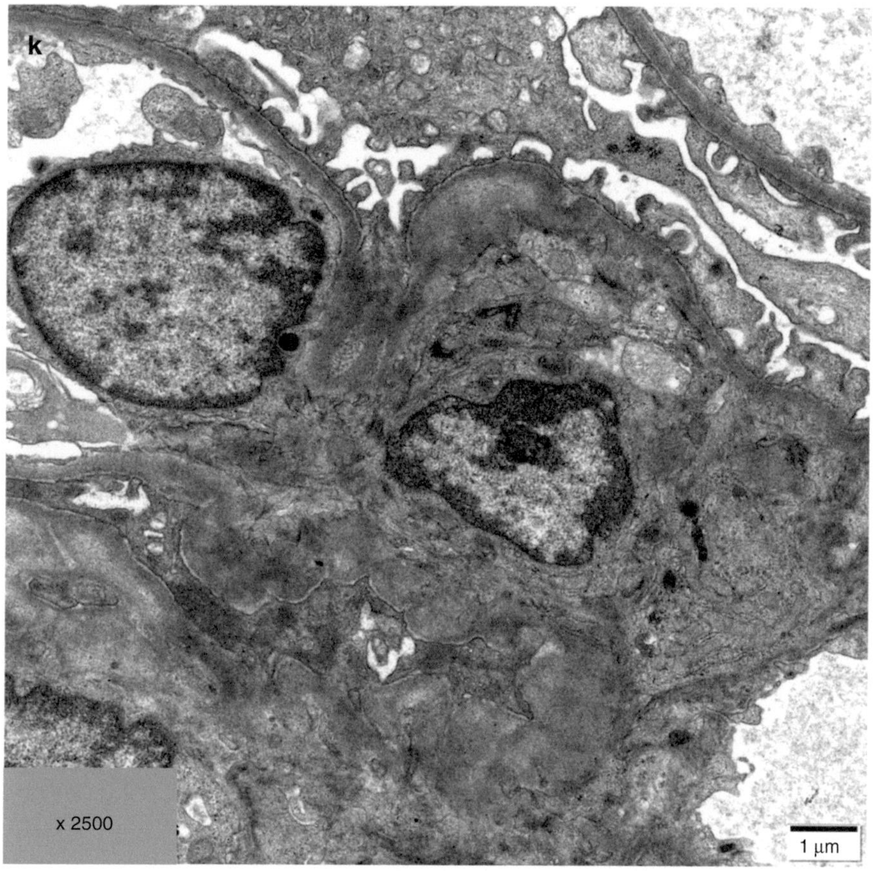

Fig. 8.1 (continued)

8.2 IgA Vasculitis: Henoch–Schonlein Purpura (HSP)

IgA vasculitis or Henoch–Schonlein Purpura (HSP) is a form of systemic vasculitis affecting small vessels including capillaries, venules, and arterioles. Most commonly it involves skin in the form of palpable purpura. Other systemic involvement is in the form of gastrointestinal involvement with patients presenting as abdominal pain or gastrointestinal bleed, glomerulonephritis, and arthritis. It can affect both children and adults, being more common in males and is seen in association with HLA-DRB1 allele. In children, it is usually seen between 2 and 10 years of age. These patients develop IgA vasculitis in short term following upper respiratory tract infection. Renal involvement is in the form of microscopic hematuria along with proteinuria; 30% of adult patients can have renal failure at the time of diagnosis.

On light microscopy, changes can range from minimal histologic changes, mesangioproliferative glomerulonephritis to crescentic glomerulonephritis. An international study group for kidney disease in children classified IgA vasculitis based on the percentage of glomeruli with crescents. Crescentic transformation and crescentic glomerulonephritis are more common in patients with IgA vasculitis than IgA nephropathy. Tubules can show the presence of red blood cells. Interstitial edema and inflammation may be seen. On Immunofluorescence IgA dominant or codominant deposits are seen in mesangium and also along GBM in many cases. It can be accompanied by C3, IgM, or IgG deposition. On electron microscopy, mesangial electron-dense deposits are seen. Frequently subendothelial and subepithelial deposits can also be seen.

In patients with IgA vasculitis, skin biopsies show evidence of leukocytoclastic vasculitis. A case of IgA vasculitis is illustrated (Fig. 8.2).

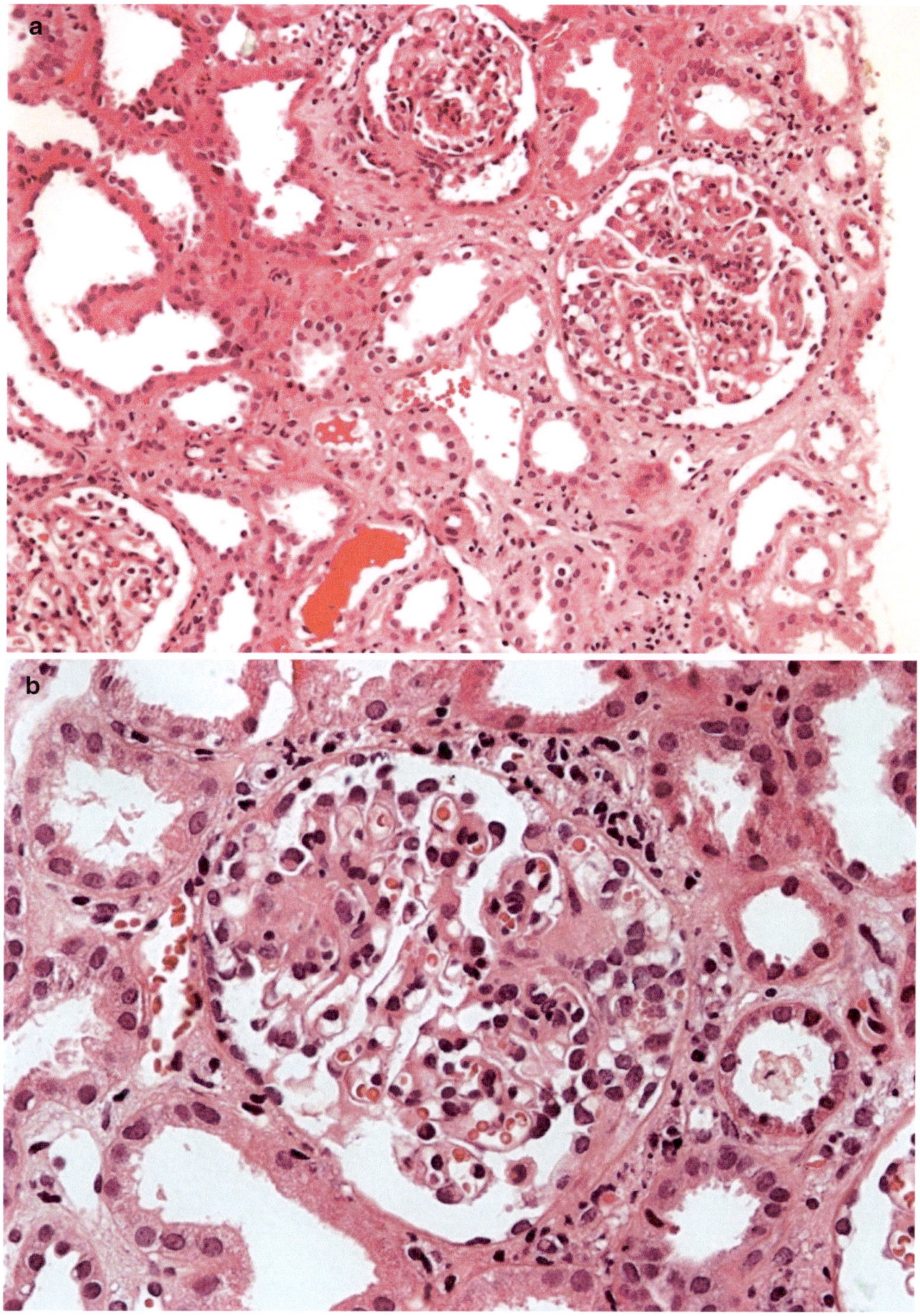

Fig. 8.2 **IgA Vasuclitis** A 17-years male patient presented with hypertension, skin rashes, swelling of both lower limbs, and puffiness of eyelids for 6 weeks. Urinary protein was 3+ with 20–30 RBC/hpf; 24 h urinary protein was 9.3 g. His serum cholesterol was 228 mg/dL and serum creatinine was 1.7 mg/dL. Serum C3 and C4 were wnl. ANA and HBsAg were negative. Renal biopsy had ten glomeruli, all of them had mild mesangial proliferation and five of them had partial cellular crescents. Some of the tubules had hyaline casts and occasional foci of tubular atrophy were present. Interstitium had edema and mild lymphocytic infiltration. Blood vessels were unremarkable. IF showed positivity for IgA (3+), C3 (3+), IgM (2+), kappa (1+) and lambda (3+) in mesangium with occasional capillary wall deposits; IgG and C1q were negative. (**a**) HE ×200, (**b**) HE ×400, (**c**) PAS ×400, (**d**) PSM ×400 and (**e–h**) IF ×400

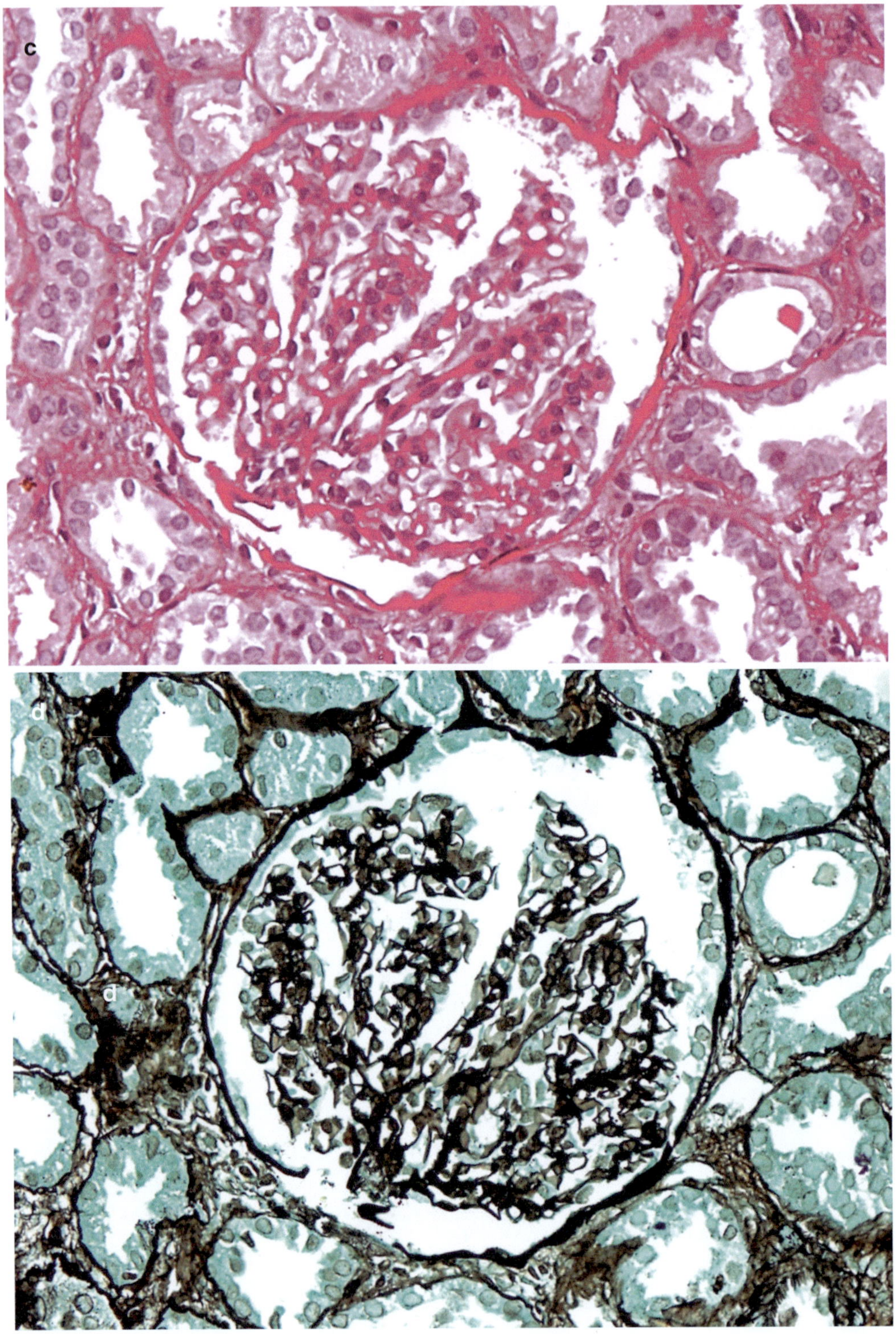

Fig. 8.2 (continued)

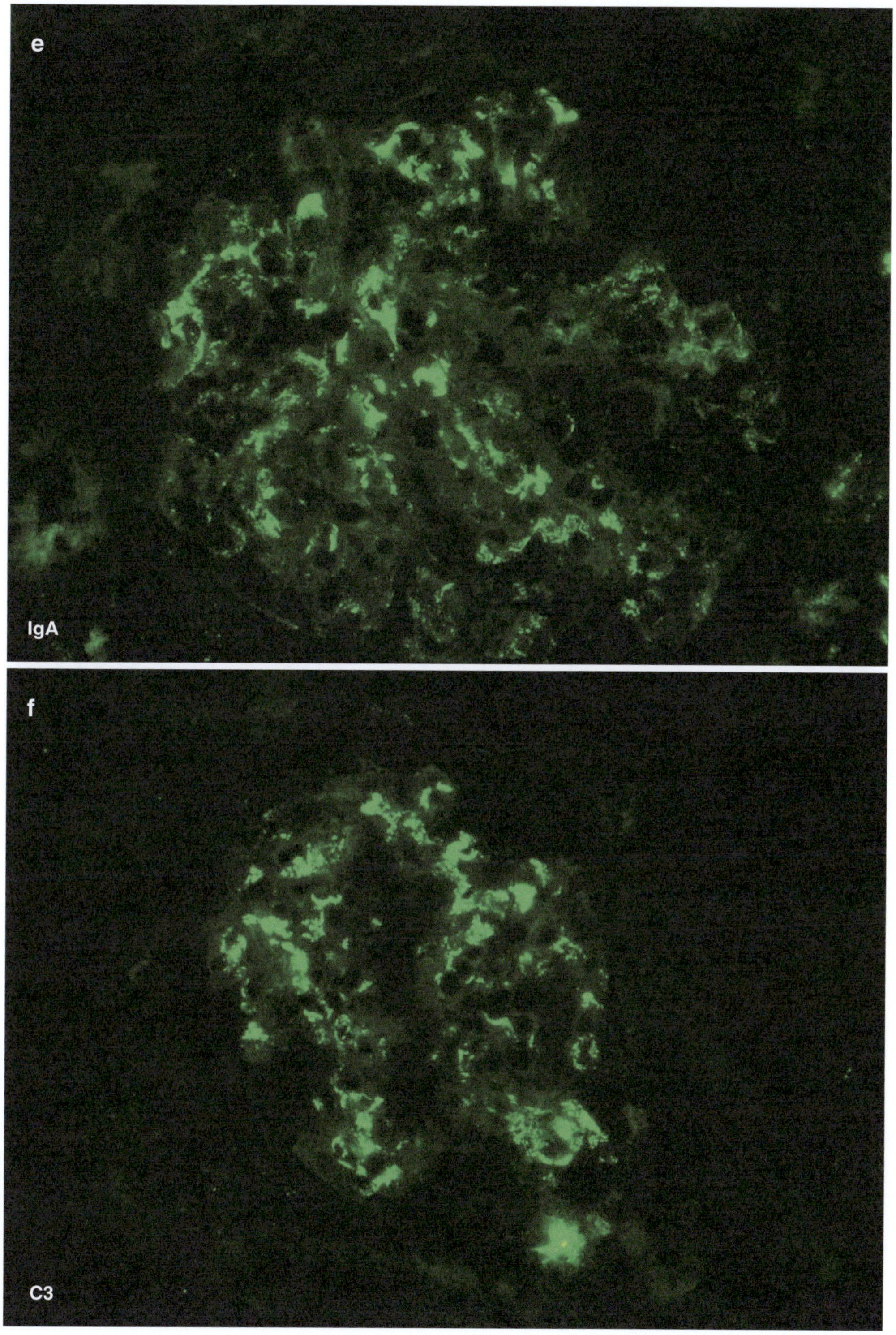

Fig. 8.2 (continued)

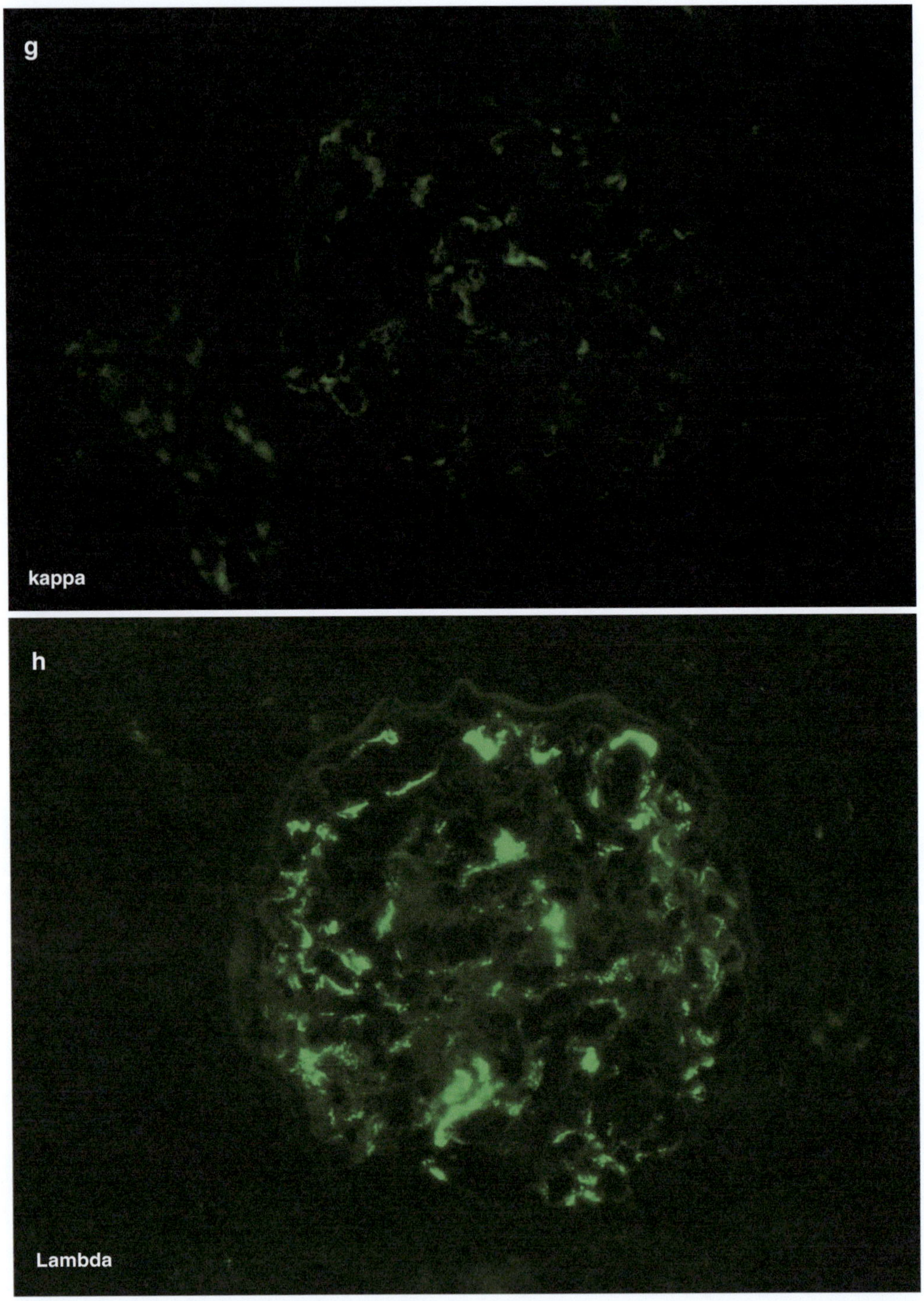

Fig. 8.2 (continued)

Further Reading

Audemard-Verger A, Pillebout E, Guillevin L, Thervet E, Terrier B. IgA vasculitis (Henoch-Shönlein purpura) in adults: diagnostic and therapeutic aspects. Autoimmun Rev. 2015;14:579–85.

Bellur SS, Troyanov S, Cook HT, Roberts IS, Working Group of International IgA Nephropathy Network and Renal Pathology Society. Immunostaining findings in IgA nephropathy: correlation with histology and clinical outcome in the Oxford classification patient cohort. Nephrol Dial Transplant. 2017;26:2533–6.

D'Agati VD, Jennette JC, Olson JL. Heptinstall's pathology of the kidney. 7th ed. Wolters Kluwer; 2014.

González-Gay MA, López-Mejías R, Pina T, Blanco R, Castañeda S. IgA vasculitis: genetics and clinical and therapeutic management. Curr Rheumatol Rep. 2018;20:24.

Perše M, Večerić-Haler Ž. The role of IgA in the pathogenesis of IgA nephropathy. Int J Mol Sci. 2019;20:6199.

Roberts IS. Pathology of IgA nephropathy. Nat Rev Nephrol. 2014;10:445–54.

Rodrigues JC, Haas M, Reich HN. IgA nephropathy. Clin J Am Soc Nephrol. 2017;12:677–86.

Selvaskandan H, Cheung CK, Muto M, Barratt J. New strategies and perspectives on managing IgA nephropathy. Clin Exp Nephrol. 2019;23:577–88.

Shi D, Chan H, Yang X, Zhang G, Yang H, Wang M, Li Q. Risk factors associated with IgA vasculitis with nephritis (Henoch-Schönlein purpura nephritis) progressing to unfavorable outcomes: a meta-analysis. PLoS One. 2019;14:e0223218.

Suzuki H, Yasutake J, Makita Y, Tanbo Y, Yamasaki K, Sofue T, Kano T, Suzuki Y. IgA nephropathy and IgA vasculitis with nephritis have a shared feature involving galactose-deficient IgA1-oriented pathogenesis. Kidney Int. 2018;93:700–5.

Trimarchi H, Barratt J, Cattran DC, Cook HT, Coppo R, Haas M, Liu ZH, Roberts IS, Yuzawa Y, Zhang H, Feehally J, IgAN Classification Working Group of the International IgA Nephropathy Network and the Renal Pathology Society; Conference Participants. Oxford classification of IgA nephropathy 2016: an update from the IgA Nephropathy Classification Working Group. Kidney Int. 2017;91:1014–21.

9 Alport's Syndrome and Thin Basement Membrane Disease

9.1 Alport's Syndrome

Alport's syndrome is a disorder characterized by hereditary familial nephritis and sensory neural deafness. It is X-linked dominant and caused by mutations in the COL4A5 gene. Mutations can also be observed in COL4A3 and CO4A4 genes. This gene encodes for α3, α4, and α5 chains of type IV collagen which is the main component of the glomerular capillary basement membrane. Patients can present at birth, infancy, or childhood with persistent hematuria, renal failure, sensory neural hearing loss, and in addition can have lenticonus and retinal flecks. Proteinuria is absent or intermittent. On light microscopy, renal biopsy may appear normal or may show focal thickening and rigidity of glomerular capillary basement membrane. Mild mesangial expansion and hypertrophy of podocytes may be seen. Focal segmental glomerulosclerosis can also be seen. Later in the course globally sclerosed glomeruli may also be seen. Tubules may show red blood cells or occasional RBC cast. Interstitial lipid-laden foam cells can be seen. It is often seen in patients with significant proteinuria. Blood vessels are unremarkable. Immunofluorescence will show the absence of immunoglobulin and complement deposits; however, occasionally scattered C3 deposits in glomerular capillary tuft may be seen. On immunohistochemistry absence of the α5 chain of type IV collagen in the GBM and tubular basement membrane can be seen in male patients with discontinuous distribution in females. Electron microscopy is essential and diagnostic and shows irregular thickening of the glomerular capillary basement membrane. Some portions of GBM show thickening with basket weave and lamellated appearance due to splitting and fragmentation of lamina densa. Patients with Alport's syndrome progress to ESRD by 20 years or 40 years of age depending on whether it is a juvenile or adult type. A case of Alport's syndrome is illustrated (Fig. 9.1).

P. Gupta, R. K. Gupta, *Pathology of Glomerular Diseases*, https://doi.org/10.1007/978-981-19-1430-0_9

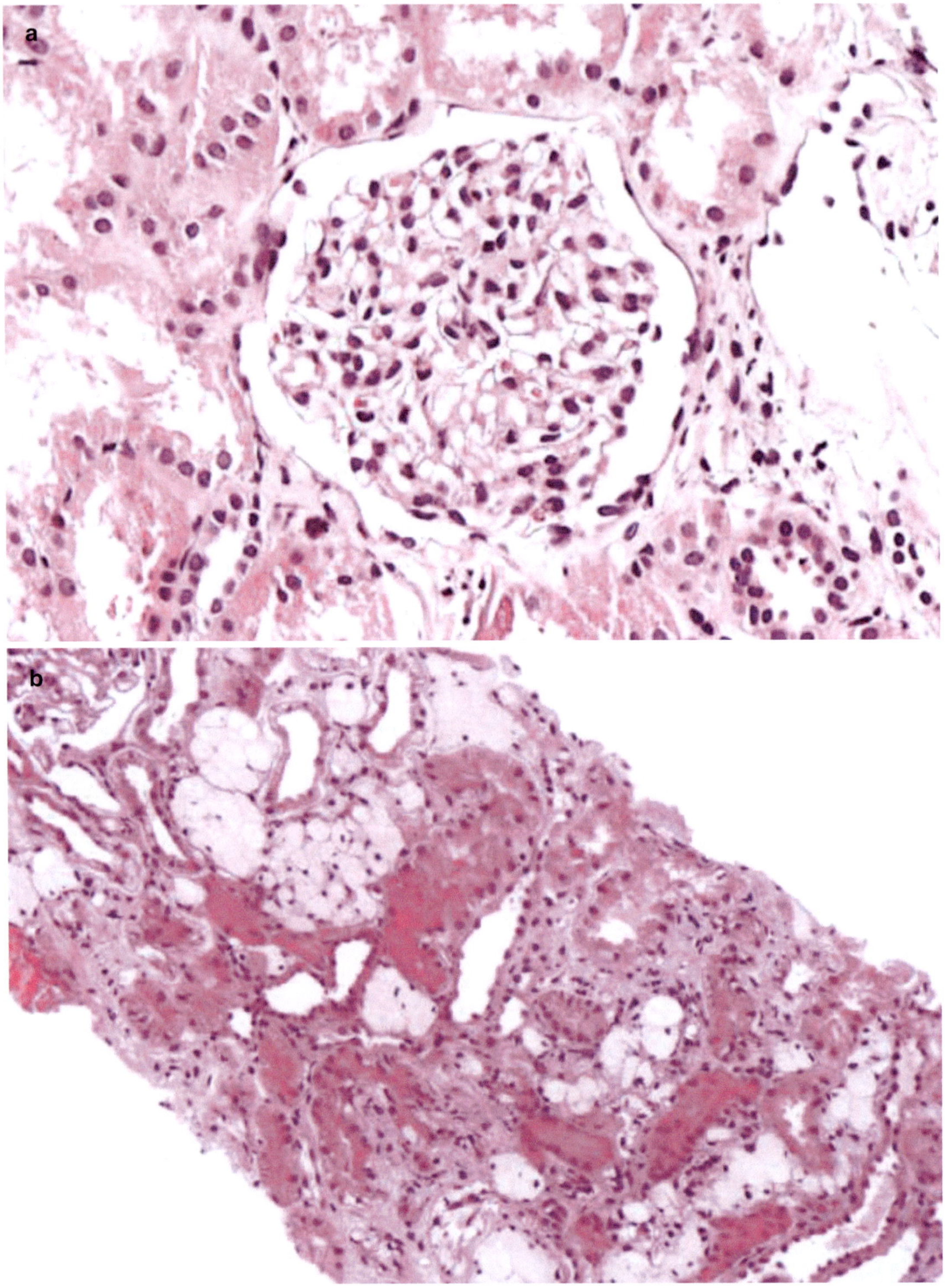

Fig. 9.1 **Alport's Syndrome** A 7-years male child with bilateral hearing impairment, presented with gross hematuria for 6 months; he also had mild pedal edema. Urinary protein was 2+ and urinary sediment had fields full of RBC and 5–6 WBC/hpf. His hemoglobin level was 9.0 g/dL. His RFT were deranged with serum creatinine of 2.3 mg/dL and P:C ratio of 6.5. Serum ANA and ANCA were negative and serum C3 and C4 were wnl. Renal biopsy had 12 glomeruli which were essentially wnl. Interstitium showed plenty of foam cells. EM showed significant effacement of foot processes of visceral epithelial cells, basement membrane showed irregular thin and thick regions (114–998 nm) along with criss-cross arrays and basket-weave pattern. (**a** and **b**) HE ×400, (**c**) PAS ×400, (**d**) PSM ×400, (**e**) EM (identity of the patient has been concealed)

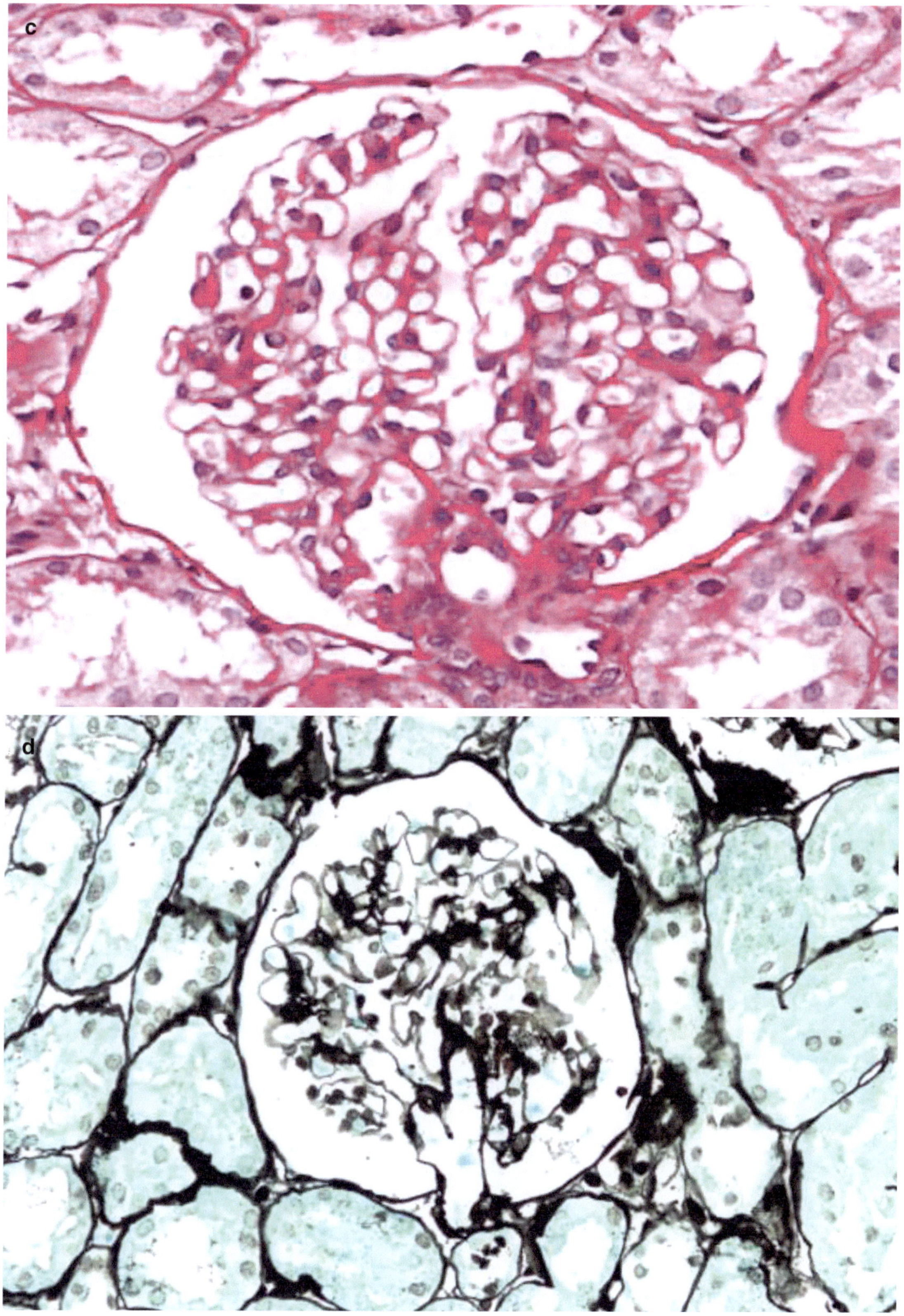

Fig. 9.1 (continued)

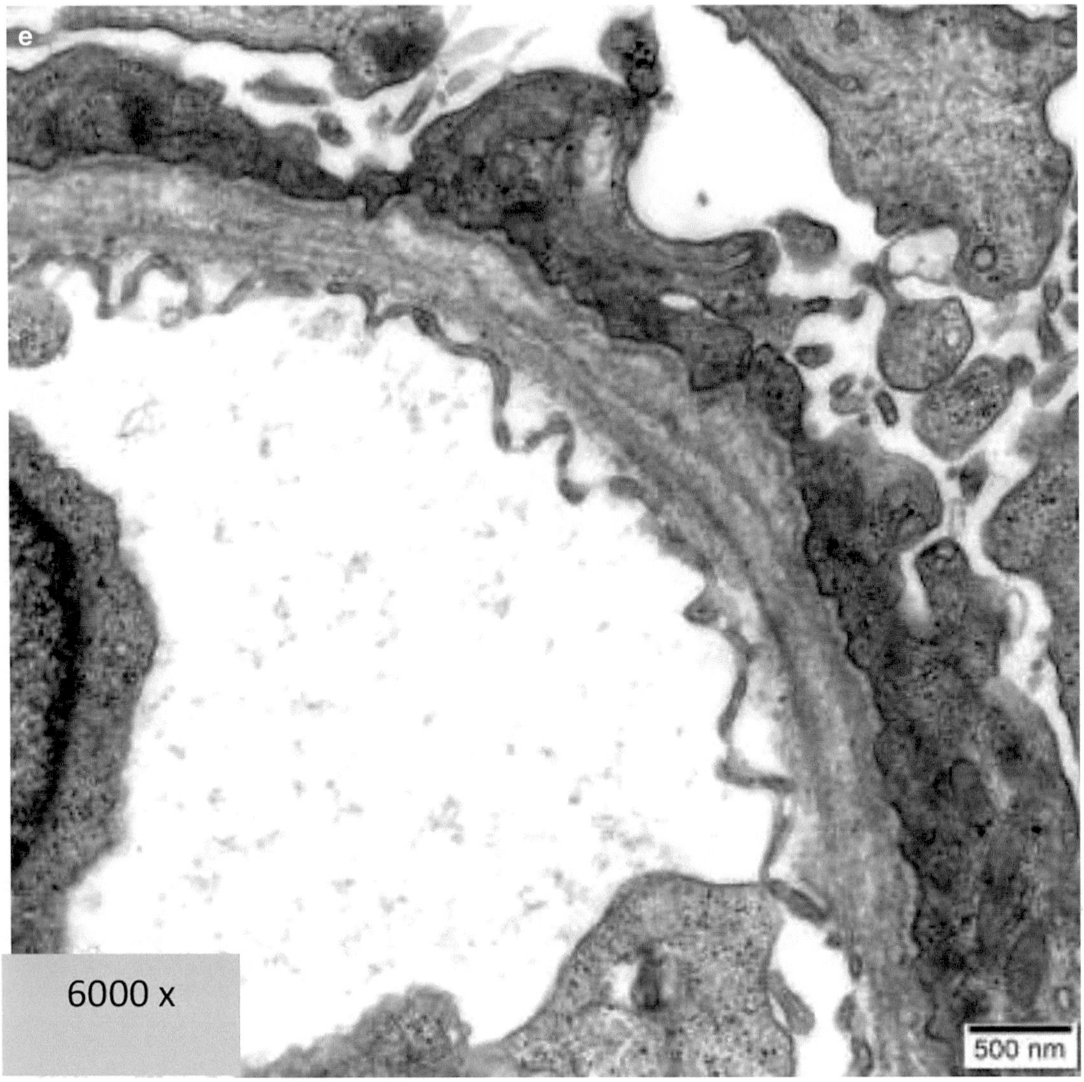

Fig. 9.1 (continued)

9.2 Thin Basement Membrane Disease

Familial benign hematuria is an autosomal dominant disorder in which patients usually have persistent hematuria and diffuse attenuation of the glomerular capillary basement membrane (thin basement membrane disease). Childhood onset is seen with most patients being detected on routine urine analysis. Family history of hematuria may be present. These children do not have significant proteinuria, renal dysfunction, hypertension, or extrarenal manifestations. Patients with thin basement membrane disease usually have heterozygous mutations in COL4A4 and COL4A3 genes. On light microscopy these patients have normal appearing glomeruli or sometimes uniform thinning of the glomerular capillary basement membrane may be appreciated on silver-stained sections. Red blood cells may be seen in Bowman's space or within lumen of renal tubules. Some authors have described a decrease in glomerular capillary lumen with smaller capillaries and an increase in extracellular mesangial matrix. No immune deposits are seen on immunofluorescence microscopy and staining for type IV collagen will be normal. On electron microscopy, glomerular capillary basement membrane thickness is generally less than 250 nm. Prognosis of patients with thin basement membrane disease is usually good but patients who develop proteinuria, hypertension, or renal dysfunction have higher chances of progression to end-stage renal disease. A case of thin basement membrane disease is illustrated (Fig. 9.2).

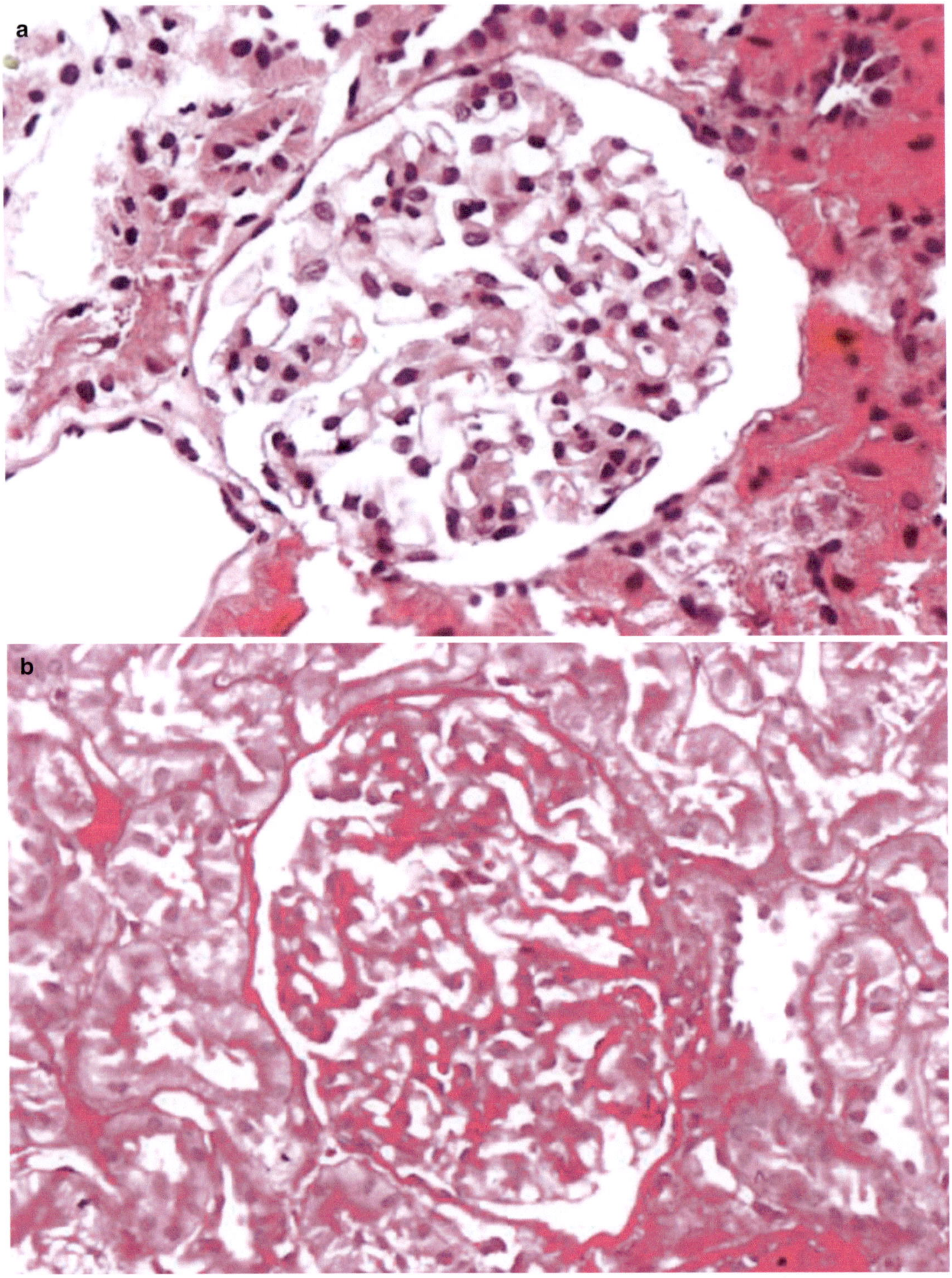

Fig. 9.2 Thin Basement Membrane Disease A 20-years female patient presented with persistent microscopic hematuria for 2.5 years. She was normotensive. She had no h/o of joint pain, rash, visual or hearing impairment. USG KUB was wnl. Urine analysis did not show any proteinuria, urine microscopy revealed 20–30 RBC/hpf. RFT and serum complements were wnl. ASO titre, Anti dsDNA, ANA and ENA profile were negative. Renal biopsy had 14 glomeruli all of which were normal on LM. EM showed thinning of basement membrane with average diameter of 157 nm, no electron-dense deposits were seen. (**a**) HE ×400, (**b**) PAS ×400, (**c**) PSM ×400 (**d** and **e**) EM (identity of the patient has been concealed)

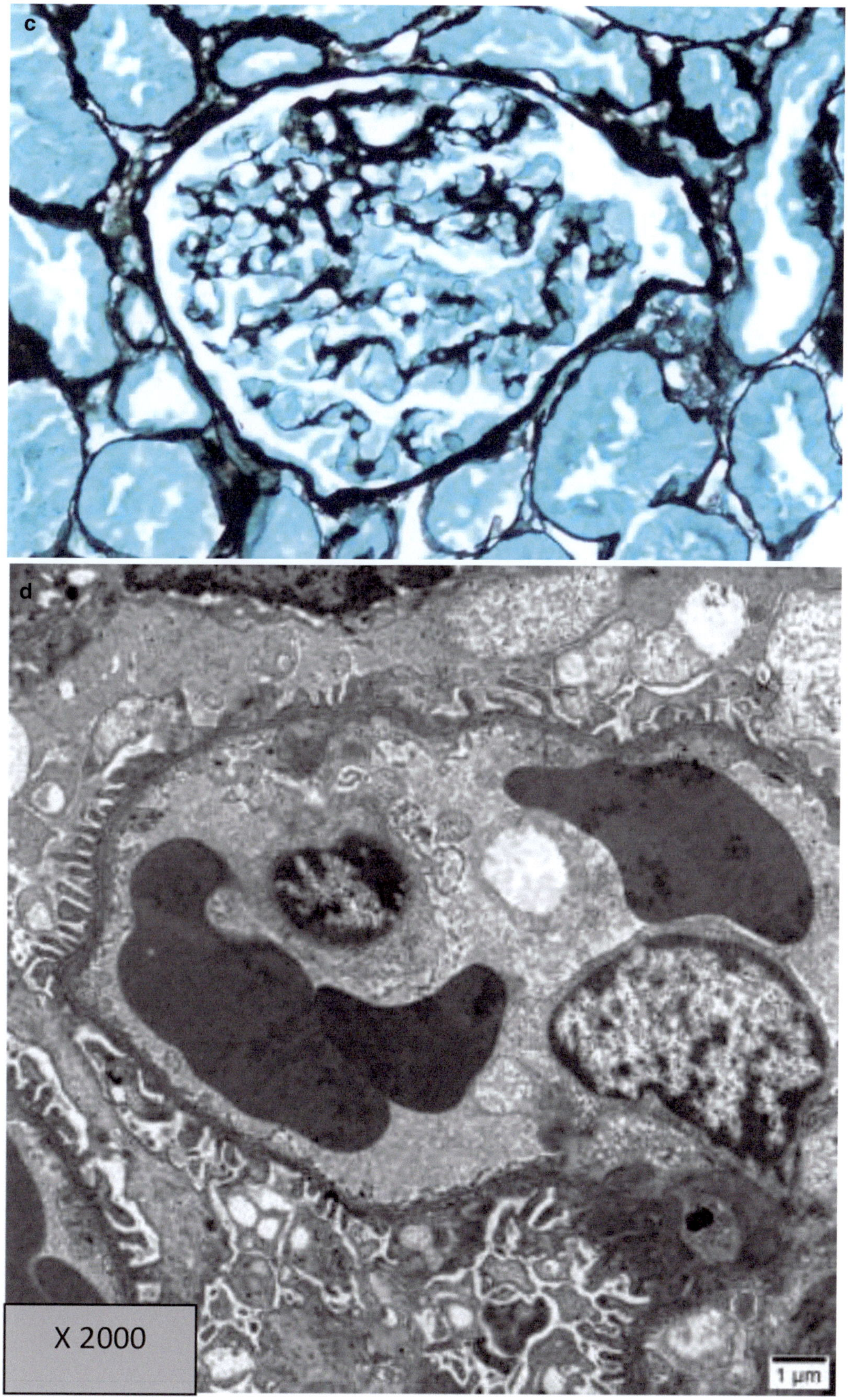

Fig. 9.2 (continued)

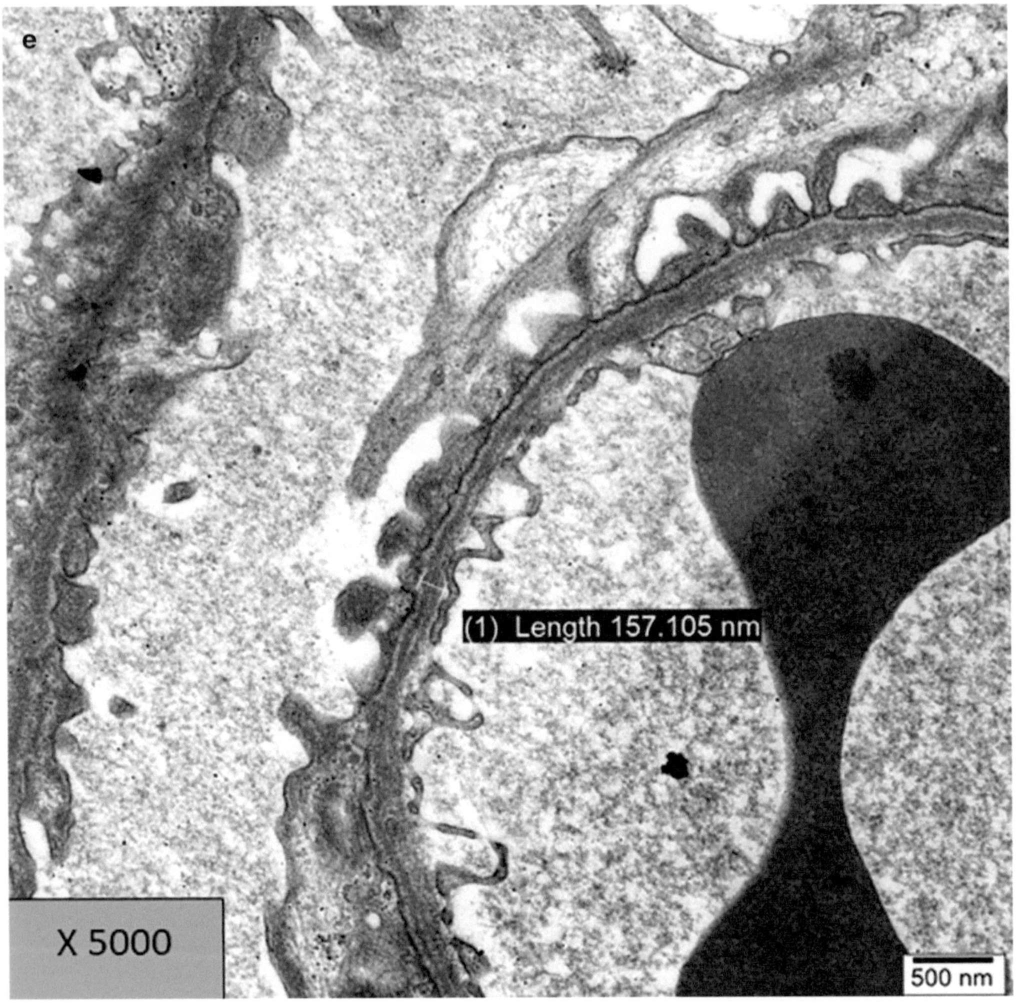

Fig. 9.2 (continued)

Further Reading

D'Agati VD, Jennette JC, Olson JL. Heptinstall's pathology of the kidney. 7th ed. Wolters Kluwer; 2014.

Frascá GM, Onetti-Muda A, Renieri A. Thin glomerular basement membrane disease. J Nephrol. 2000;13:15–9.

Frascà GM, Balestra E, Fanciulli E, Freddi P, Mazzucchelli R, Montironi R, D'Arezzo M, Sagripanti S. La nefropatia a membrane basali sottili [Thin glomerular basement membrane disease]. G Ital Nefrol. 2008;25:49–56.

Kajimoto Y, Endo Y, Terasaki M, Kunugi S, Igarashi T, Mii A, Terasaki Y, Shimizu A. Pathologic glomerular characteristics and glomerular basement membrane alterations in biopsy-proven thin basement membrane nephropathy. Clin Exp Nephrol. 2019;23:638–49.

Kashtan CE, Ding J, Garosi G, Heidet L, Massella L, Nakanishi K, Nozu K, Renieri A, Rheault M, Wang F, Gross O. Alport syndrome: a unified classification of genetic disorders of collagen IV α345: a position paper of the Alport Syndrome Classification Working Group. Kidney Int. 2018;93:1045–51.

Kruegel J, Rubel D, Gross O. Alport syndrome–insights from basic and clinical research. Nat Rev Nephrol. 2013;9:170–8.

Savige J, Gregory M, Gross O, Kashtan C, Ding J, Flinter F. Expert guidelines for the management of Alport syndrome and thin basement membrane nephropathy. J Am Soc Nephrol. 2013;24:364–75.

10 Congenital Nephrotic Syndrome and Diffuse Mesangial Sclerosis

10.1 Congenital Nephrotic Syndrome

Congenital nephrotic syndrome is characterized by nephrotic syndrome in the first 3 months of life. It is caused usually by genetic mutations in the structural proteins forming the glomerular filtration barrier namely NPHS-1, NPHS-2, WT-1, INF-2, CD2AP, LAMB-2, and PLCE-1. However, it can also be caused by infections like congenital syphilis, cytomegalovirus, or toxoplasmosis. Other causes include maternal systemic lupus erythematosus, renal vein thrombosis, and mercury poisoning. Children present in the first 3 months of life with edema, massive hypoalbuminemia, and hyperlipidemia. Congenital nephrotic syndrome (Finnish type/congenital nephrotic syndrome type 1) is caused by mutations in NPHS-1 that encodes for nephrin. It is an autosomal recessive disorder and is the most common type of congenital nephrotic syndrome. The patients have proteinuria at birth and it can be accompanied by hematuria, aminoaciduria, and glucosuria. These children usually are born as premature births with large placenta. Muscular hypotonia and cardiac hypertrophy can also be seen in neonates. Creatinine is normal at presentation. On renal biopsy, these patients have cystic dilation of proximal tubules. Glomerular findings are nonspecific and include fetal glomeruli, mesangial sclerosis, and global glomerulosclerosis later in life. Electron microscopy will show widespread effacement of the podocyte foot processes with an absent slit diaphragm between adjacent pedicels. End-stage renal disease is seen early in the course of life. Congenital nephrotic syndrome caused by an autosomal recessive mutation in NPHS-2 that codes for podocin, presents with focal segmental glomerulosclerosis. Patients with congenital nephrotic syndrome are steroid unresponsive and require renal replacement therapy for survival. A case of congenital nephrotic syndrome is illustrated (Fig. 10.1).

P. Gupta, R. K. Gupta, *Pathology of Glomerular Diseases*, https://doi.org/10.1007/978-981-19-1430-0_10

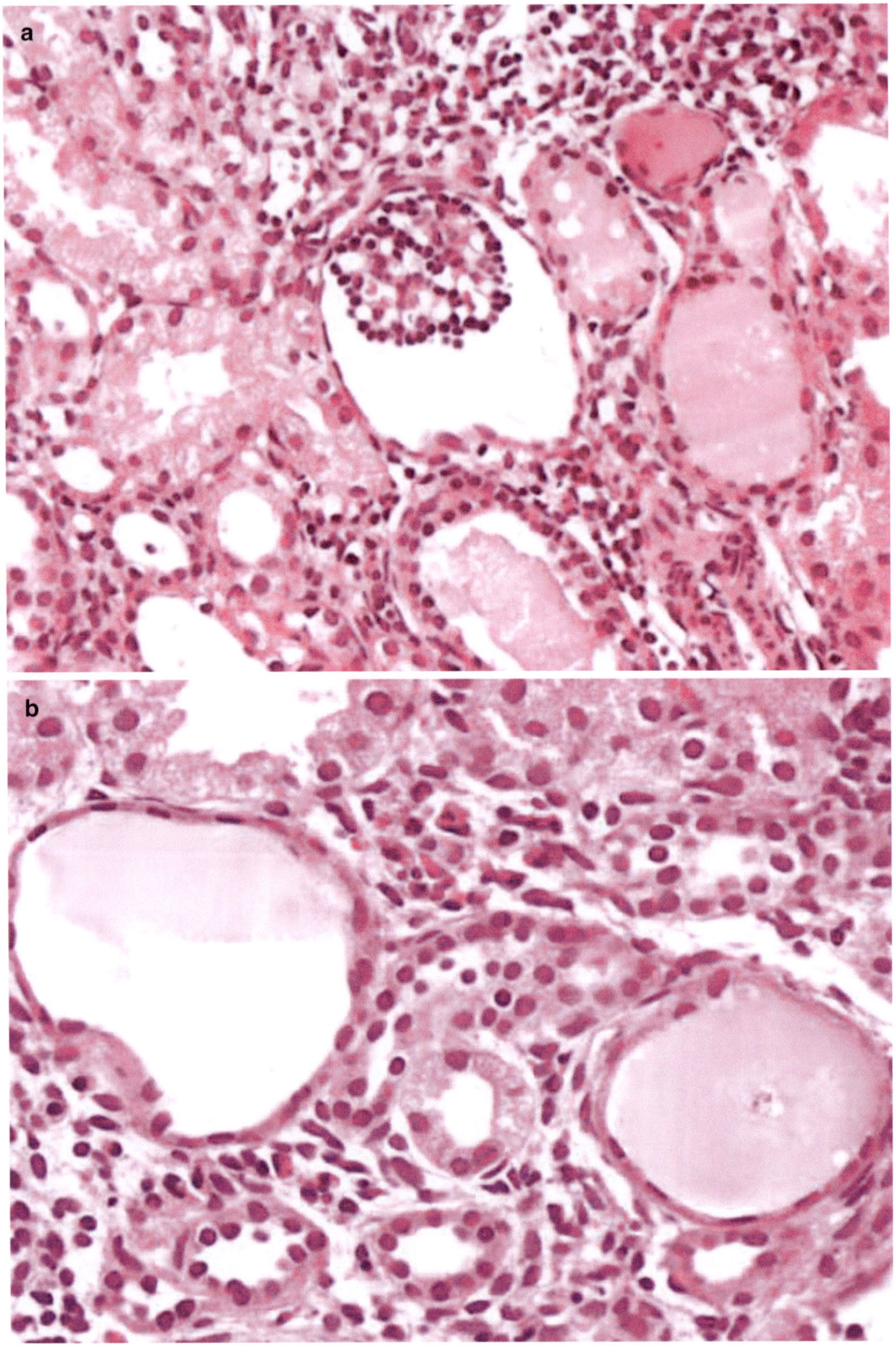

Fig. 10.1 **Congenital Nephrotic Syndrome** A 2-months male child presented with abdominal distention and scrotal swelling. Urine analysis revealed albumin 3+ with 24 h urinary albumin 3 g. Total serum protein was 3 g/dL with serum albumin 0.41 g/dL. Serum cholesterol was 125 mg/dL and serum creatinine was 0.9 mg/dL. Renal biopsy had 48 fetal appearing glomeruli with shrunken glomerular tuft, prominent podocytes, and enlarged and dilated Bowman's space. Renal tubules were cystically dilated and the interstitium had mild lymphocytic infiltration; blood vessels were wnl. IF for IgG, IgM, IgA, C3, C1q and kappa and lambda light chains was negative. (**a** and **b**) HE ×400. Post biopsy genetic evaluation showed NPHS-1 gene mutation

10.2 Diffuse Mesangial Sclerosis (DMS)

Diffuse mesangial sclerosis can be seen as an isolated condition or as a part of Denys-Drash syndrome both of which are caused by WT-1 missense mutations in exons 8 and 9. Apart from WT-1 mutations, it can also be seen in patients with mutations LAMB2 (Pierson syndrome). It is a distinct form of glomerular disease seen in congenital or infantile nephrotic syndrome patients with rapid progression to end-stage renal disease usually by 5 years of age. Patients may have parental consanguinity or history of familial involvement. On renal biopsy initially diffuse increase in mesangial matrix is seen followed by mesangial sclerosis and thickening of glomerular capillary basement membrane. Accumulation of extracellular mesangial matrix leads to obliteration of capillary lumen. Glomerular capillary tuft contraction is seen with hypertrophy and mild hyperplasia of the visceral epithelial cells. Podocytes can show increased expression of Ki-67 proliferation markers. Increased cytokeratin expression can also be seen in podocyte suggestive of a dedifferentiated phenotype. Dilated and atrophic tubules can be seen. If diffuse mesangial sclerosis presents at birth, congenital nephrotic syndrome Finnish type (Type I) is considered as a differential diagnosis. On Immunofluorescence microscopy nonspecific deposits of C3 and IgM are seen in mesangium. On electron microscopy, zones of subepithelial lucent widening with wavy appearance of glomerular capillary basement membrane are seen along with increased mesangial collagen fibrils. A case of diffuse mesangial sclerosis is illustrated (Fig. 10.2).

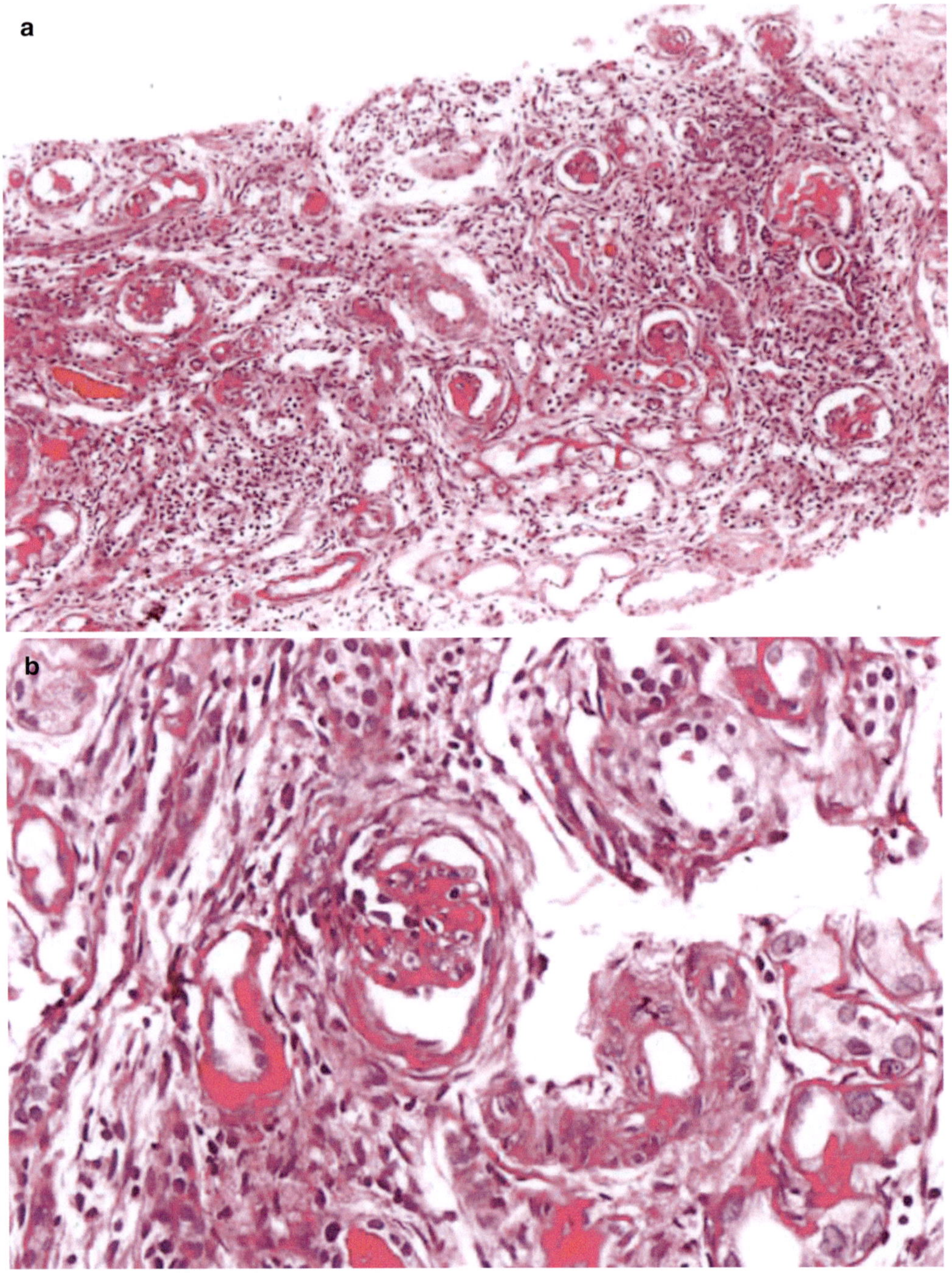

Fig. 10.2 **Diffuse Mesangial Sclerosis** A 3-months female child presented with hypertension; she was dialysis-dependent. USG abdomen revealed that both kidneys had a loss of cortico-medullary demarcation, any cysts were not seen. Urine analysis revealed proteinuria 3+ with 20–30 RBC and 5–10 WBC/hpf. Blood urea and serum creatinine were raised. Renal biopsy had nine glomeruli, all had shrunken tuft with mesangial sclerosis, few showed prominent podocytes. Some of the proximal tubules were dilated and the interstitium had mild fibrosis. IF for IgG, IgM, IgA, C3, C1q, kappa and lambda was uniformly negative. EM showed the shrunken glomerular capillary tuft with effacement of podocyte foot processes and prominent mesangial matrix, no electron-dense deposits were seen. (**a**) PAS ×100, (**b**) PAS ×400, (**c**) HE ×400 and (**d**) EM (identity of the patient has been concealed)

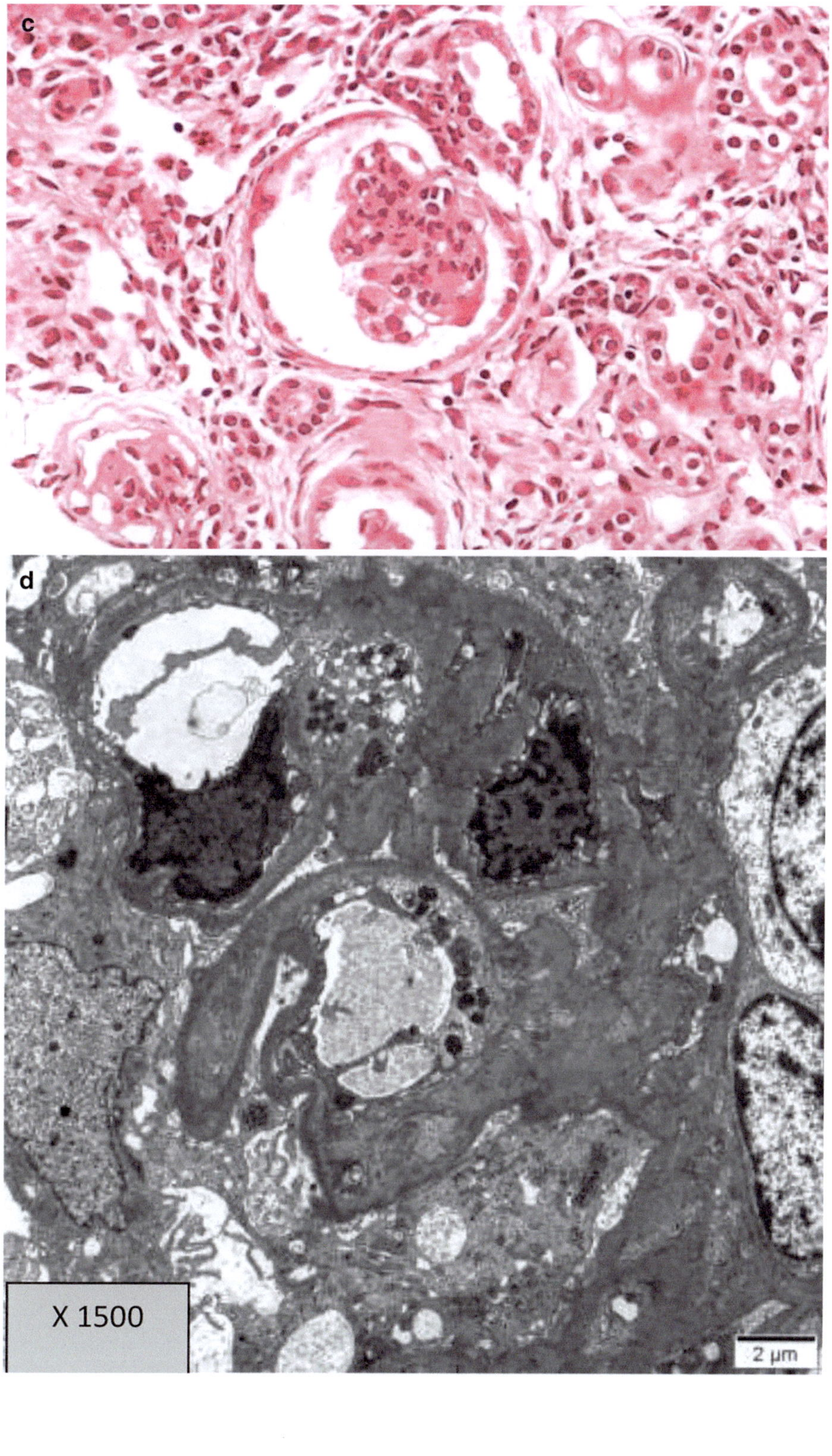

Fig. 10.2 (continued)

Further Reading

Barisoni L, Schnaper HW, Kopp JB. A proposed taxonomy for the podocytopathies: a reassessment of the primary nephrotic diseases. Clin J Am Soc Nephrol. 2007;2:529–42.

Bérody S, Heidet L, Gribouval O, Harambat J, Niaudet P, Baudouin V, Bacchetta J, Boudaillez B, Dehennault M, de Parscau L, Dunand O, Flodrops H, Fila M, Garnier A, Louillet F, Macher MA, May A, Merieau E, Monceaux F, Pietrement C, Rousset-Rouvière C, Roussey G, Taque S, Tenenbaum J, Ulinski T, Vieux R, Zaloszyc A, Morinière V, Salomon R, Boyer O. Treatment and outcome of congenital nephrotic syndrome. Nephrol Dial Transplant. 2019;34:458–67.

D'Agati VD, Jennette JC, Olson JL. Heptinstall's pathology of the kidney. 7th ed. Wolters Kluwer; 2014.

Heptinstalls textbook of the Kidney. 7th ed. Wolters Kluwer; 2014.

Jalanko H. Congenital nephrotic syndrome. Pediatr Nephrol. 2009;24:2121–8.

Nagatani K, Hayashi M. Combination therapy improves pathology indices in diffuse mesangial sclerosis. Pediatr Int. 2019;61(5):517–20.

Wang JJ, Mao JH. The etiology of congenital nephrotic syndrome: current status and challenges. World J Pediatr. 2016;12:149–58.

Yang Y, Zhang SY, Sich M, Béziau A, van den Heuvel LP, Gubler MC. Glomerular extracellular matrix and growth factors in diffuse mesangial sclerosis. Pediatr Nephrol. 2001;16(5):429–38.

11 Lupus Nephritis and Lupus Podocytopathy

11.1 Lupus Nephritis

Renal involvement in patients with SLE manifests as a varying degree of proteinuria, hematuria, and renal dysfunction depending on the pathologic changes seen in renal biopsy. Multiple pathogenic mechanisms are involved in the development of lupus nephritis and include autoantibody production, immune complex formation, and complement activation. Renal involvement in lupus nephritis is an important predictor of morbidity and mortality.

ISN/RPS classification of lupus nephritis 2003 described six classes based on light microscopy, immunofluorescence, and electron microscopic findings. The latest revision to this classification with updates on definition of various lesions has been made in the year 2018.

Class I lupus nephritis is characterized by the absence of any changes on light microscopy with minimal mesangial immune complex deposits of immunoglobulins and complements on immunofluorescence microscopy or electron microscopy. No renal dysfunction, significant proteinuria, or hematuria is seen.

Class II lupus nephritis is characterized by an increase in mesangial cellularity (≥4 mesangial cells surrounded by matrix/mesangial area excluding hilar region) and mesangial matrix. There is no endocapillary hyperplasia, neutrophilic infiltration, wire loop lesions, fibrinoid necrosis or crescents. On immunofluorescence mesangial granular deposits of all immunoglobulins (IgG, IgM, and IgA) and complements (C3 and C1q) are seen. Electron microscopy also shows mesangial immune complex deposits. Patients present with microscopic hematuria with sub-nephrotic range proteinuria and with minimally reduced or normal GFR.

Class III focal proliferative lupus nephritis is characterized by the involvement of less than 50% glomeruli present in the biopsy. Segmental endocapillary hypercellularity, fibrinoid necrosis, polymorphonuclear cell infiltration, wire loop lesions/hyaline thrombi, and crescents can be seen. Changes are more often segmental than global. Segmental areas of scarring can also be seen in chronic lesions. Tubulointerstitial changes are also observed. On immunofluorescence full house pattern is seen with subendothelial capillary wall deposits of all immunoglobulins (IgG, IgM, IgA) and complements (C3, C1q). Mesangial deposits may also be seen. Electron microscopy shows predominantly subendothelial and some mesangial immune deposits. For combined class III and Class V, membranous pattern should be seen in 50% of the glomerular capillary surface of at least 50% of the glomeruli present in the biopsy. Patients of class III lupus nephritis present with hematuria with significant proteinuria often in the nephritic range with an acute reduction in GFR.

Class IV diffuse proliferative lupus nephritis is characterized by similar changes as seen in class III but with involvement of ≥50% of the total glomeruli present in the biopsy. The lesions can be segmental or global. In the latest update on lupus nephritis, subclassification of lupus nephritis into class IV-G/S has been abolished. Like class III, full house pattern on immunofluorescence with subendothelial capillary wall deposits of immunoglobulins and complements. Mesangial deposits may also be seen. Electron microscopy shows predominantly subendothelial and some mesangial immune deposits. For combined class IV and Class V, membranous patterns should be seen in 50% of the glomerular capillary surface of at least 50% of the glomeruli present in the biopsy.

Class V lupus nephritis is characterized by severe proteinuria which often manifests as nephrotic syndrome with a gradual reduction in GFR. Membranous pattern of glomerular involvement is seen on light microscopy. Mesangial proliferation may also be seen. On immunofluorescence, subepithelial deposits of immunoglobulins (IgG, IgM and IgA) and complements (C3, C1q) are seen. There can be accompanying mesangial deposits. Electron microscopy shows subepithelial electron-dense deposits often accompanied by mesangial deposits. As class V progresses to chronicity, segmental or globally sclerosed glomeruli may be seen.

Class VI advanced lupus nephritis is characterized by global glomerulosclerosis involving ≥90 glomeruli present in the biopsy which can be attributed to lupus nephritis and not caused by other disease processes. Classes II, III, IV, and class V can progress to advanced class VI lupus nephritis. This is the least encountered class in renal biopsies.

P. Gupta, R. K. Gupta, *Pathology of Glomerular Diseases*, https://doi.org/10.1007/978-981-19-1430-0_11

11.1.1 Lupus Nephritis Class I (Fig. 11.1)

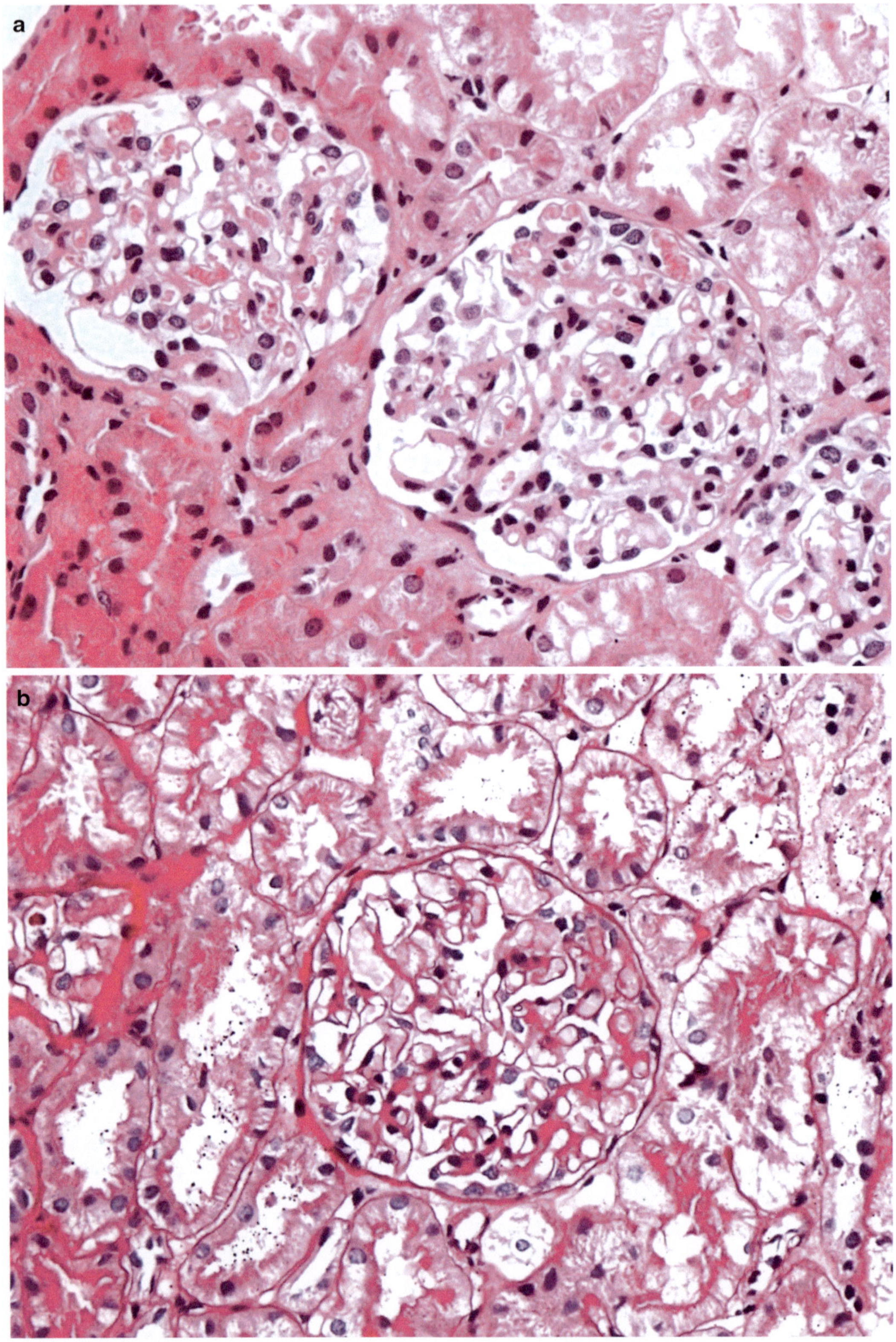

Fig. 11.1 **Class I lupus nephritis.** An 8-years female child, known case of lupus, presented with an episode of mild intermittent hematuria. Urine analysis revealed 1+ protein with bland urinary sediment; 24 h urinary protein was 1.2 g. Serum complement C3 and C4 were wnl. Renal bx had ten glomeruli which were almost unremarkable; tubules, interstitium, and blood vessels were also unremarkable. IF showed minimal mesangial granular deposits of IgG (1+), similar mesangial deposits of IgM, IgA, C3, C1q were also seen. EM showed few mesangial electron-dense deposits. (**a**) HE ×200, (**b**) PAS ×400, (**c**) IF ×400 and (**d**) EM (identity of the patient has been concealed)

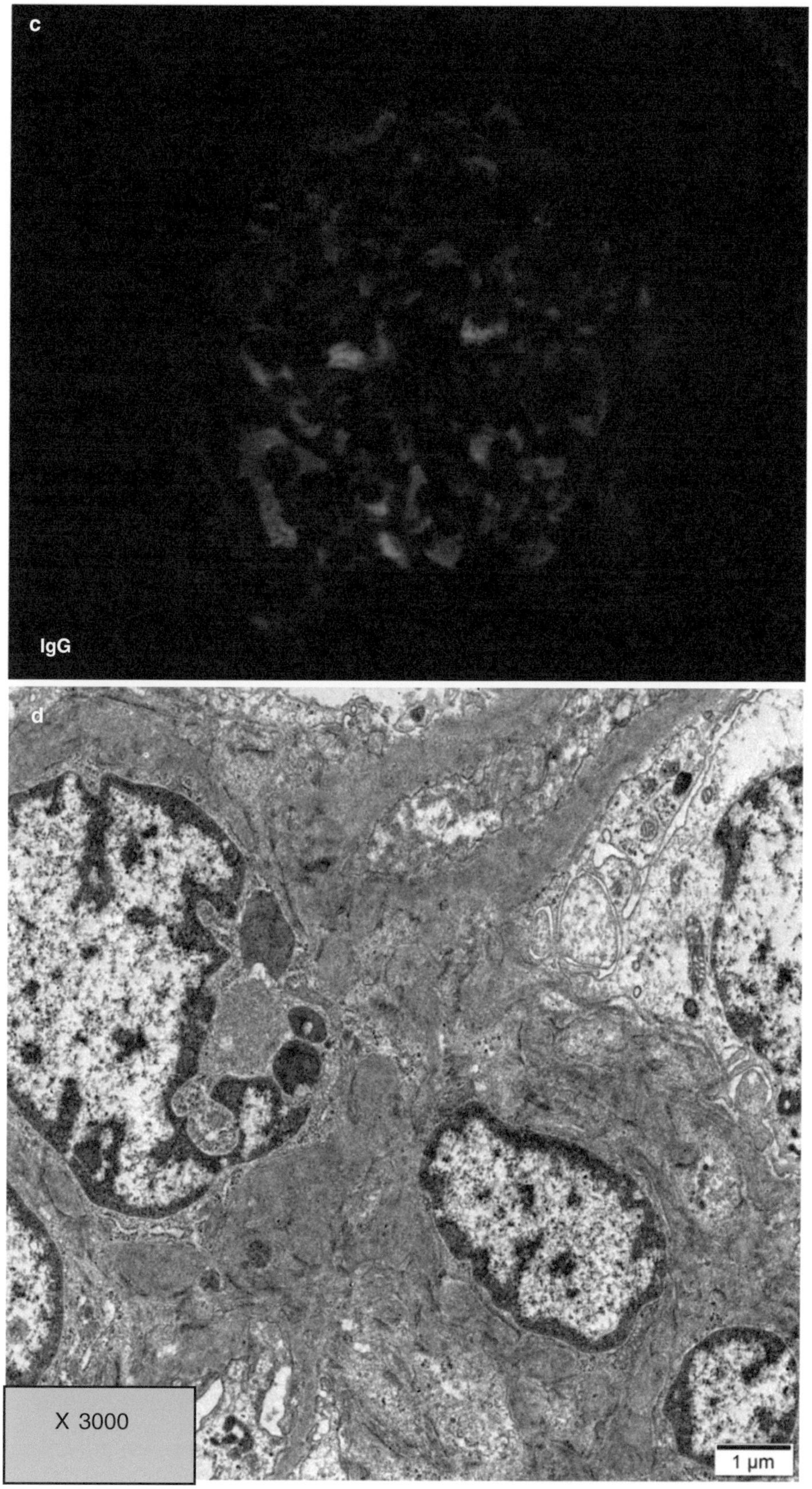

Fig. 11.1 (continued)

11.1.2 Lupus Nephritis Class II (Fig. 11.2)

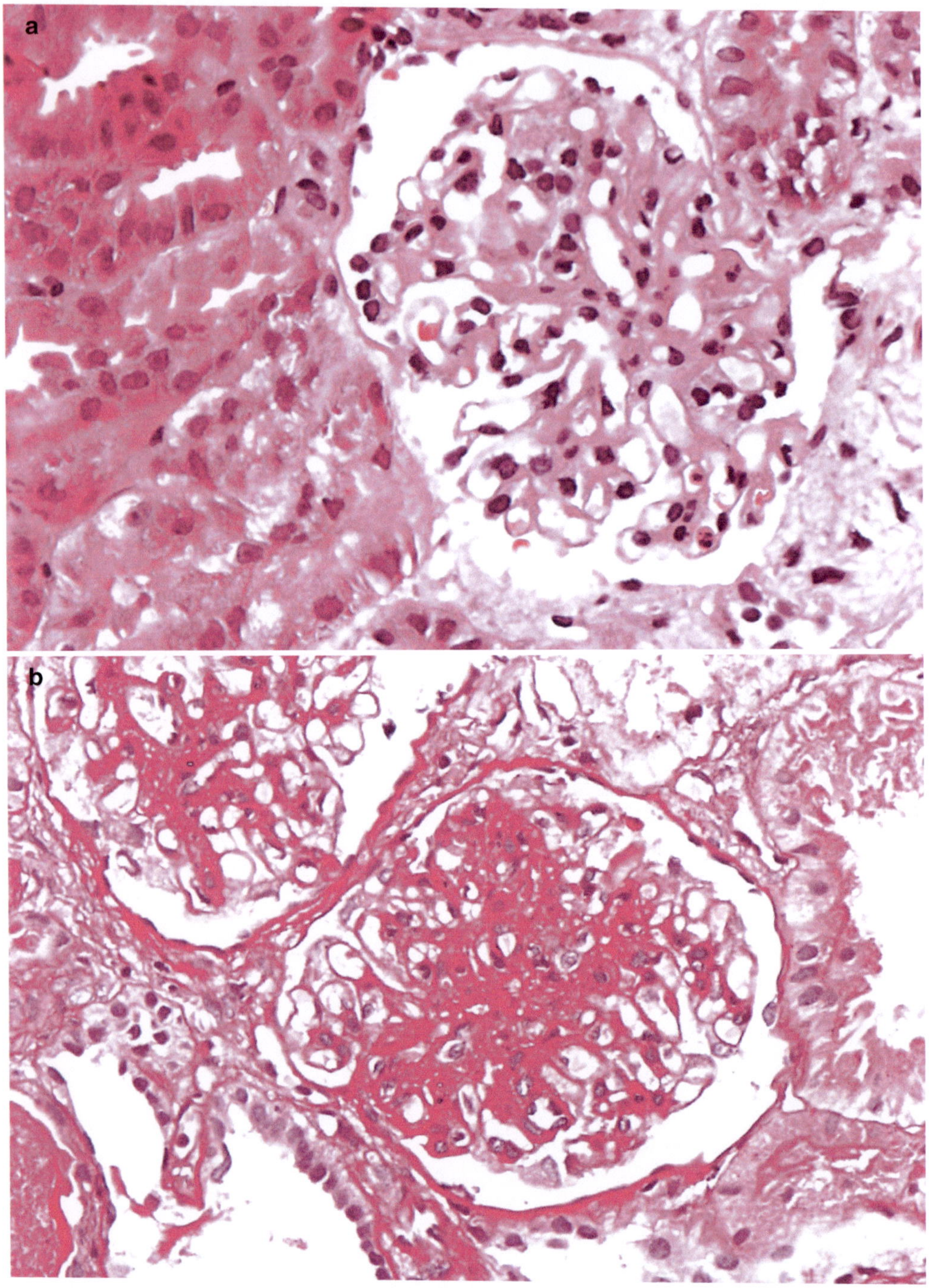

Fig. 11.2 Class II lupus nephritis A 6-years female child presented with subnephrotic range proteinuria. There was no h/o hematuria, rash or joint pain; she did not have any family history of kidney disease. Urine analysis revealed protein 2+ with bland urinary sediment, 24 h urinary protein was 1.1 g and serum creatinine was 0.6 mg/dL. Serology for HIV, HCV, and HBsAg was negative, ANA was 2+ homogeneous and serum complements were wnl. Kidney biopsy revealed nine glomeruli, one of which showed segmental sclerosis, and other glomeruli showed mild mesangial expansion and an increase in mesangial cellularity. IF showed 3+ granular mesangial positivity for IgG, IgM, IgA, C3, C1q, and kappa and lambda. EM showed focal effacement of visceral epithelial foot processes with electron-dense deposits (conventional) in mesangial and paramesangial areas. (**a**) HE ×400, (**b**) PAS ×400, (**c**) PSM ×400, (**d**)–(**h**) IF ×400, (**i**) EM (identity of the patient has been concealed)

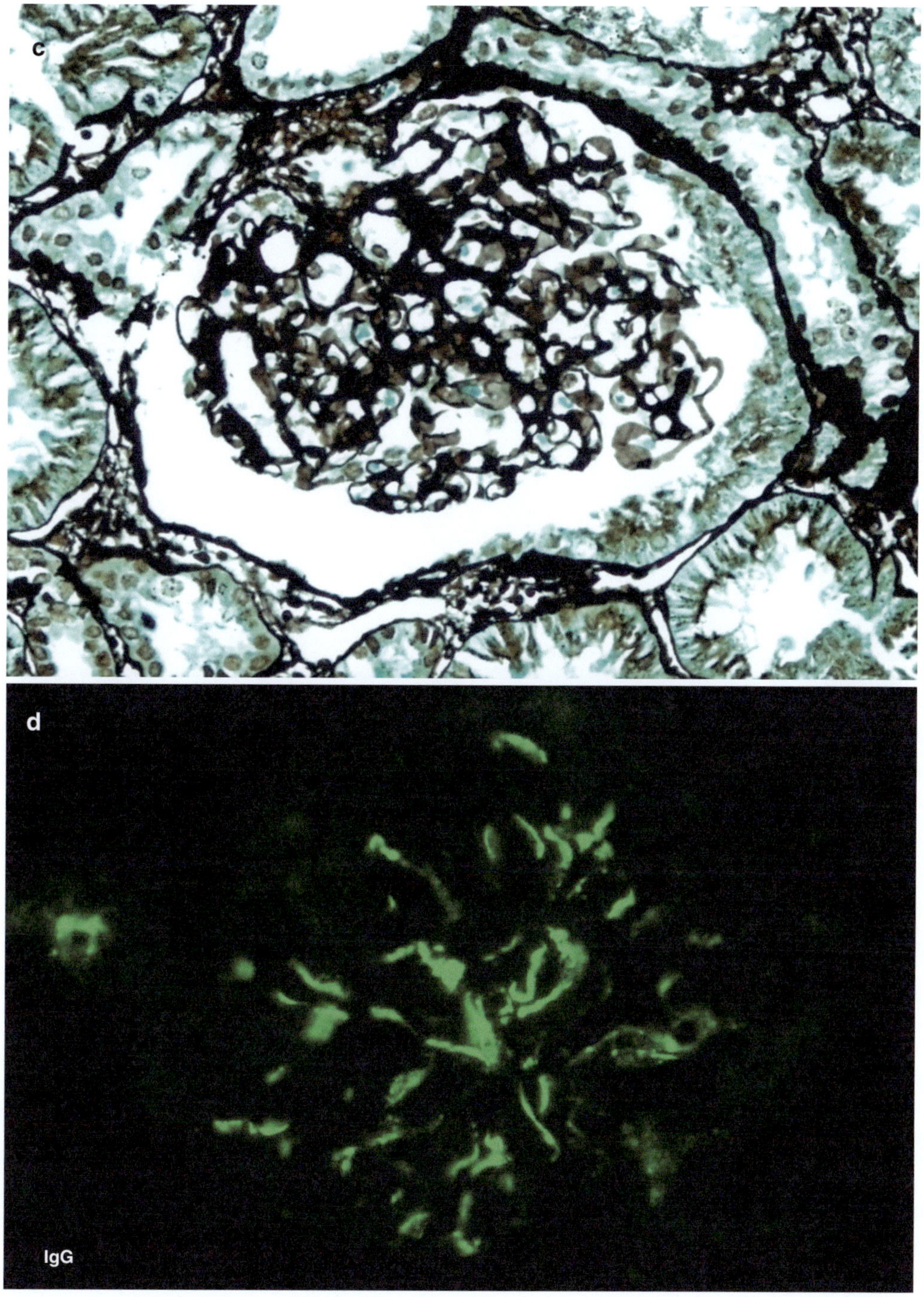

Fig. 11.2 (continued)

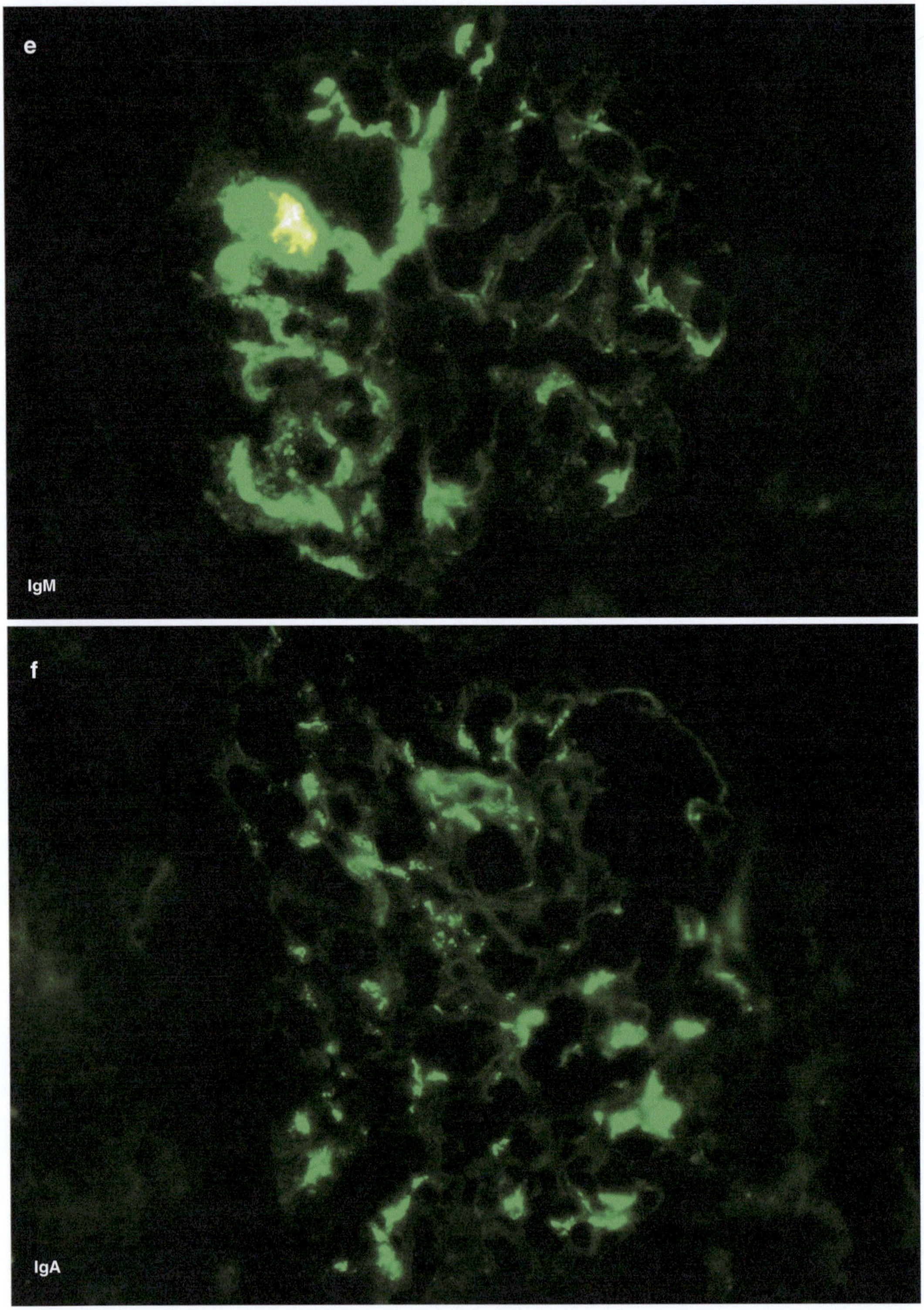

Fig. 11.2 (continued)

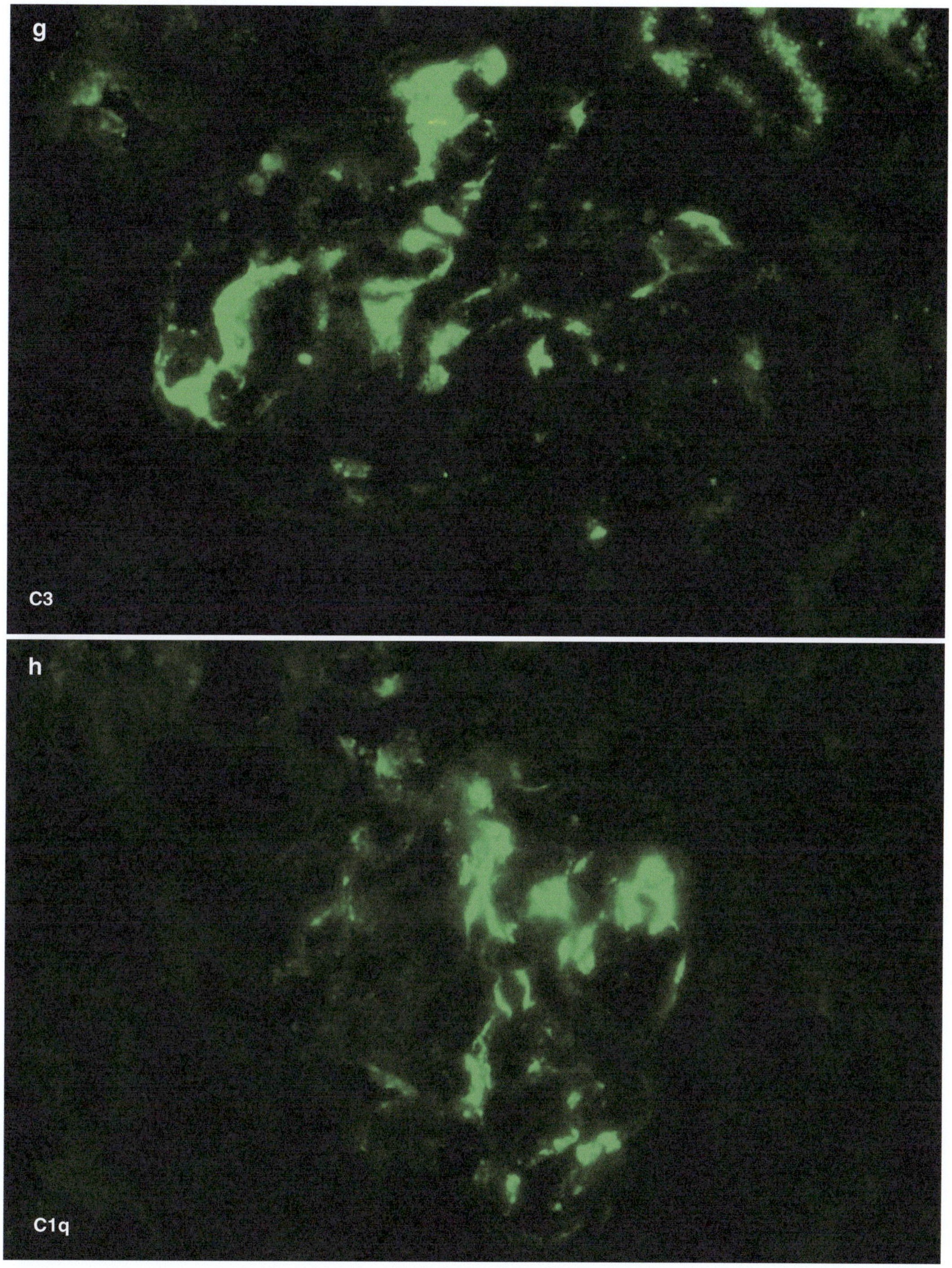

Fig. 11.2 (continued)

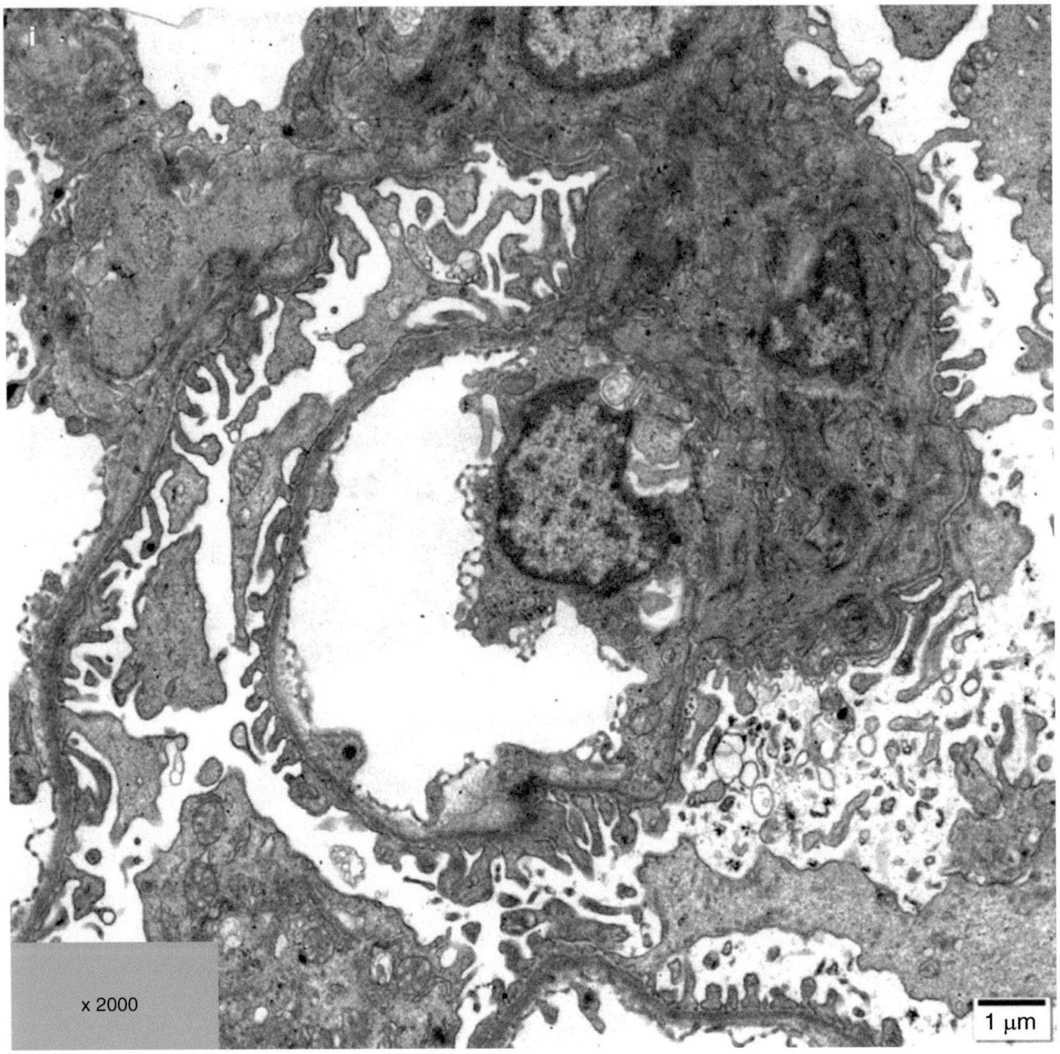

Fig. 11.2 (continued)

11.1.3 Lupus Nephritis Class III (Fig. 11.3)

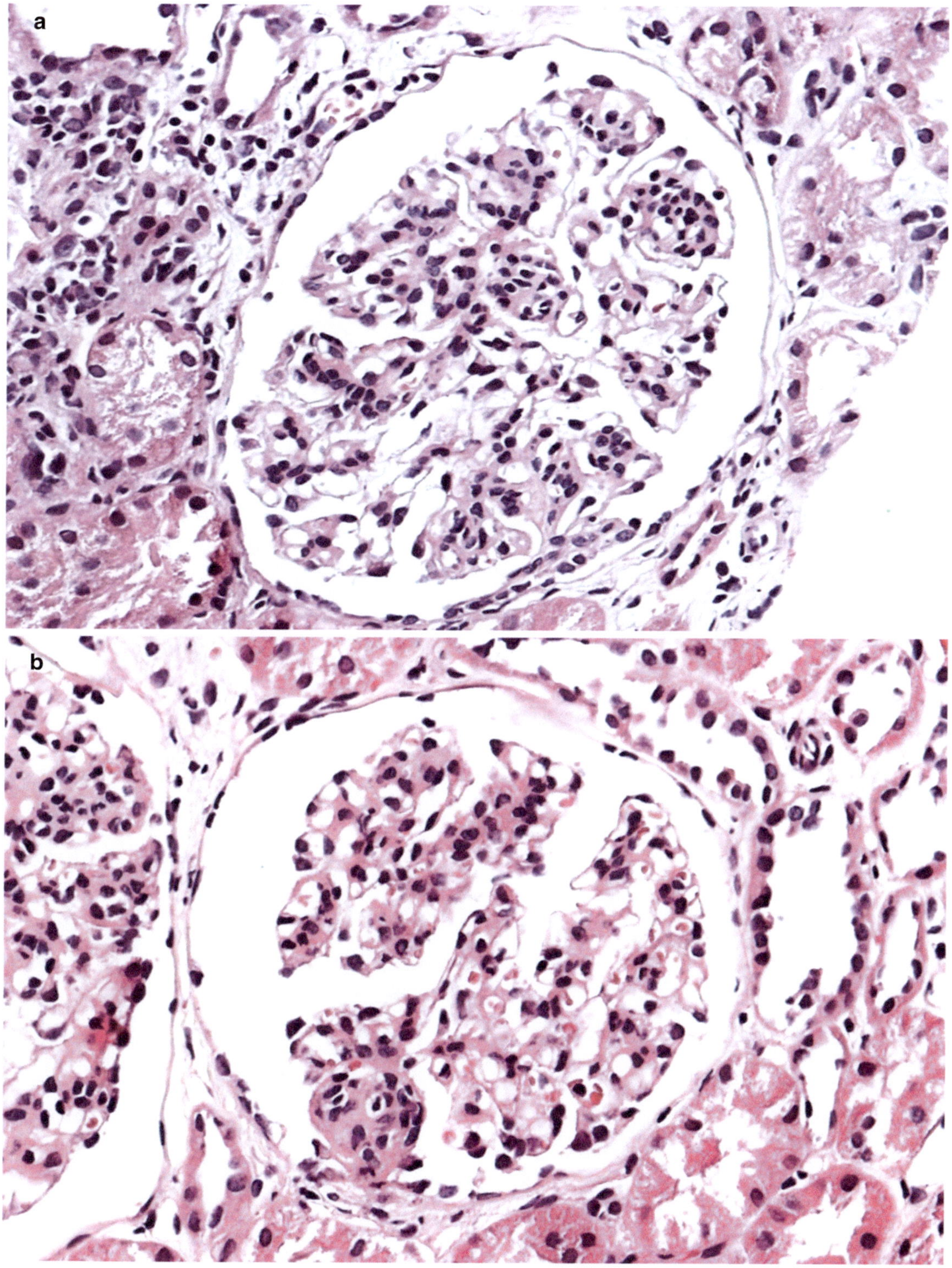

Fig. 11.3 **Class III Lupus Nephritis.** A 14-years female patient presented with malar rash and pedal edema for 3 months. Laboratory workup revealed that she had pancytopenia with Hb of 9.1 g/dL, total WBC count was 2300 per cu mm and platelets were 90,000 per cu mm. Urinary protein was 3+ with 24 h urinary protein of 3.3 g, microscopic examination showed 10–12 RBC/hpf. On serological evaluation the ANA was 3+ homogeneous and anti-ds-DNA was also elevated (>100 IU/mL); C3 was low (760 mg/L). Renal biopsy had ten glomeruli, four showed segmental endocapillary hyperplasia and mild neutrophilic infiltration; any fibrinoid necrosis, crescents, or wireloop lesions were not seen. Interstitium showed mild lymphocytic infiltrate. Activity score 4/24 and chronicity score was 0/12. IF showed full house pattern with granular capillary wall and mesangial positivity for IgG, IgM, IgA, C3 and C1q in glomeruli and also in the wall of blood vessels. EM showed subendothelial electron-dense deposits with occasional mesangial deposits. (**a** and **b**) HE ×400, (**c**) PAS ×400, (**d**) PSM ×400, (**e**)–(**j**) IF ×400, (**k**) EM (identity of the patient has been concealed)

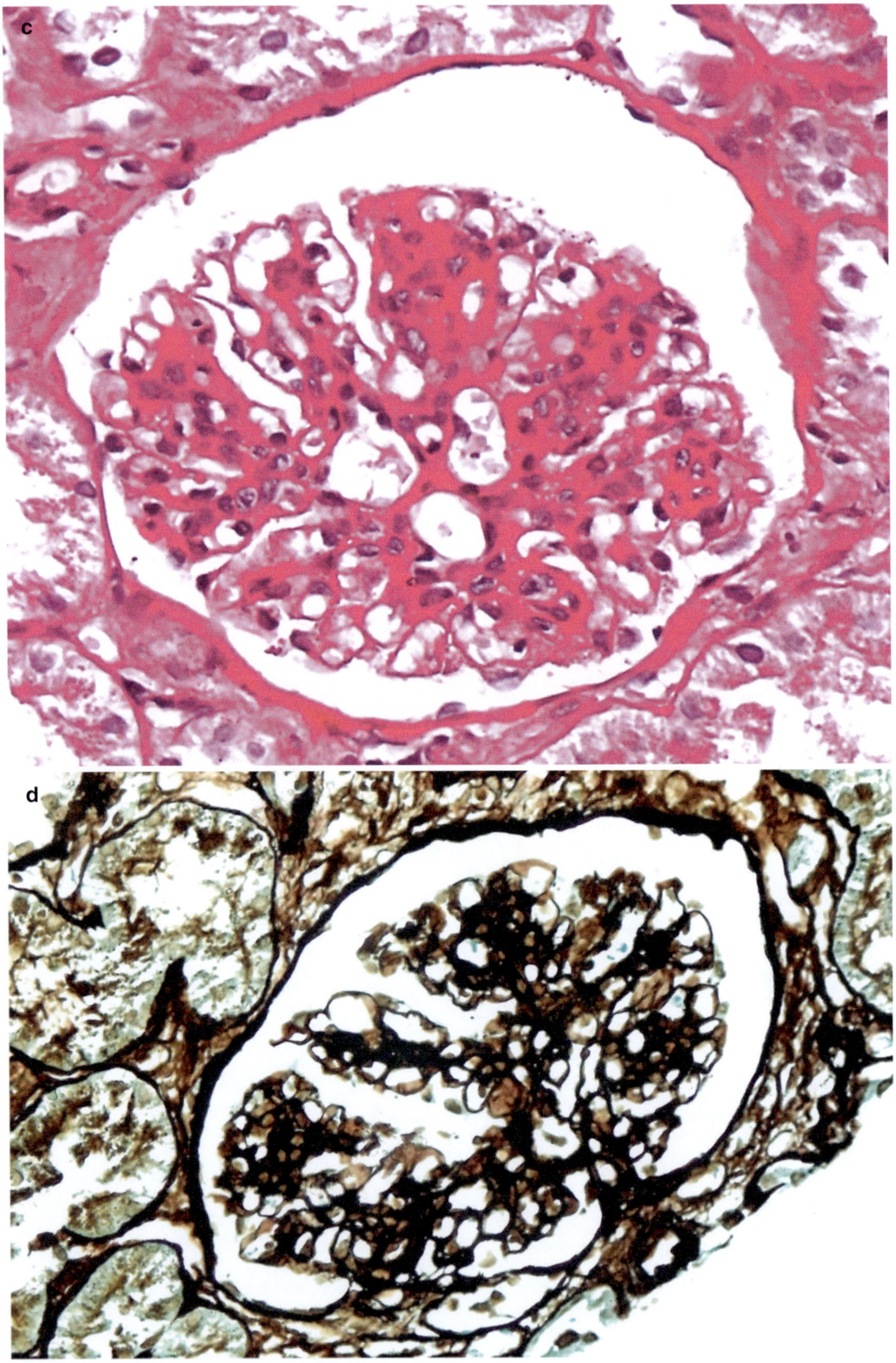

Fig. 11.3 (continued)

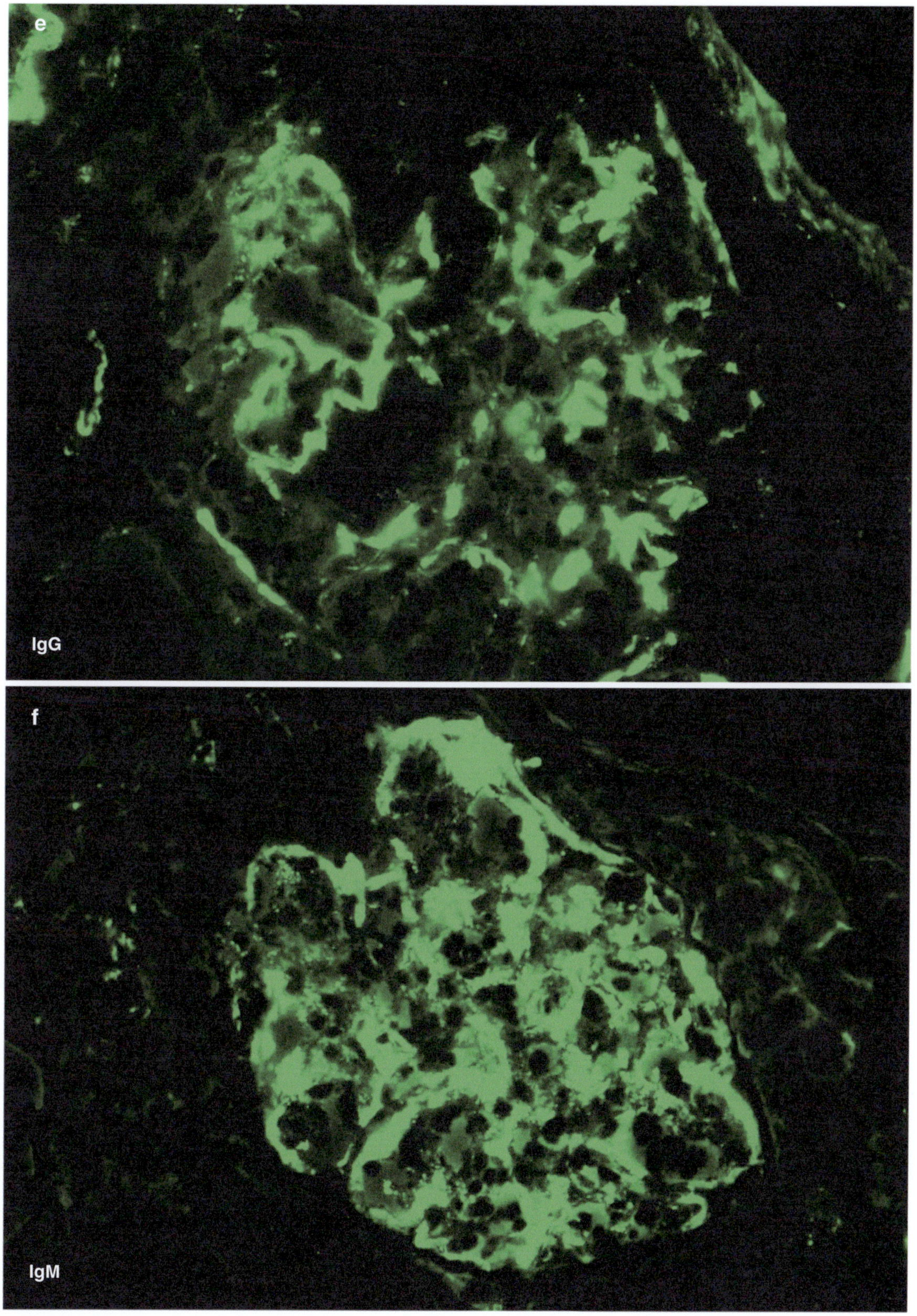

Fig. 11.3 (continued)

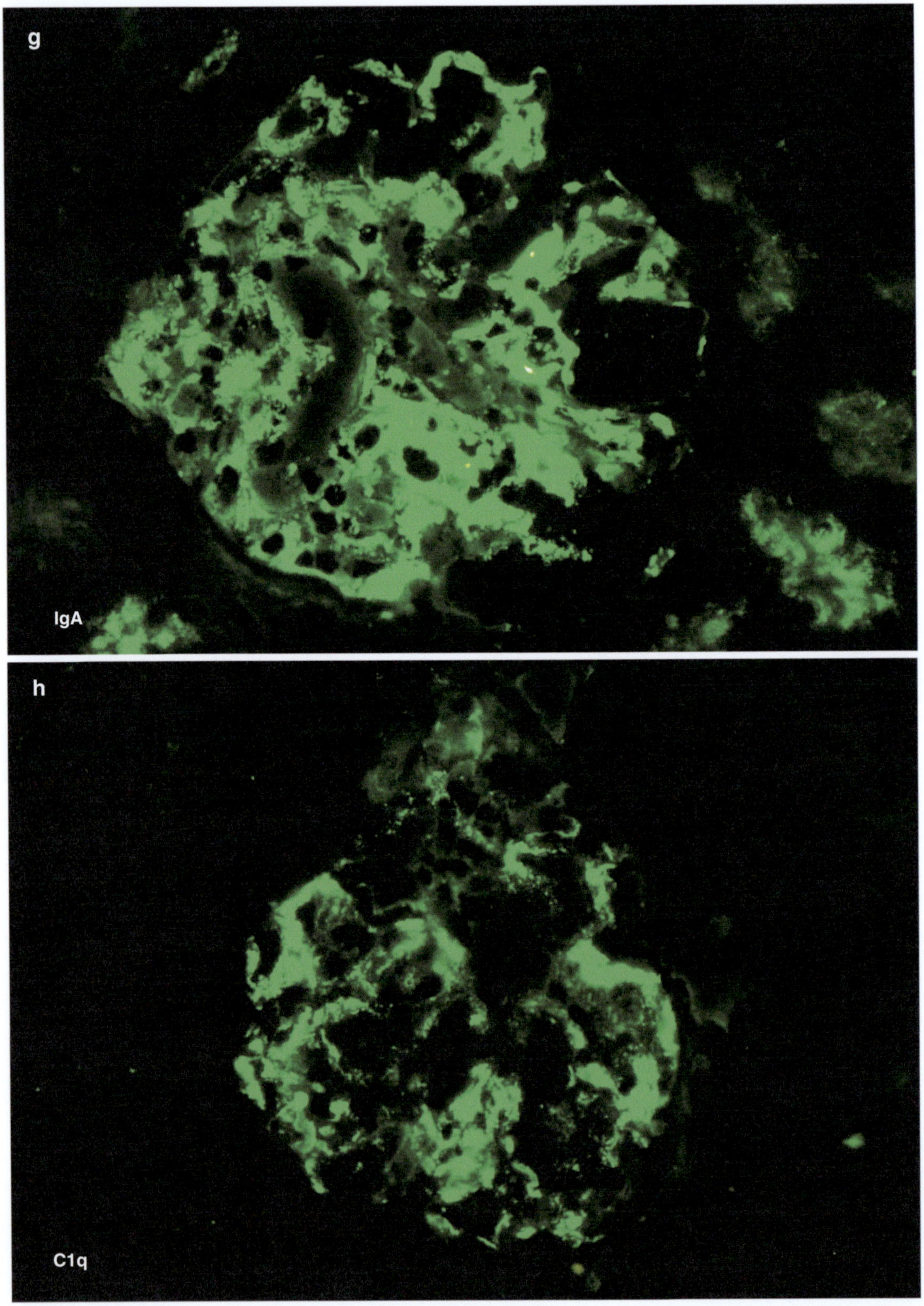

Fig. 11.3 (continued)

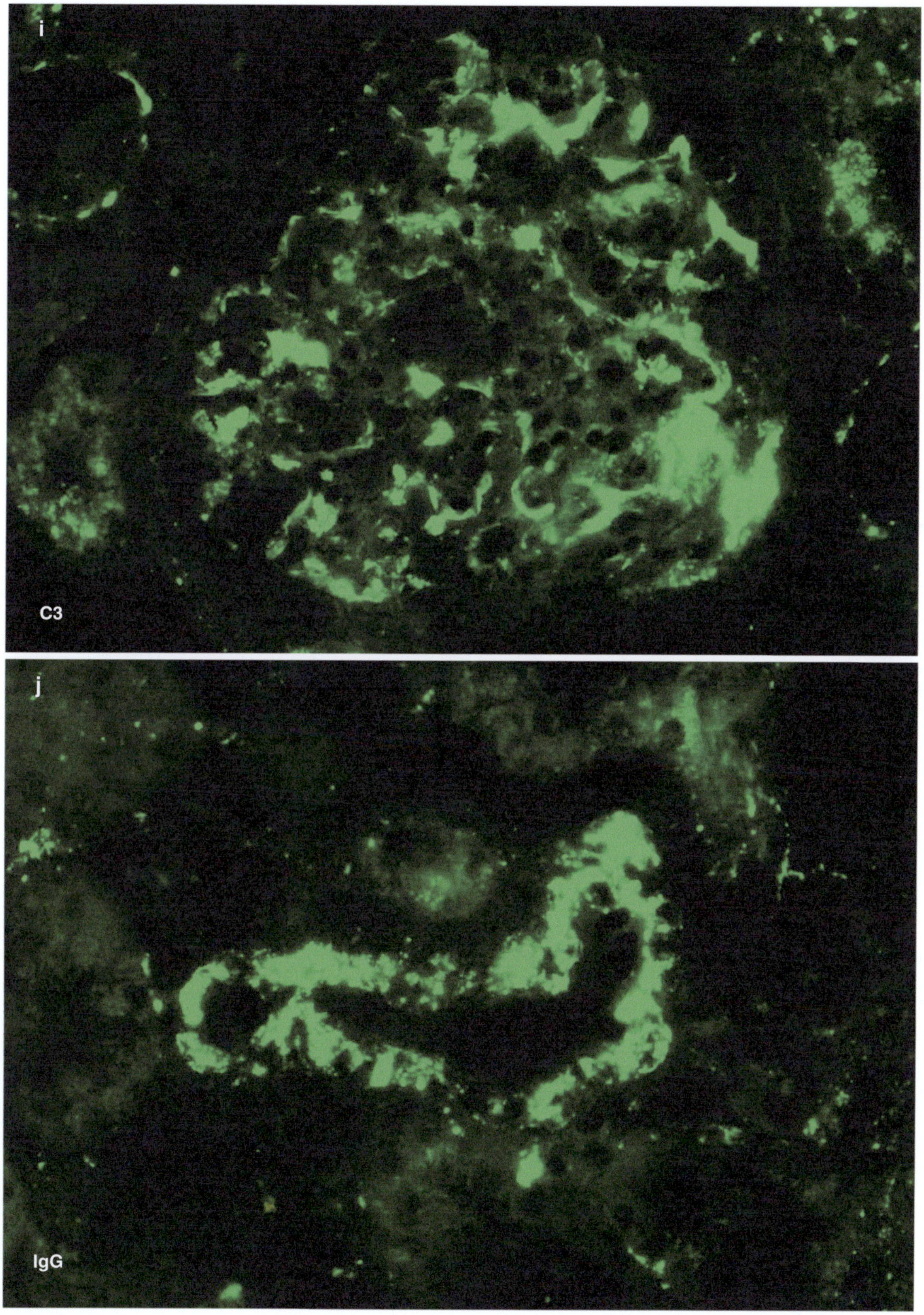

Fig. 11.3 (continued)

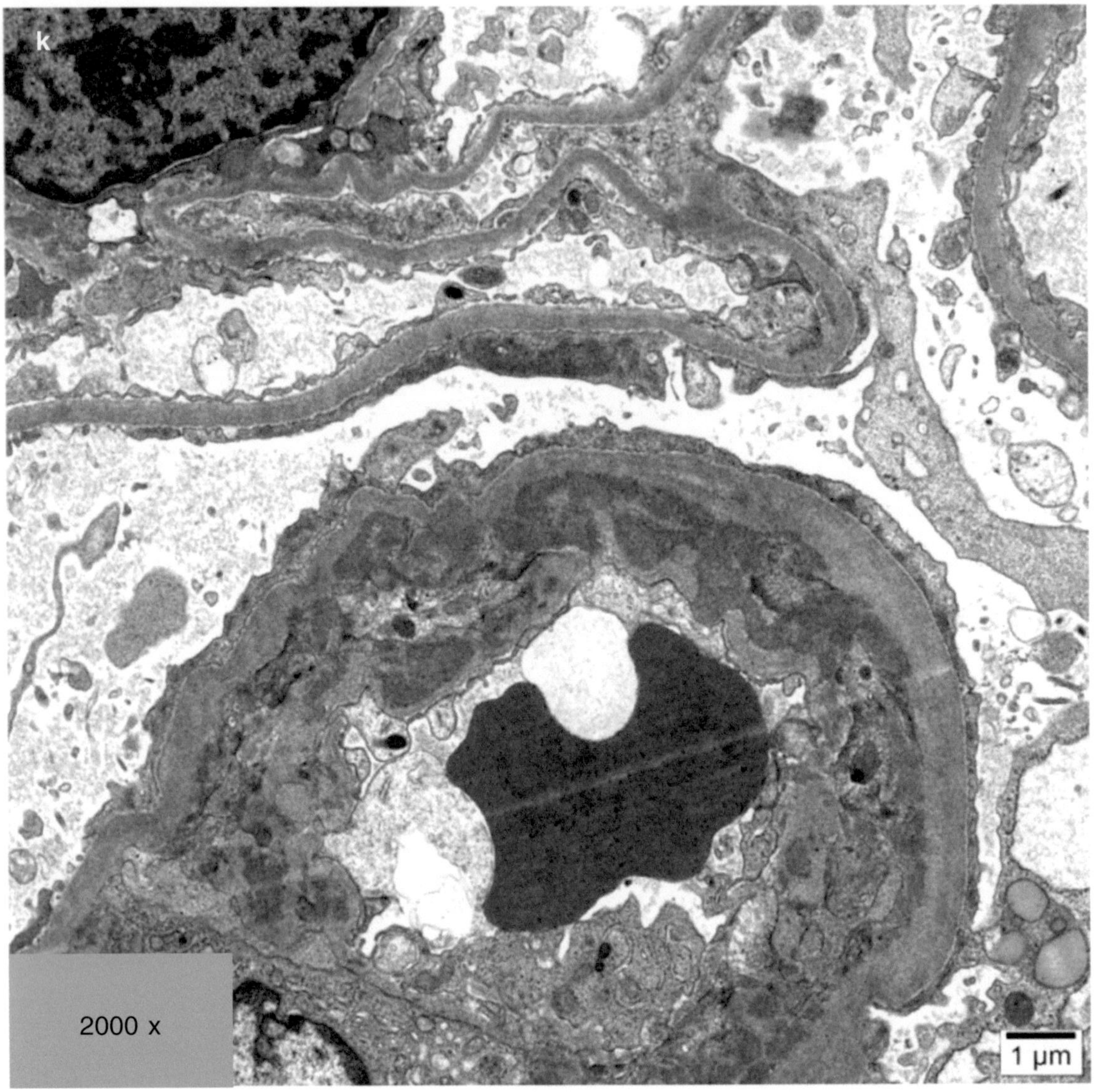

Fig. 11.3 (continued)

11.1.4 Lupus Nephritis Class III + V (Fig. 11.4)

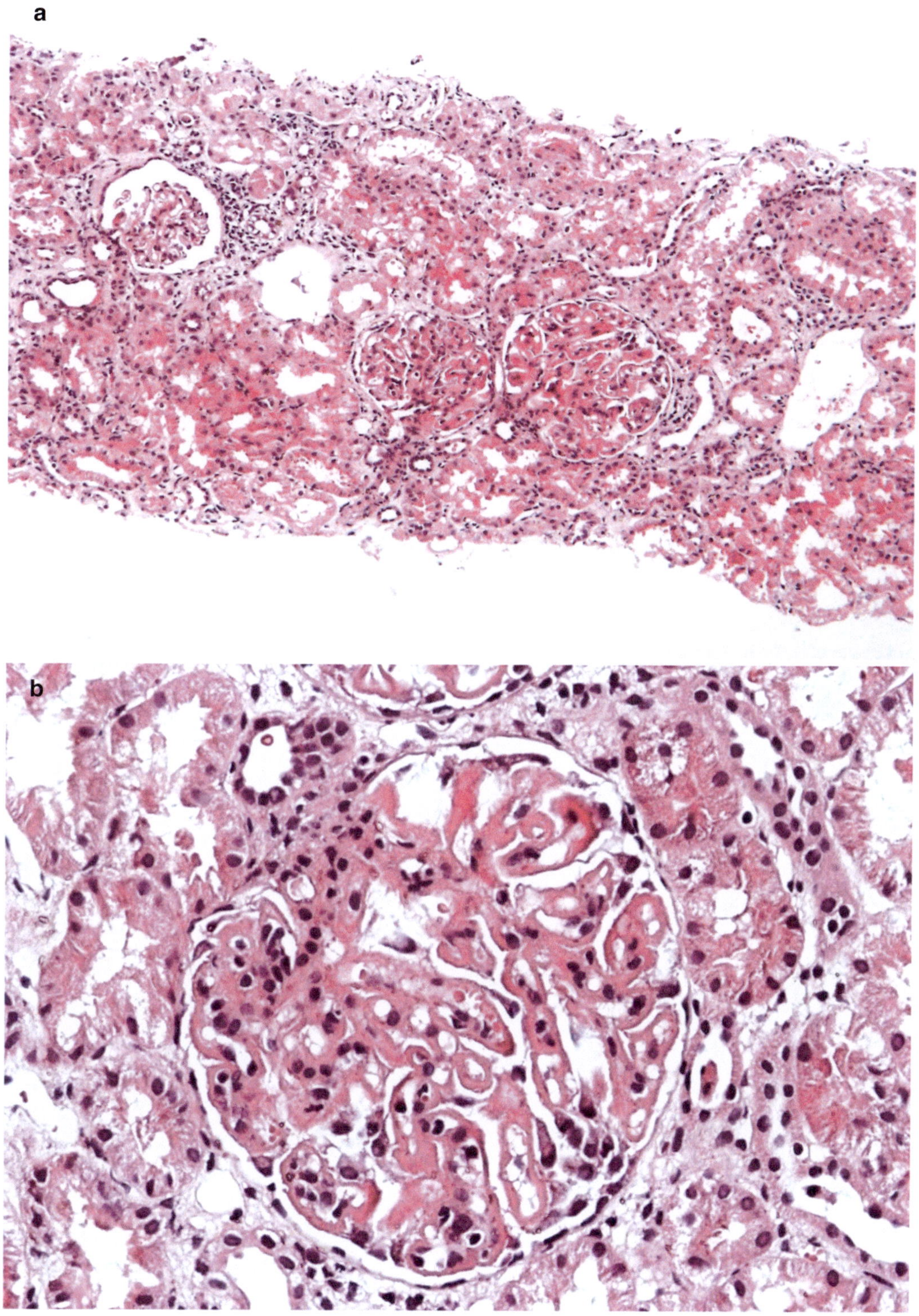

Fig. 11.4 **Class III + V lupus nephritis.** A 26-years male patient presented with swelling of both lower limbs for 1 year and was also hypertensive for the past 1 year. Laboratory workup revealed that his hemoglobin was 10.2 g/dL with total WBC count of 8900 per cu mm and platelet count of 274,000 per cu mm. Urine spot PC ratio was 3.6 and serum creatinine was 0.65 mg/dL. Patient was hypoproteinemic with total serum protein being 3.77 g/dL and serum albumin was 1.35 g/dL with serum globulin being 2.42 g/dL. Serum complement C3 and C4 were reduced being 545 mg/L and 66 mg/L respectively. Anti-ds-DNA was >1000 IU/mL. Renal biopsy had ten glomeruli, four of them showed segmental endocapillary proliferation and all the glomeruli showed thickening of GBM with the presence of argyrophilic epimembranous spikes. Disease activity score was 4/24 and chronicity score was 0/12. IF for IgG, IgM, IgA, Complement C3 and C1q showed granular positivity along GBM with full house pattern (both endothelial and outer aspect of GBM). (**a**) HE ×100, (**b**) HE ×400, (**c**) PAS ×400, (**d**) PSM ×400, (**e**)–(**i**). IF ×400

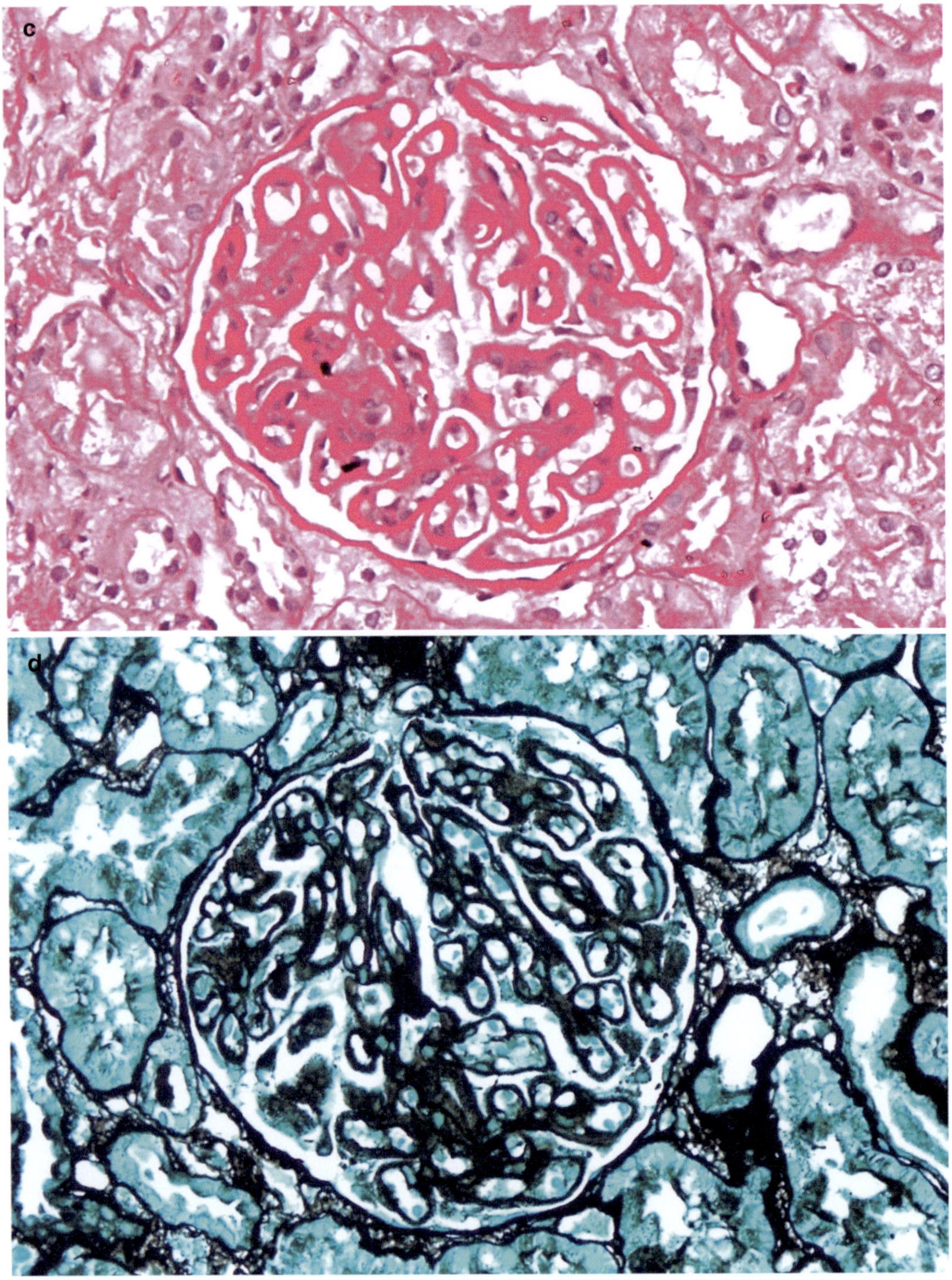

Fig. 11.4 (continued)

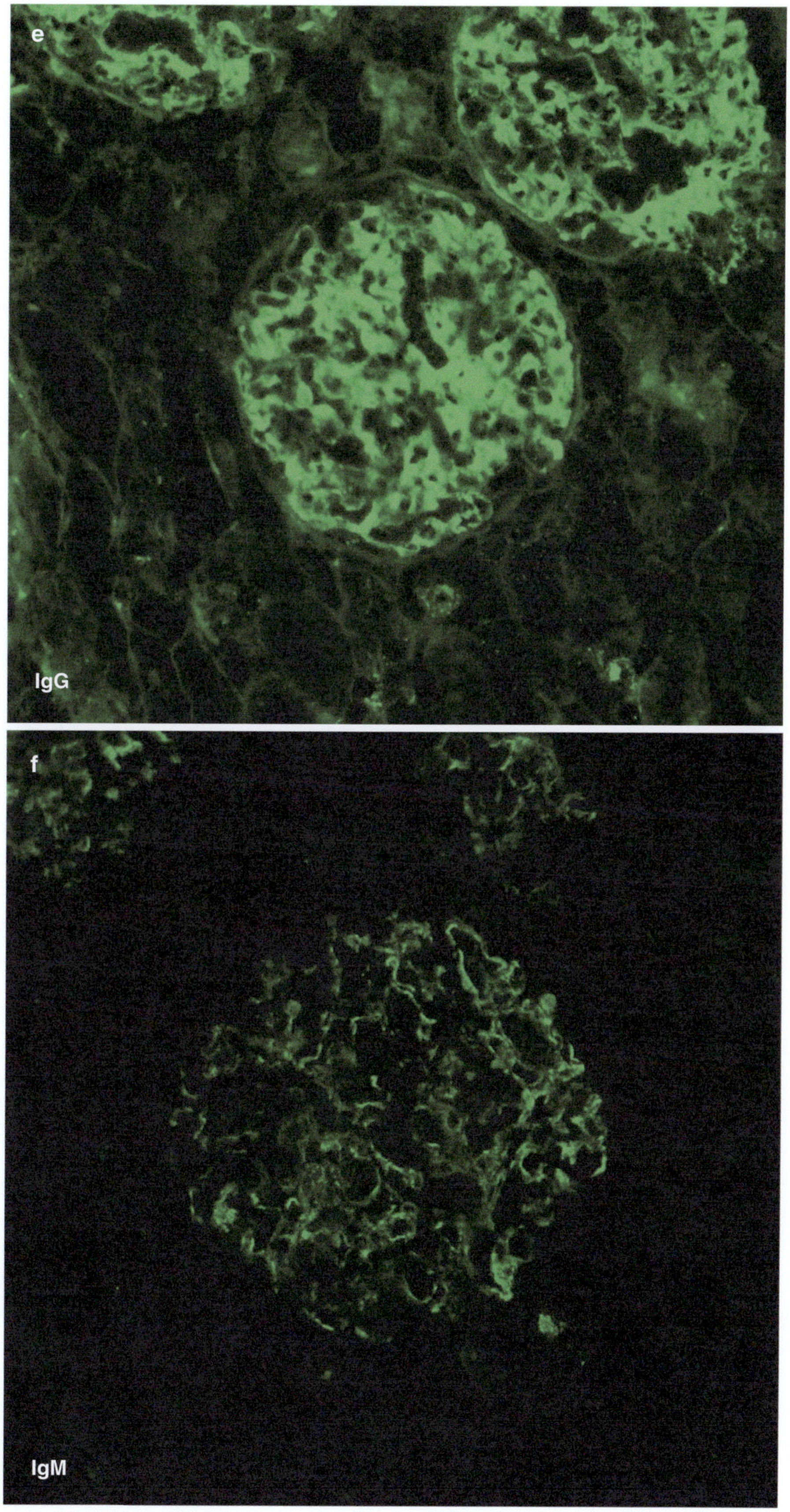

Fig. 11.4 (continued)

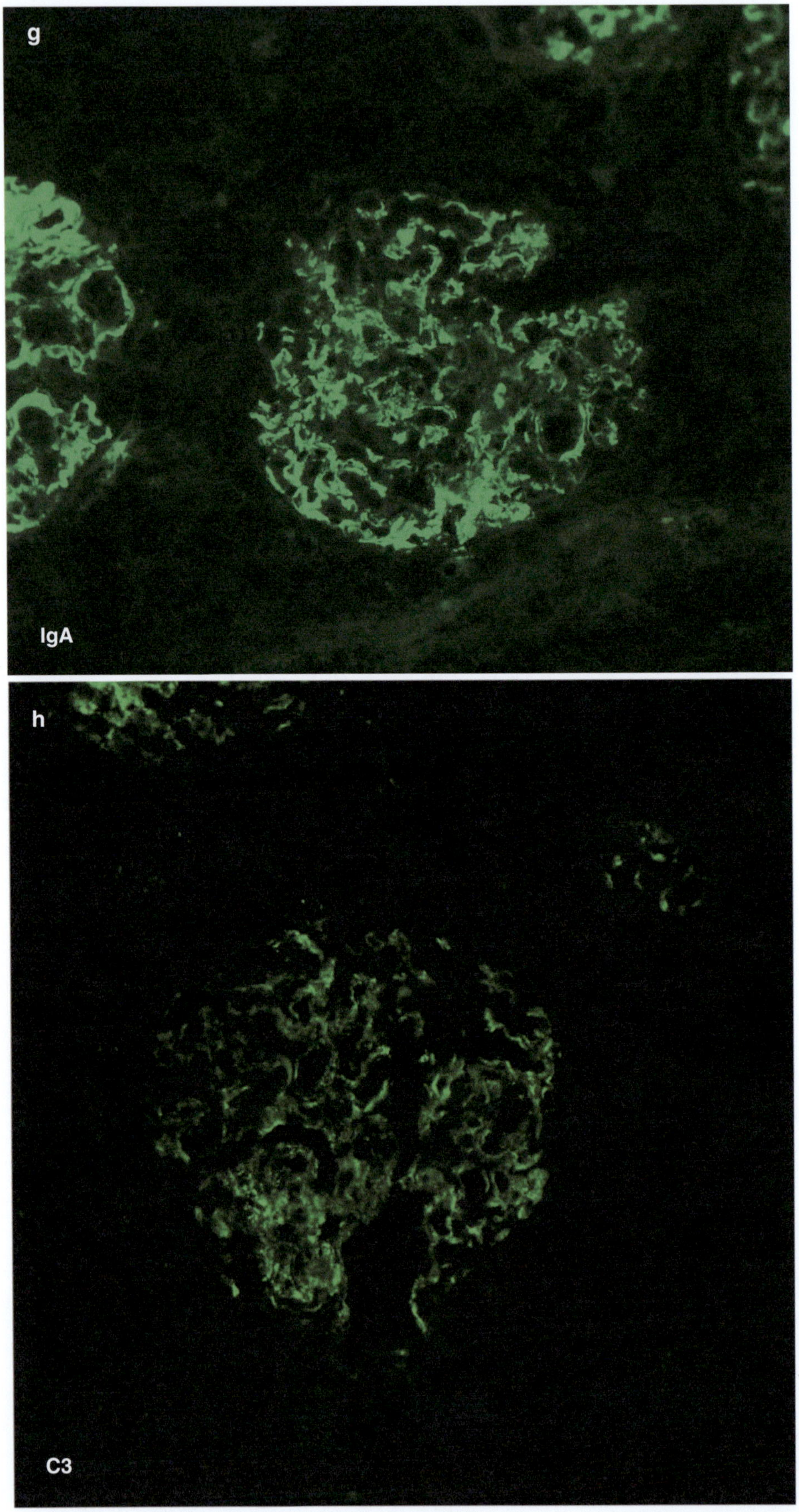

Fig. 11.4 (continued)

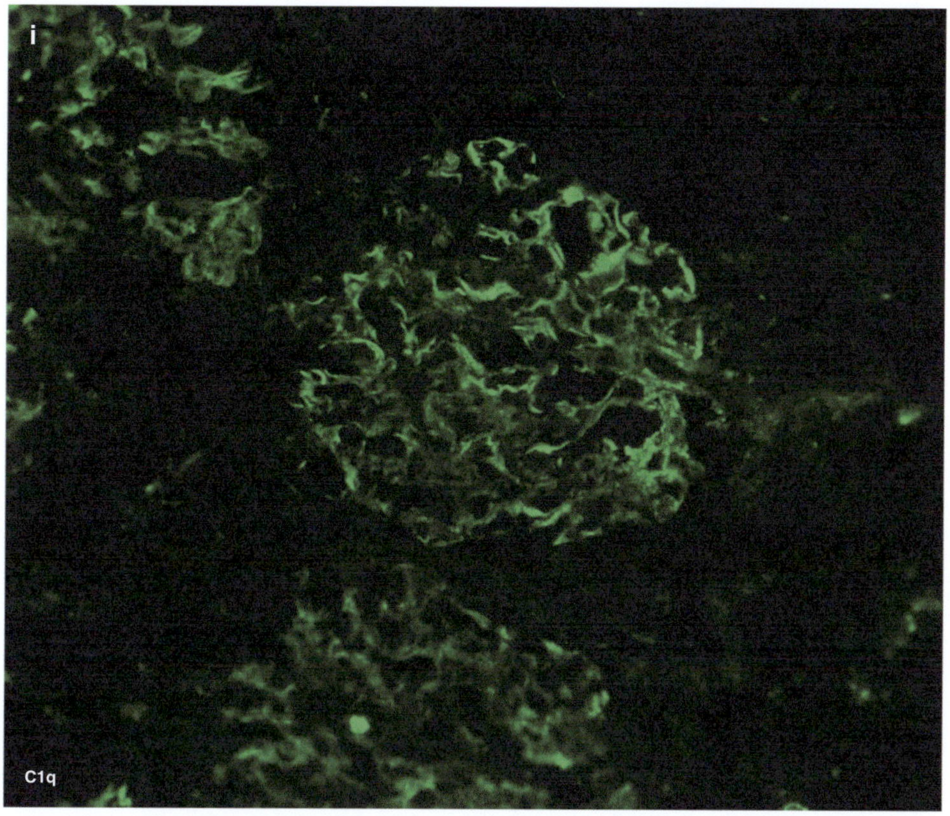

Fig. 11.4 (continued)

11.1.5 Lupus Nephritis Class IV (Fig. 11.5)

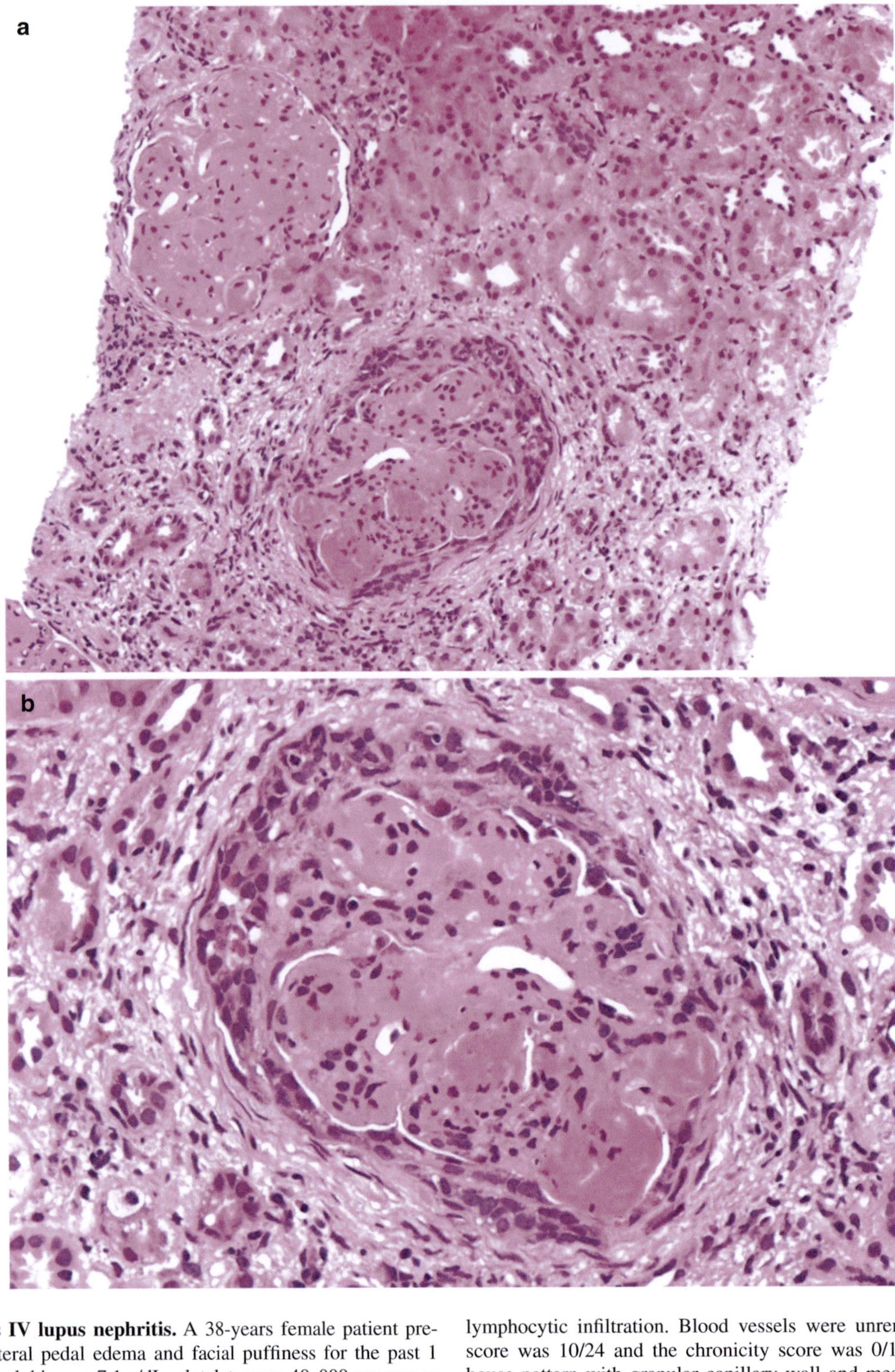

Fig. 11.5 **Class IV lupus nephritis.** A 38-years female patient presented with bilateral pedal edema and facial puffiness for the past 1 month. Her hemoglobin was 7.1 g/dL, platelets were 40, 000 per cu mm and ESR was 60 mm (Westergren). Urinary protein was 3+ with 5–10 RBC/hpf and urine PC ratio was 8.37. Both serum C3 and C4 were markedly reduced being 195 mg/L and 35 mg/L respectively. Serum ANA was 3+. Renal biopsy had 28 glomeruli, all were enlarged and all of them showed subendothelial hyaline deposits (wireloop lesions) with segmental endocapillary hyperplasia; 4 glomeruli had cellular/fibrocellular crescents. Some of the glomeruli also had neutrophilic infiltration. Some of the tubules had hyaline casts and the interstitium had mild lymphocytic infiltration. Blood vessels were unremarkable. Activity score was 10/24 and the chronicity score was 0/12. IF showed full house pattern with granular capillary wall and mesangial deposits of IgG, IgM, IgA, C3, C1q; interstitial and tubular deposits were also seen. EM showed subendothelial, mesangial and occasional subepithelial/intramembranous electron-dense deposits with focal effacement of visceral epithelial cell foot processes along with tubuloreticular inclusions in endothelial cell cytoplasm of glomerular capillaries. (**a**) HE ×200, (**b**)–(**d**) HE ×400, (**e**) MT ×400, (**f**) PSM ×400, (**g**)–(**k**) IF ×400, (**l**) and (**m**) EM (identity of patient has been concealed)

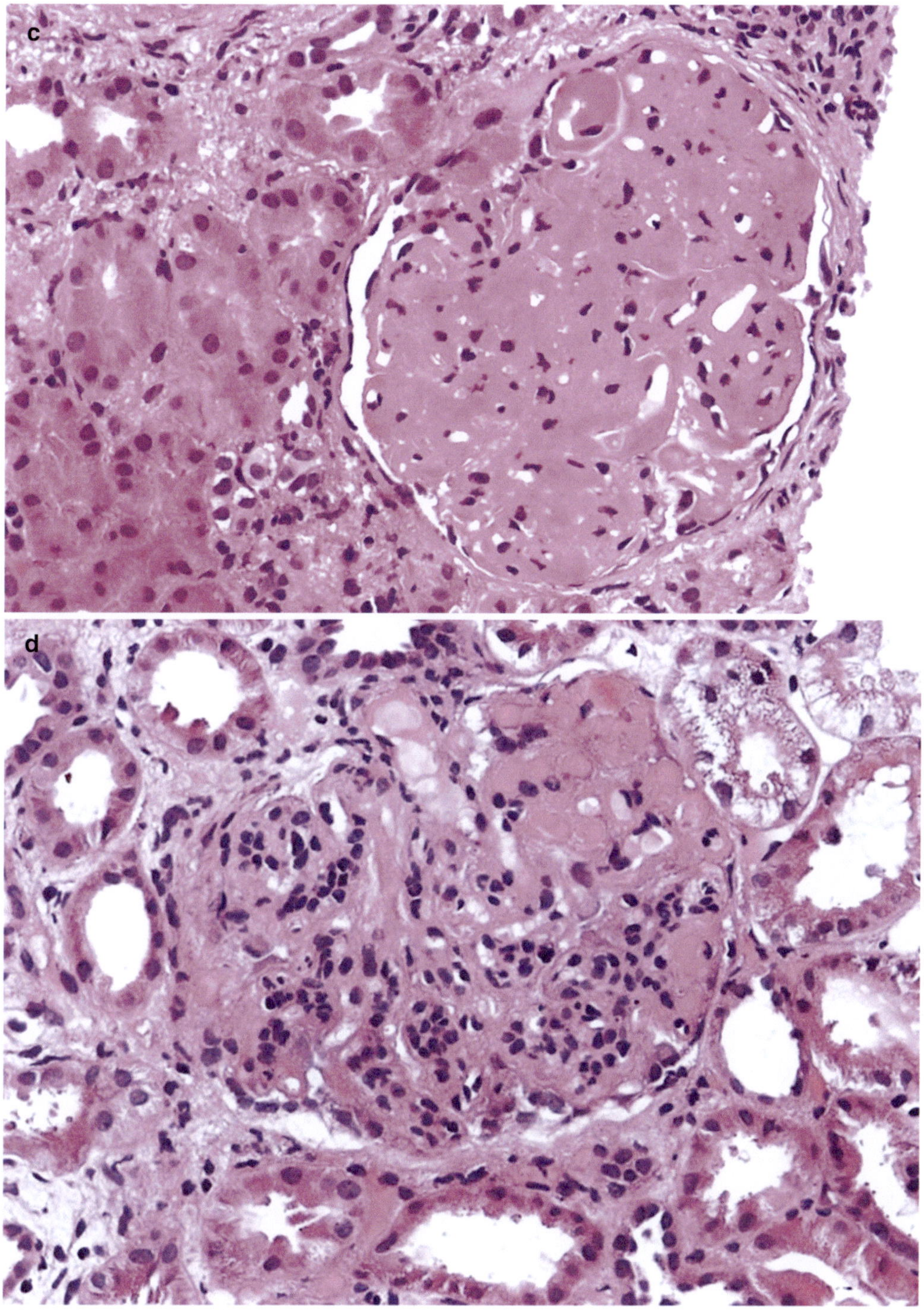

Fig. 11.5 (continued)

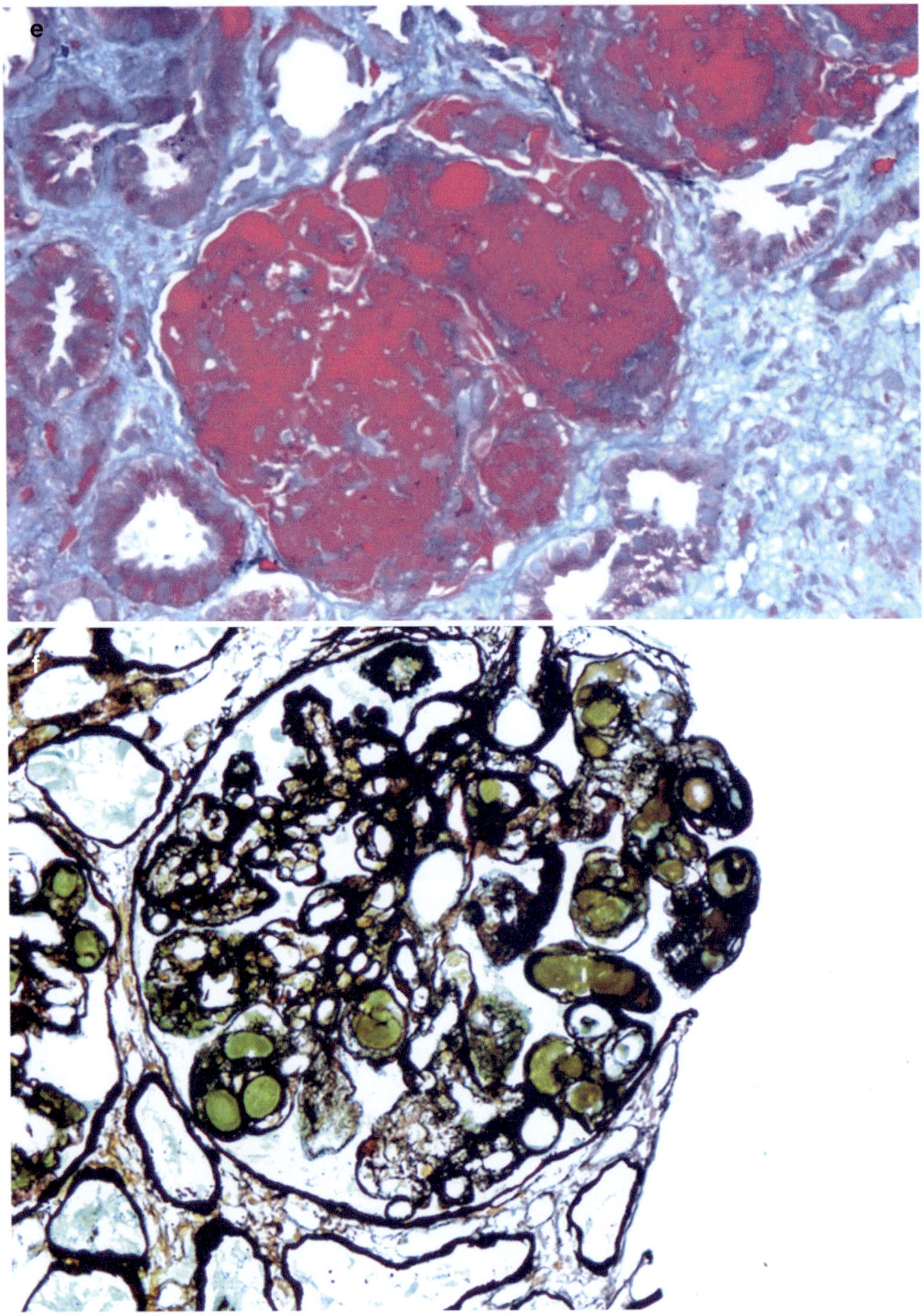

Fig. 11.5 (continued)

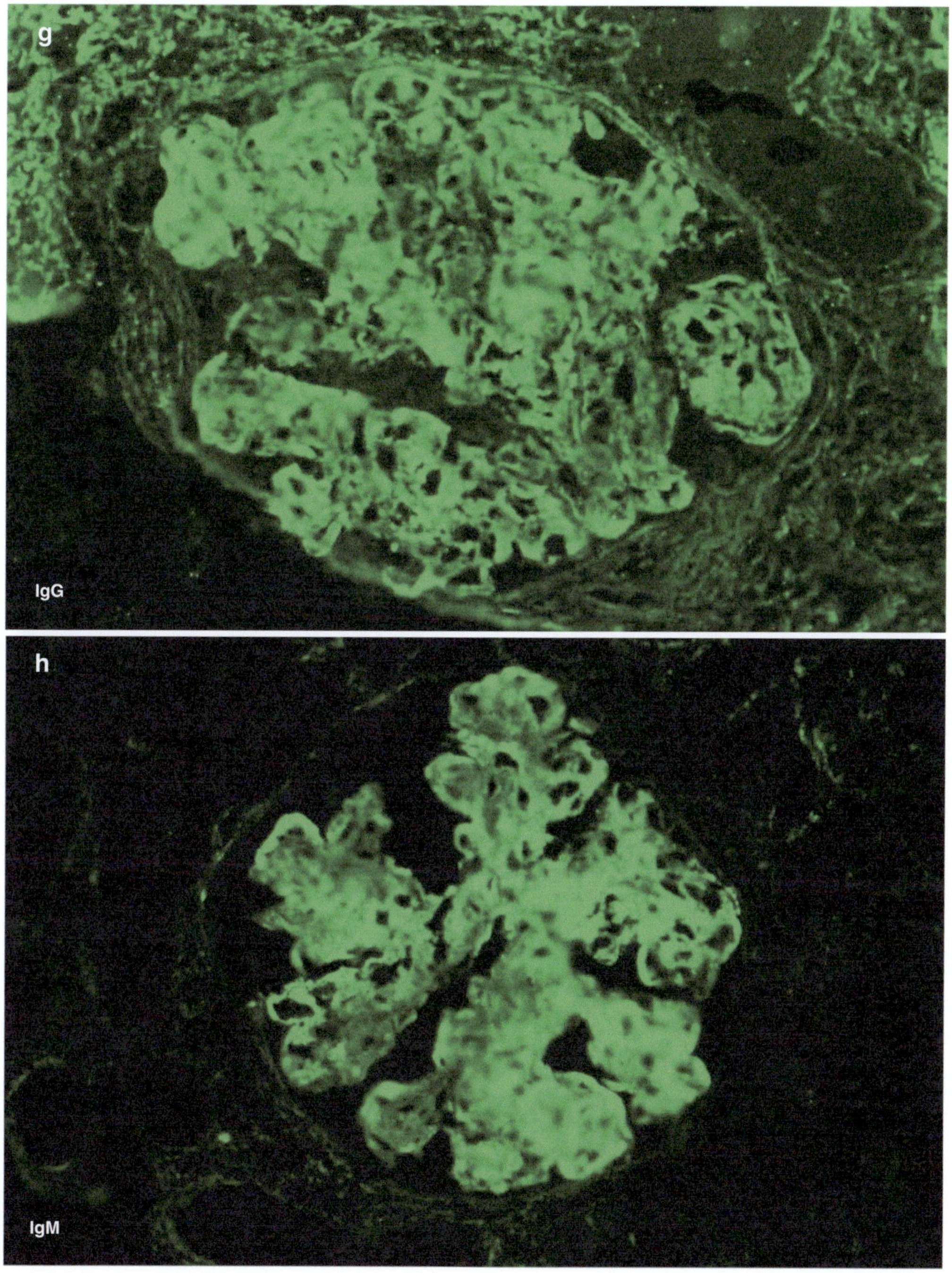

Fig. 11.5 (continued)

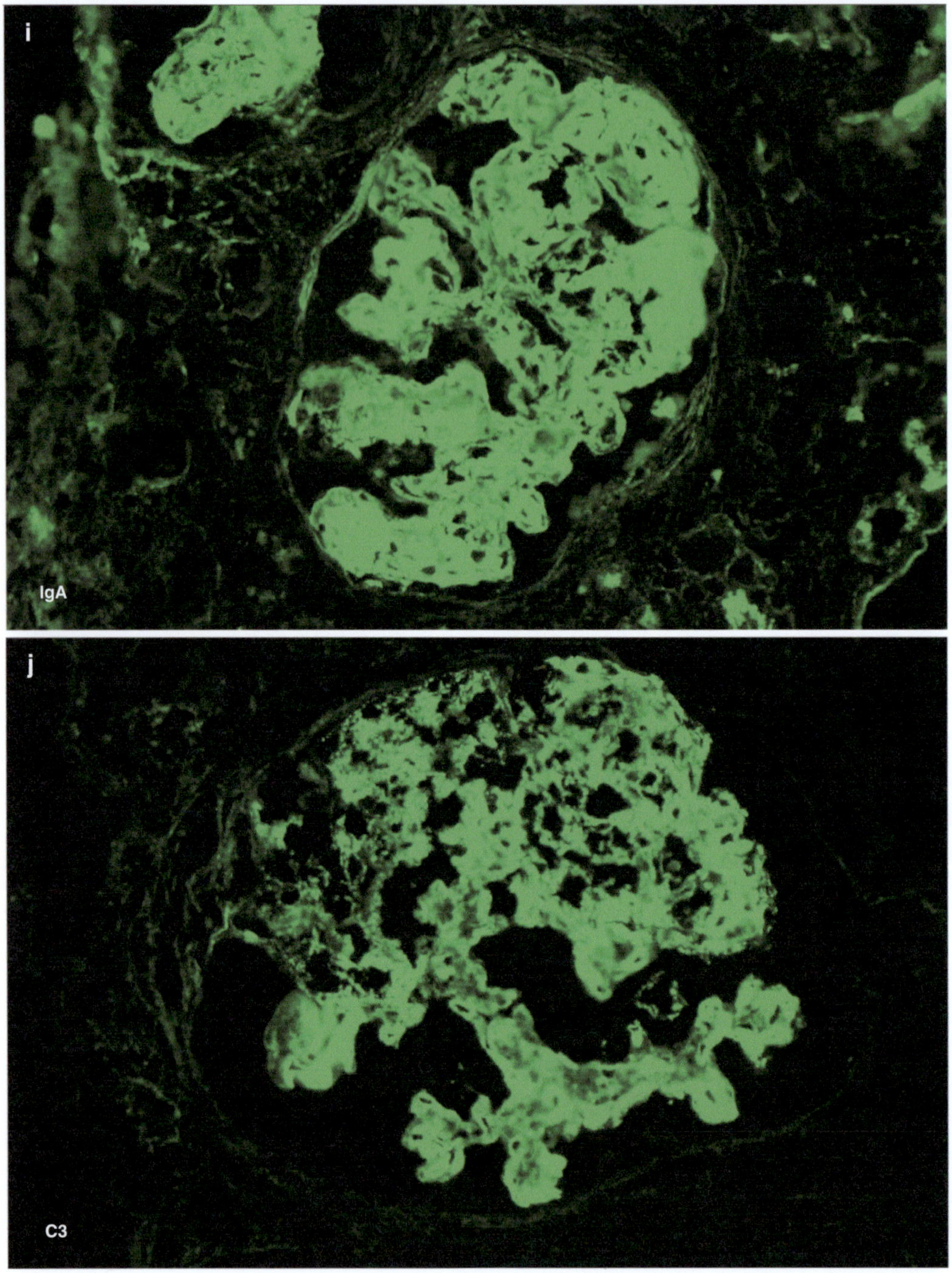

Fig. 11.5 (continued)

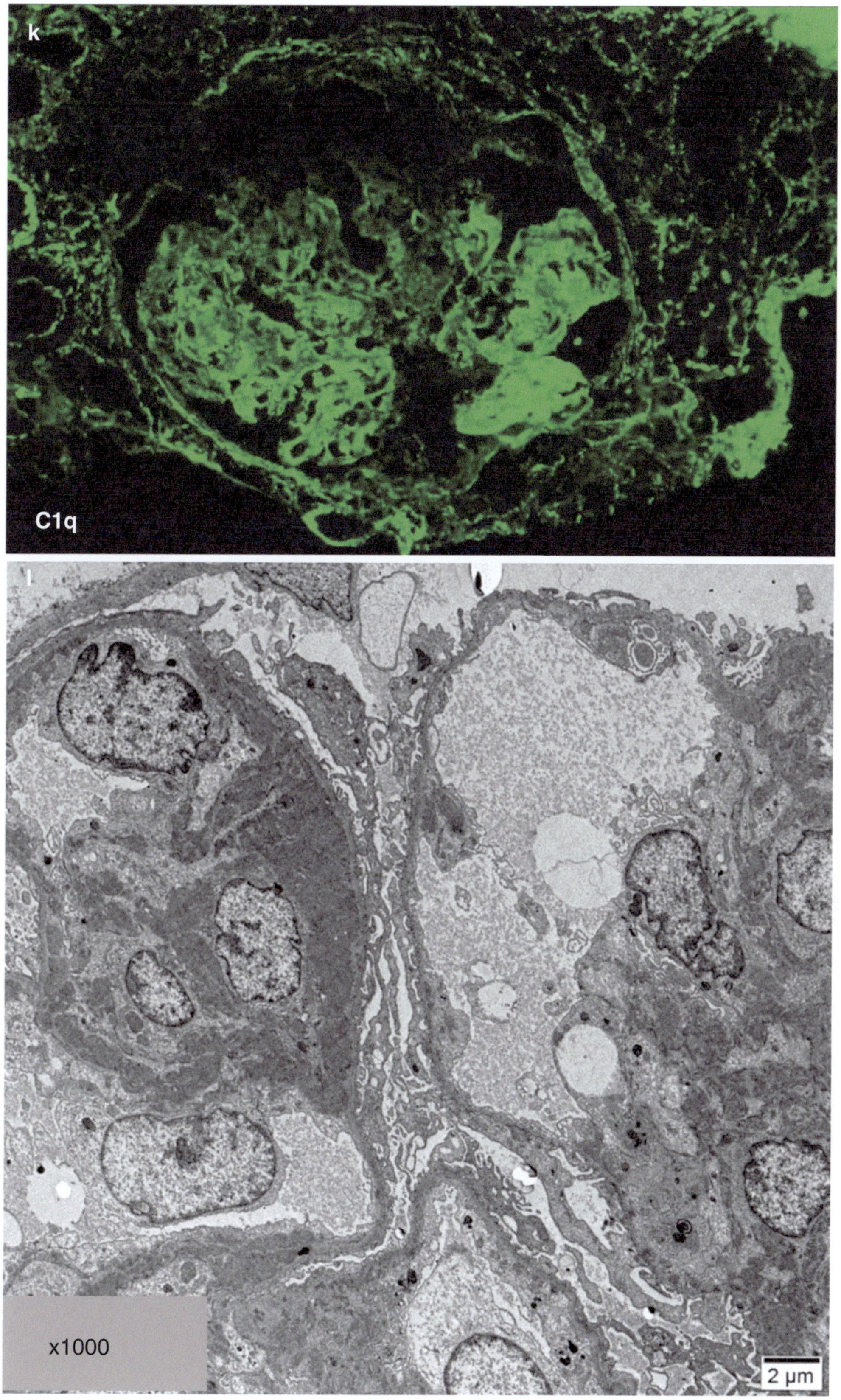

Fig. 11.5 (continued)

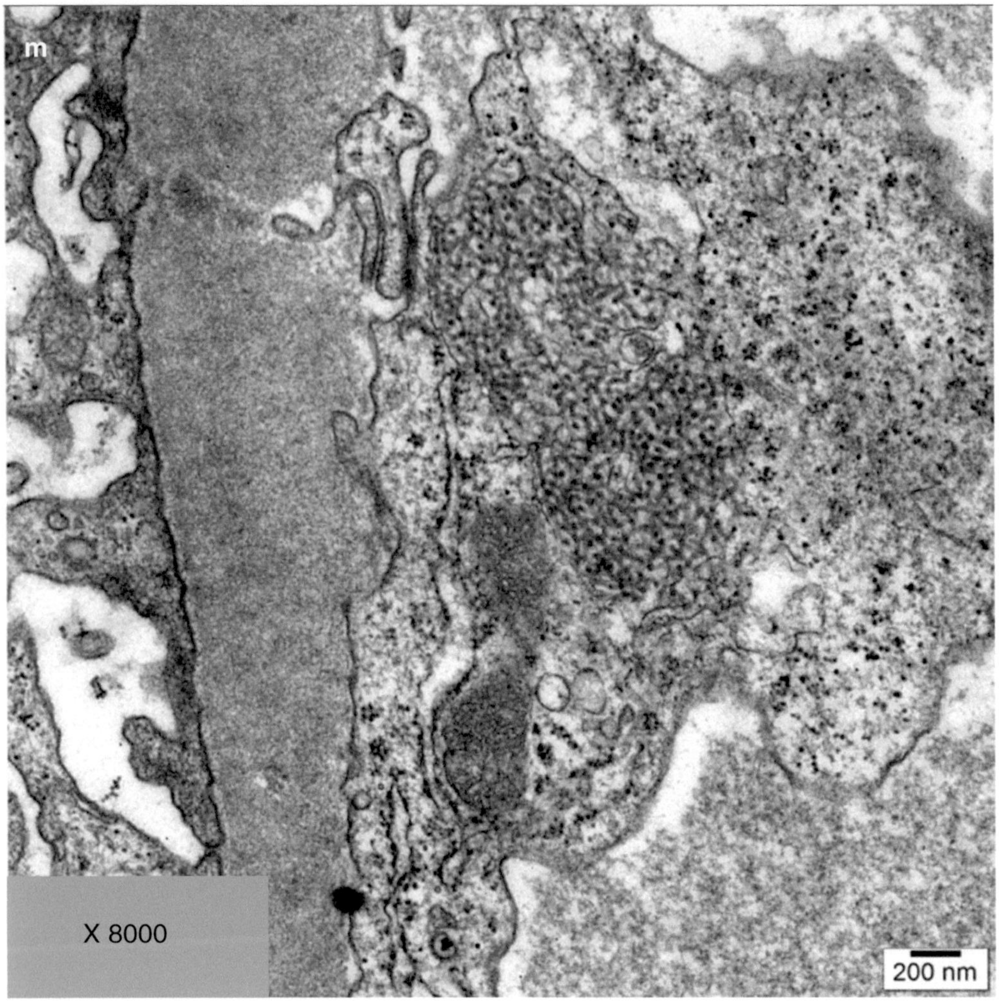

Fig. 11.5 (continued)

11.1.6 Lupus Nephritis Class IV (Fig. 11.6)

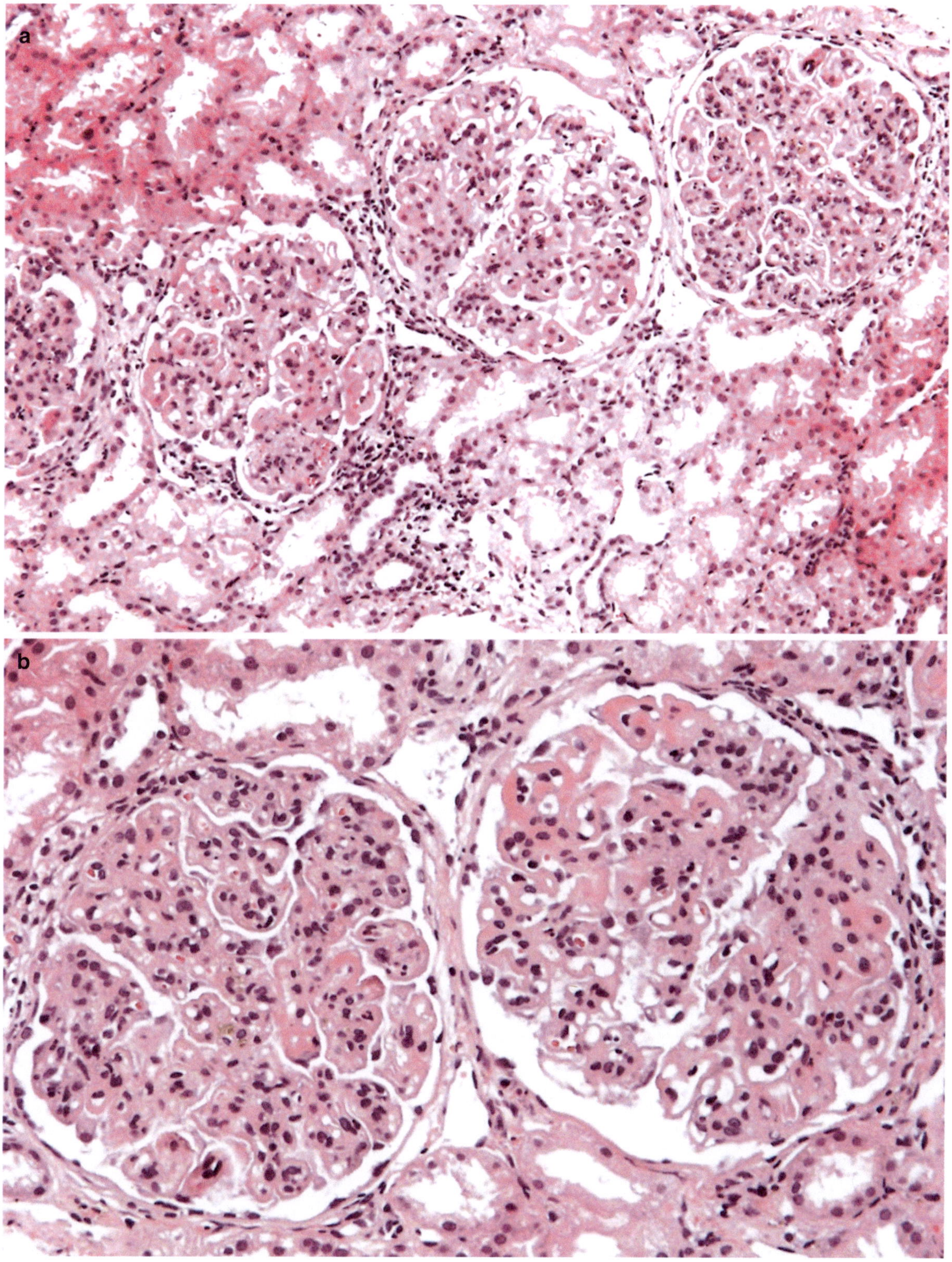

Fig. 11.6 **Class IV lupus nephritis.** A 32-years female patient presented with pedal edema and ulceration of legs for 6 weeks. Urinary protein was 2+ with 5–8 RBC/phf and 15–20 WBC/phf; urinary PC ratio was 14. Her hemoglobin was 7.5 g/dL and the platelets were 118,000 per cu mm. Serum creatinine was 0.54 mg/dL. ANA was positive and anti-ds-DNA was 183.6 IU/mL. Renal biopsy had 24 glomeruli, all of them were enlarged and showed endocapillary hyperplasia with the presence of wire loop lesions in all glomeruli. Some of the glomeruli also had neutrophilic infiltration. Any fibrinoid necrosis or crescents were not seen. Interstitium had focal lymphocytic infiltration while the tubules and the blood vessels were unremarkable. IF showed intense (3+) granular positivity for IgG, IgM, IgA, C3, C1q, kappa and lambda (full house pattern) along the capillary loops and the mesangium. (**a**) HE ×100, (**b**) HE ×200, (**c**) HE ×400, (**d**) PAS ×400, (**e**) PSM ×400, (**f**)–(**j**) IF ×400

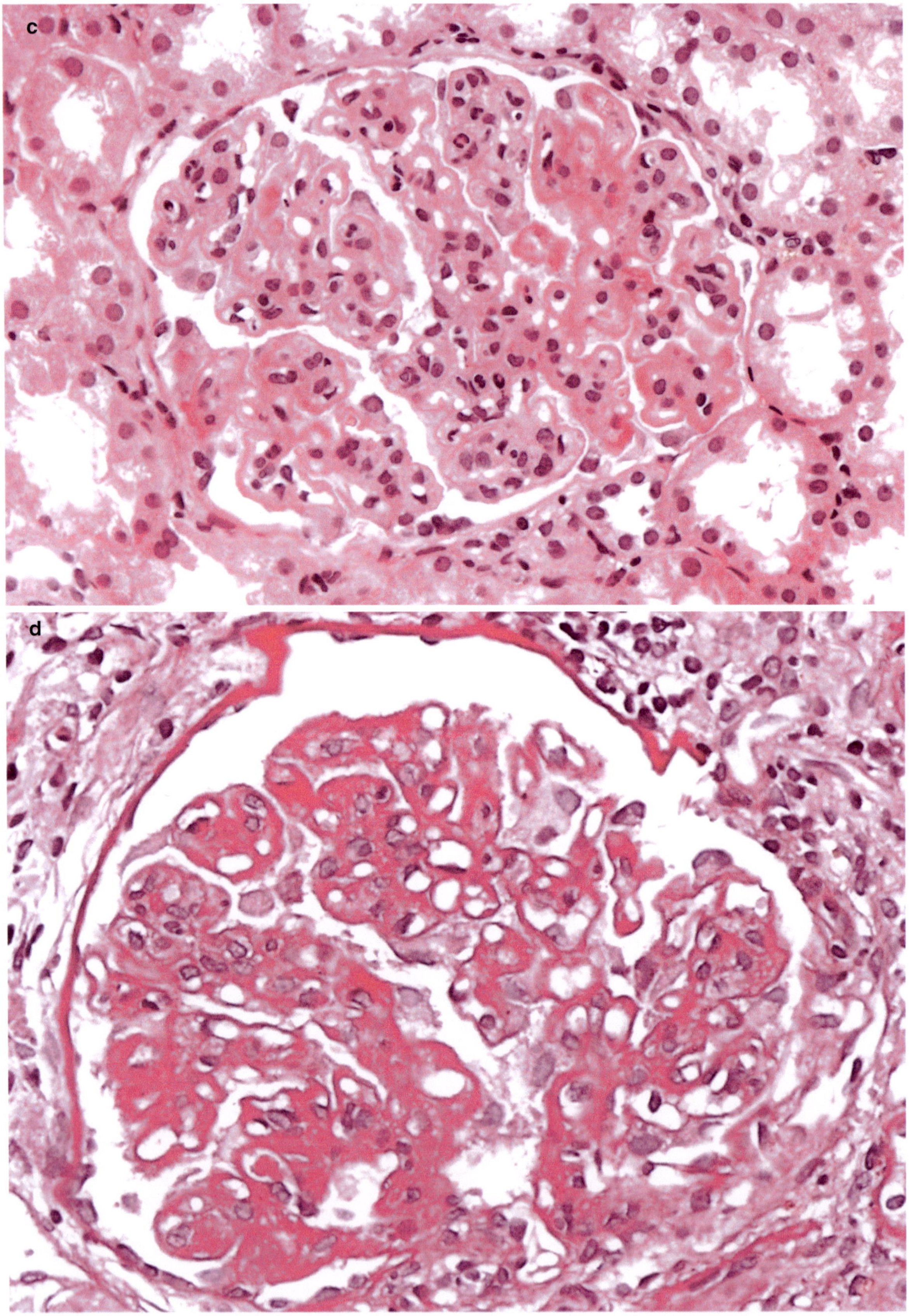

Fig. 11.6 (continued)

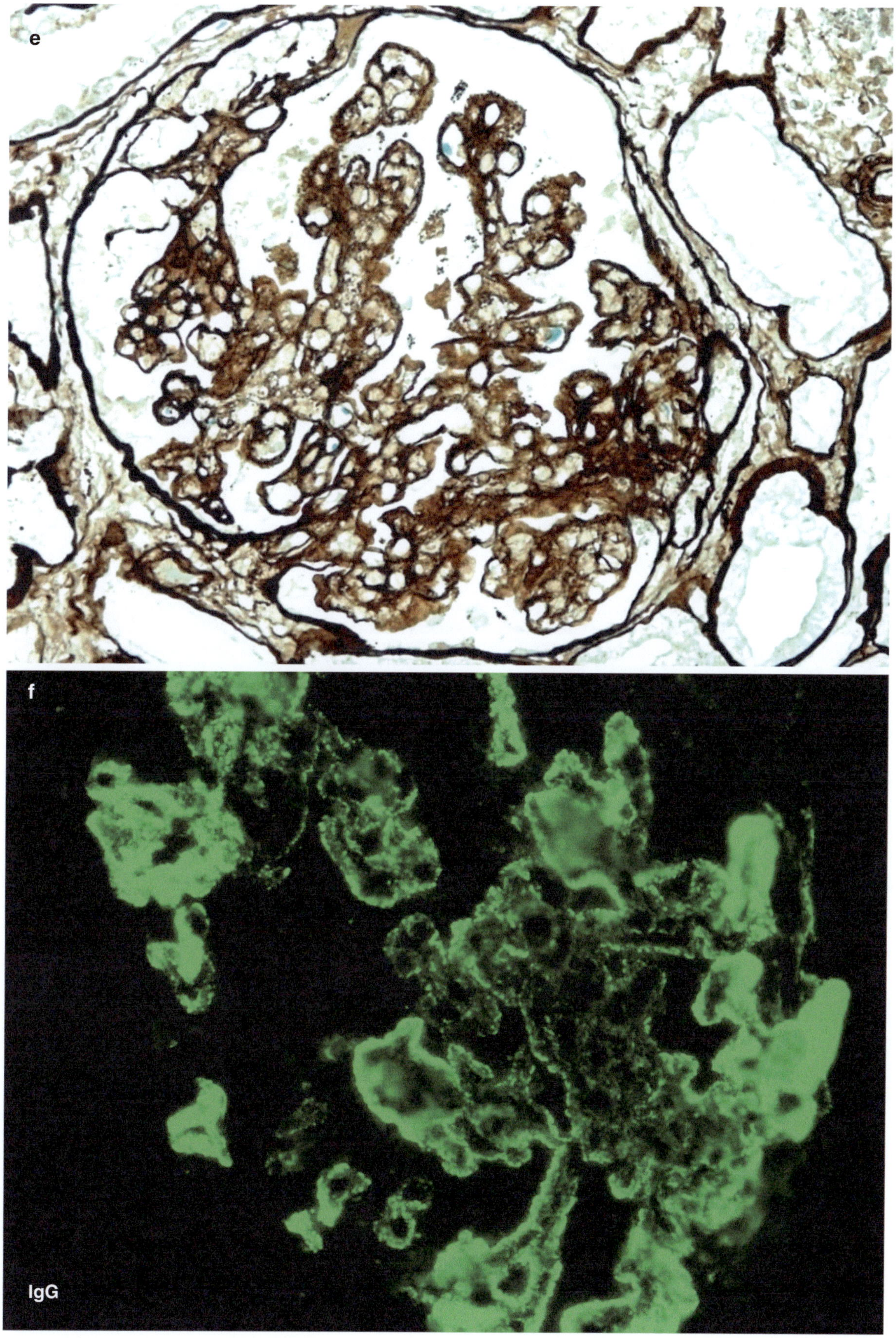

Fig. 11.6 (continued)

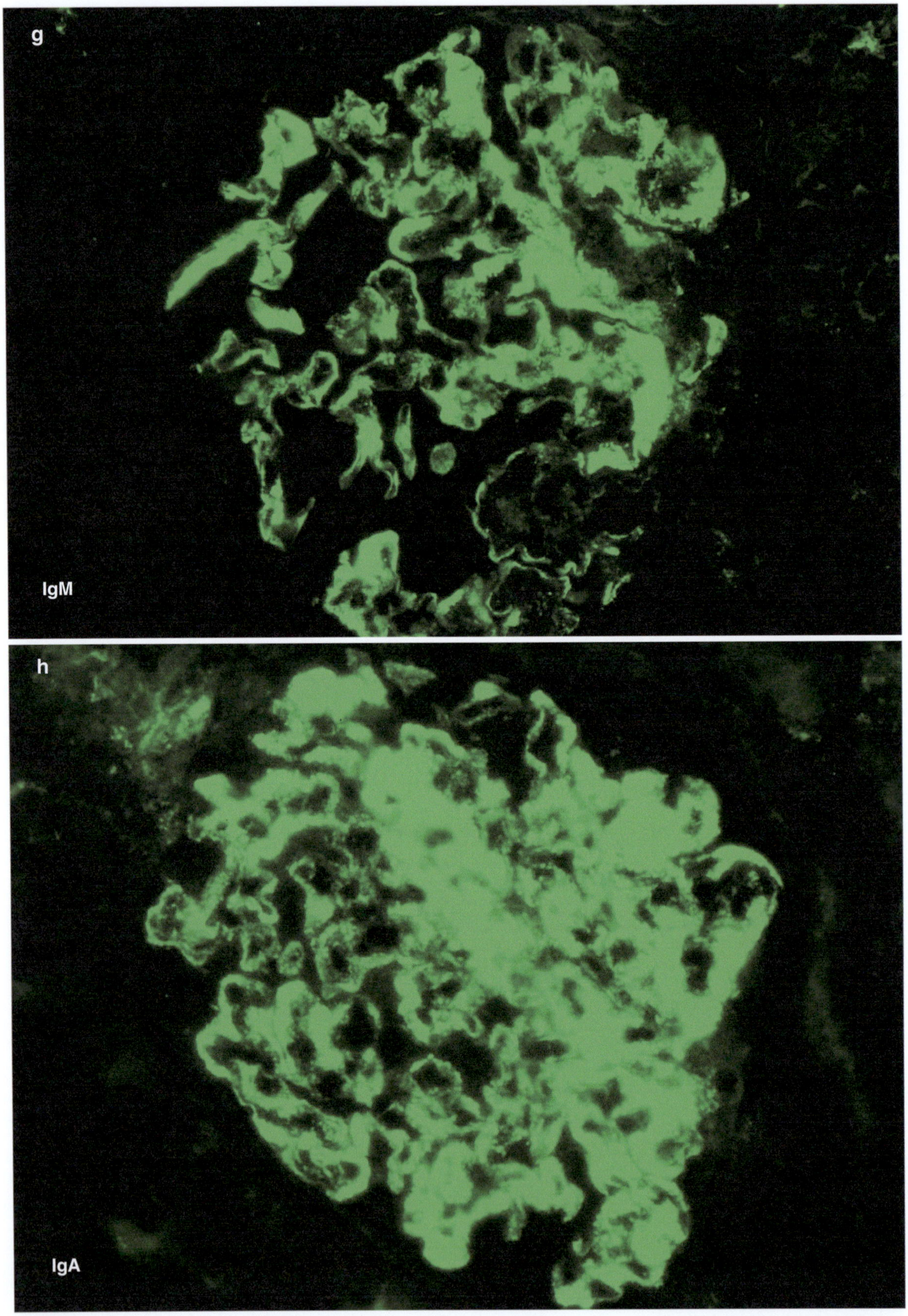

Fig. 11.6 (continued)

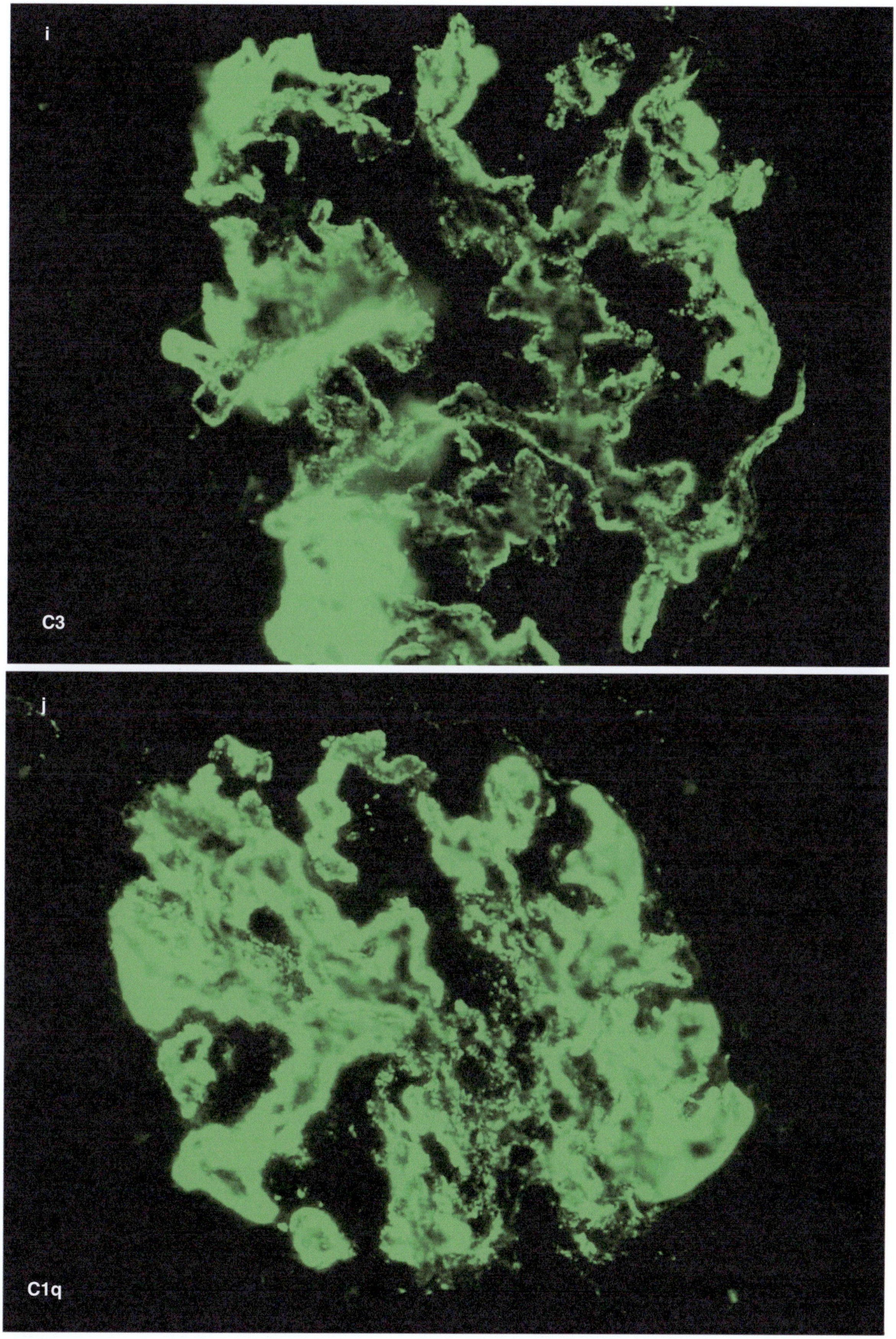

Fig. 11.6 (continued)

11.1.7 Lupus Nephritis Class IV (Immune Complex Mediated Crescentic Glomerulonephritis) (Fig. 11.7)

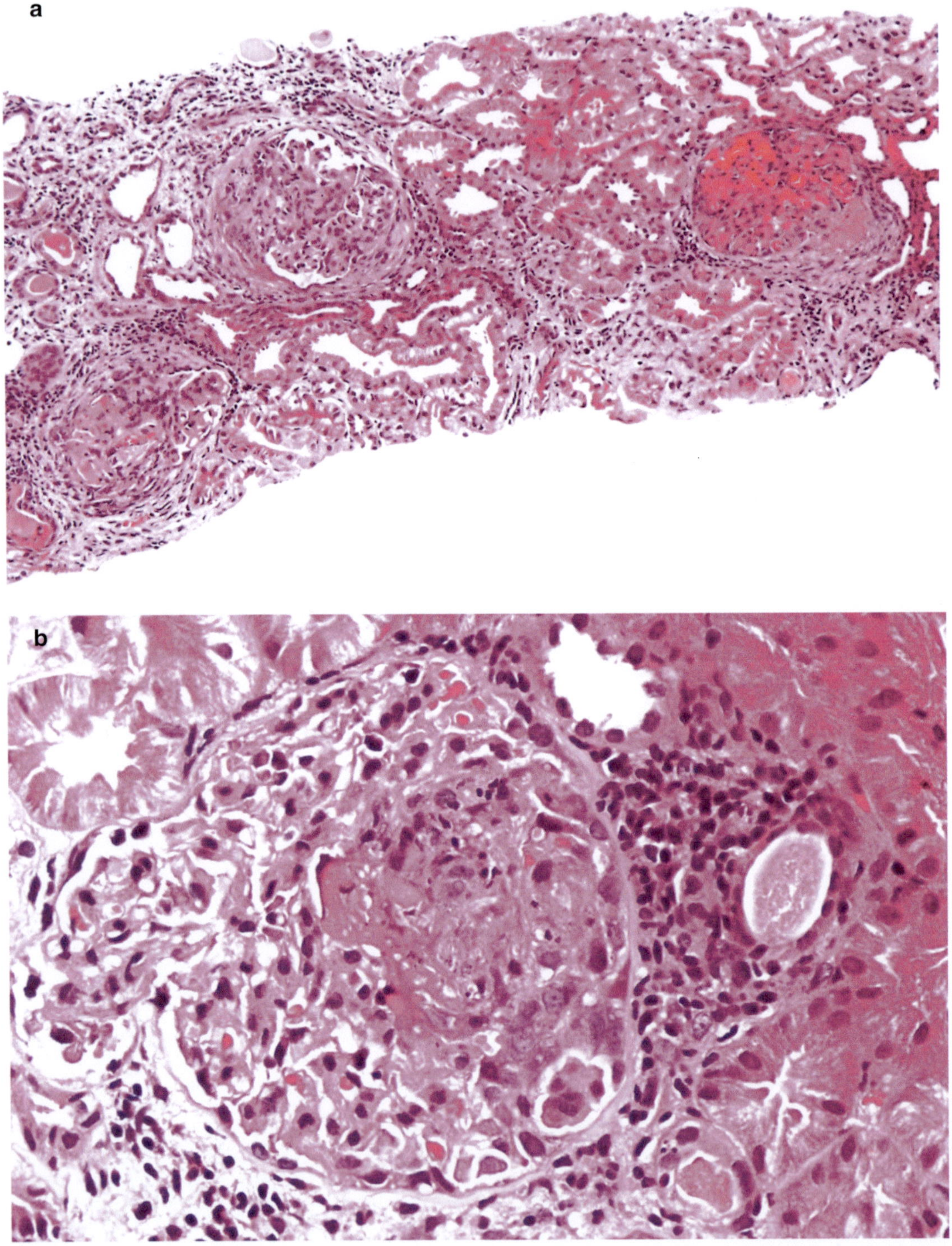

Fig. 11.7 **Class IV lupus (crescentic).** A 29-years female patient presented with nephrotic range proteinuria, Urine examination revealed protein 2+, numerous RBC and 20–30 WBC/hpf; urinary PC ratio was 7.6. Serum creatinine was 2.5 mg/dL. Serum complement levels were reduced with C3 being 456 mg/L and C4 at 83 mg/L, CRP was 63 mg/L and anti-ds-DNA was >1500 IU/mL. Renal biopsy showed 22 glomeruli, all of them were enlarged and showed proliferative lesions with varied morphology. All the glomeruli showed endothelial cell hyperplasia along with infiltration of polymorphonuclear inflammatory cells; segmental fibrinoid necrosis of the glomerular capillary loops was also observed, 17 glomeruli had crescents (cellular 12/fibrocellular 5). Tubular atrophy with interstitial infiltration of inflammatory cells was also present. Disease activity score was 14/24 and chronicity score was 2/12. IF showed full house pattern with both glomerular capillary wall and mesangial positivity. (**a**) HE ×100, (**b**)–(**d**) HE ×400, (**e**)–(**i**) IF ×400

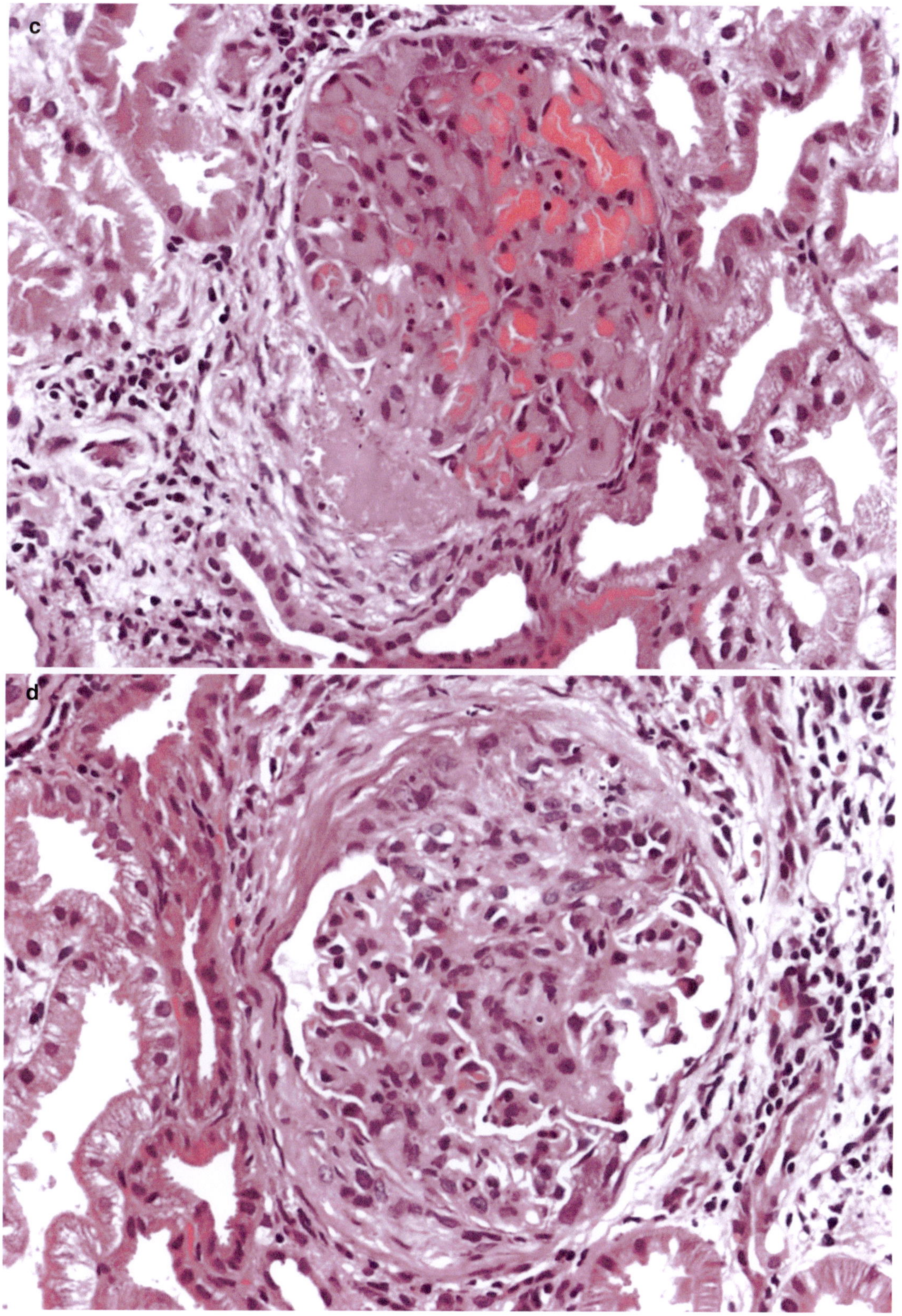

Fig. 11.7 (continued)

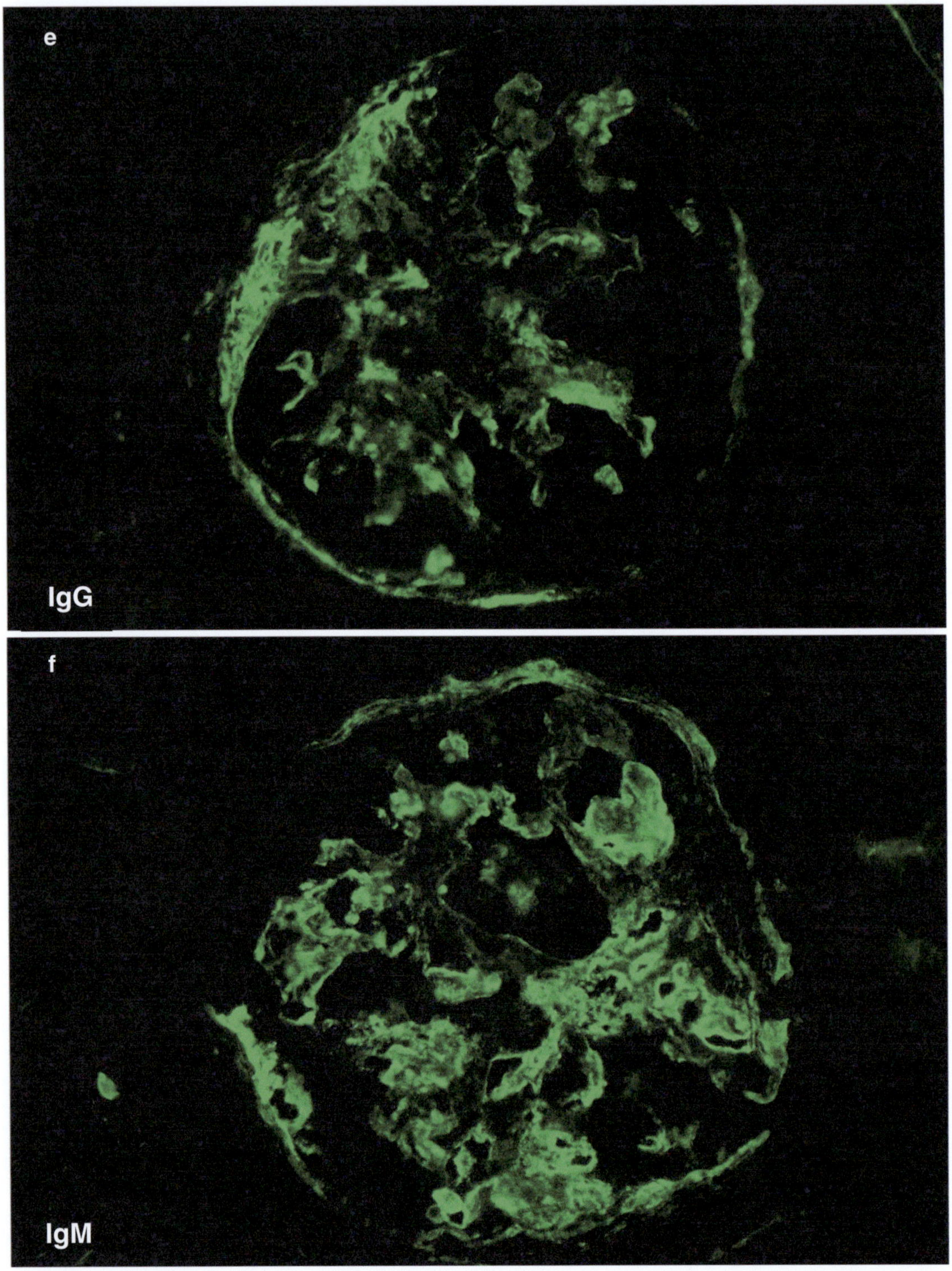

Fig. 11.7 (continued)

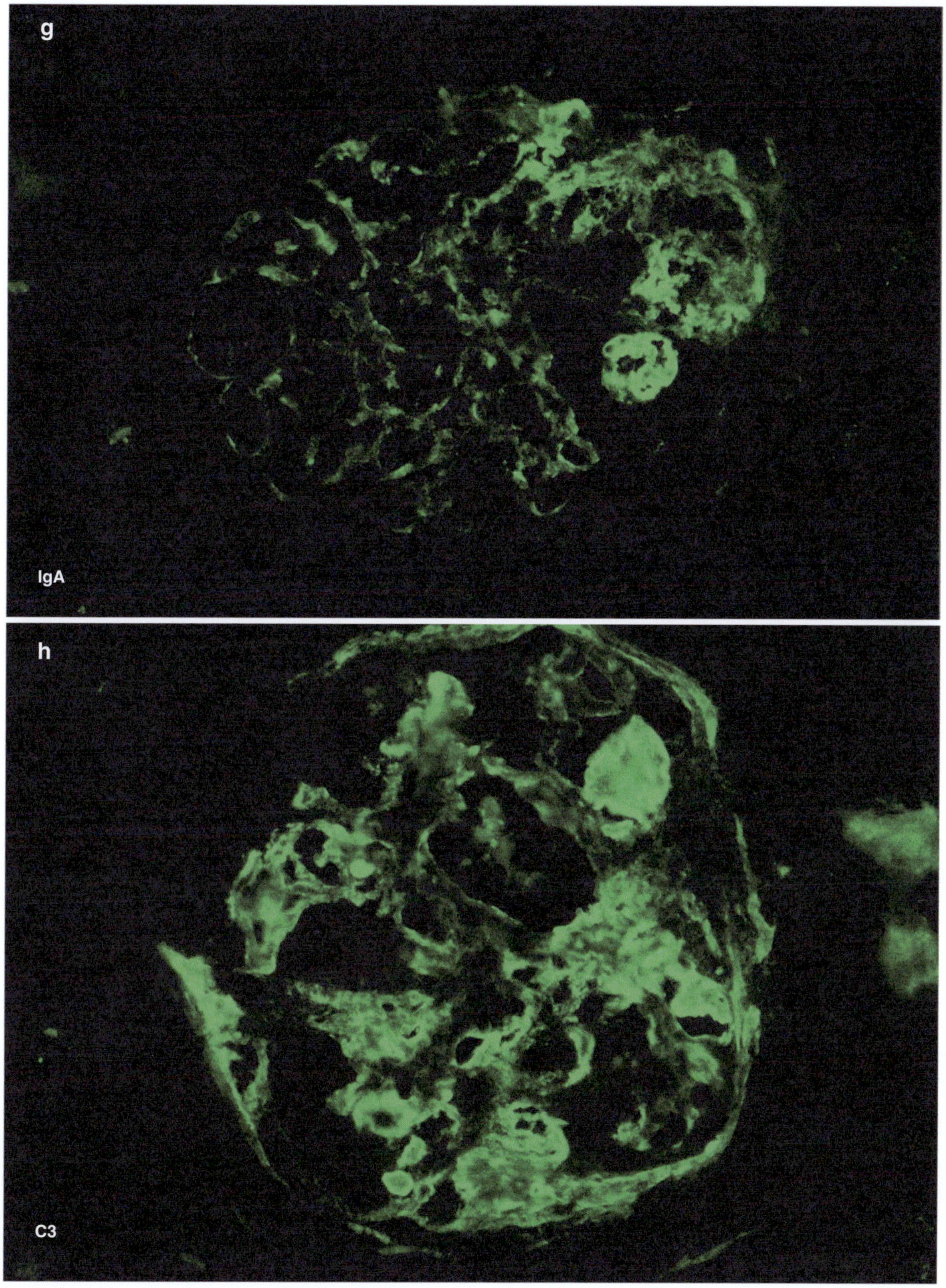

Fig. 11.7 (continued)

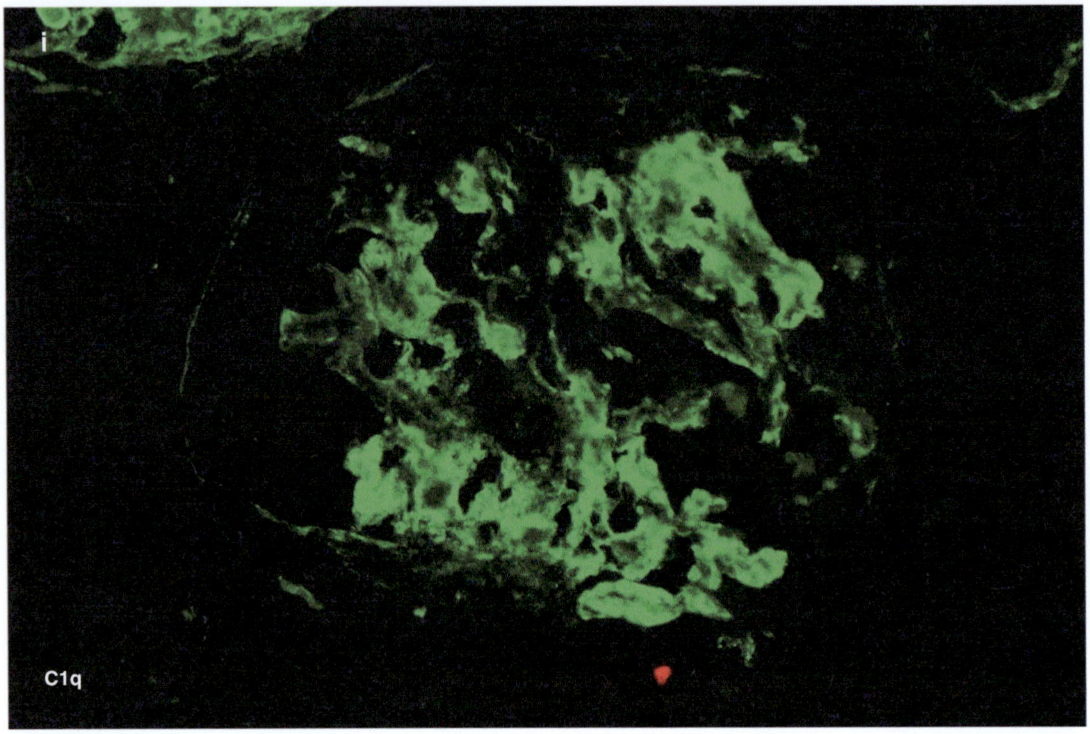

Fig. 11.7 (continued)

11.1.8 Lupus Nephritis Class IV + V (Fig. 11.8)

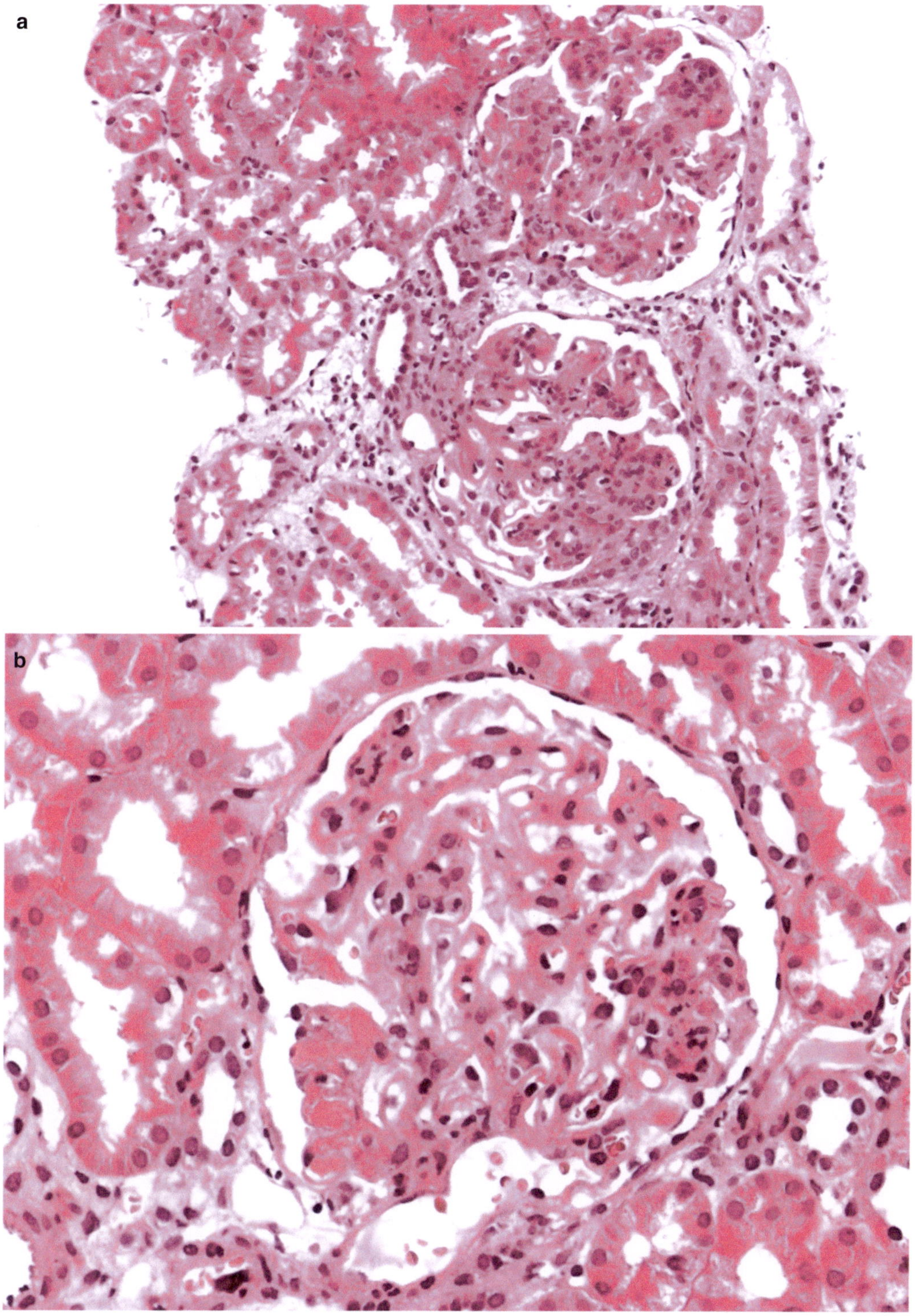

Fig. 11.8 Class IV + V lupus nephritis. A 23-years male patient presented with fever, facial puffiness, and dry cough for 3–4 months. He had no history of skin rashes or hematuria. Laboratory workup revealed that the blood counts were within normal limits with ESR of 23 mm for first hour (Westergren). Urinary protein was 4+, pus cells 2–3/hpf, occasional RBC and a few granular casts and 24 h urinary protein was 18 g. Serum complements were low, C3 being 338 mg/L and serum C4 was 89 mg/L. Antibodies to ds-DNA were present (1133 IU/ml). USG revealed that both kidneys were of normal size. Renal biopsy had 11 glomeruli, all of them were enlarged with accentuated lobular pattern and showed endocapillary hyperplasia, with the presence of neutrophils, cellular crescents and fibrin thrombi in capillary loops. There was no fibrinoid necrosis and none of the glomeruli had segmental or global sclerosis. Activity score was 8/24 and the chronicity score was 0/12. Intramembranous immune deposits with wire loop lesions were also present. Silver stain showed thickening of GBM with argyrophilic epimembranous spikes in >50% glomeruli. IF showed granular deposits of IgG, IgM, IgA, C3, C1q, kappa and lambda along GBM as well as mesangium (full house pattern). (**a**) HE ×200, (**b**) HE ×400, (**c**) PAS ×400, (**d**) MT ×400, (**e**) PSM ×400, (**f**)–(**j**) IF ×400

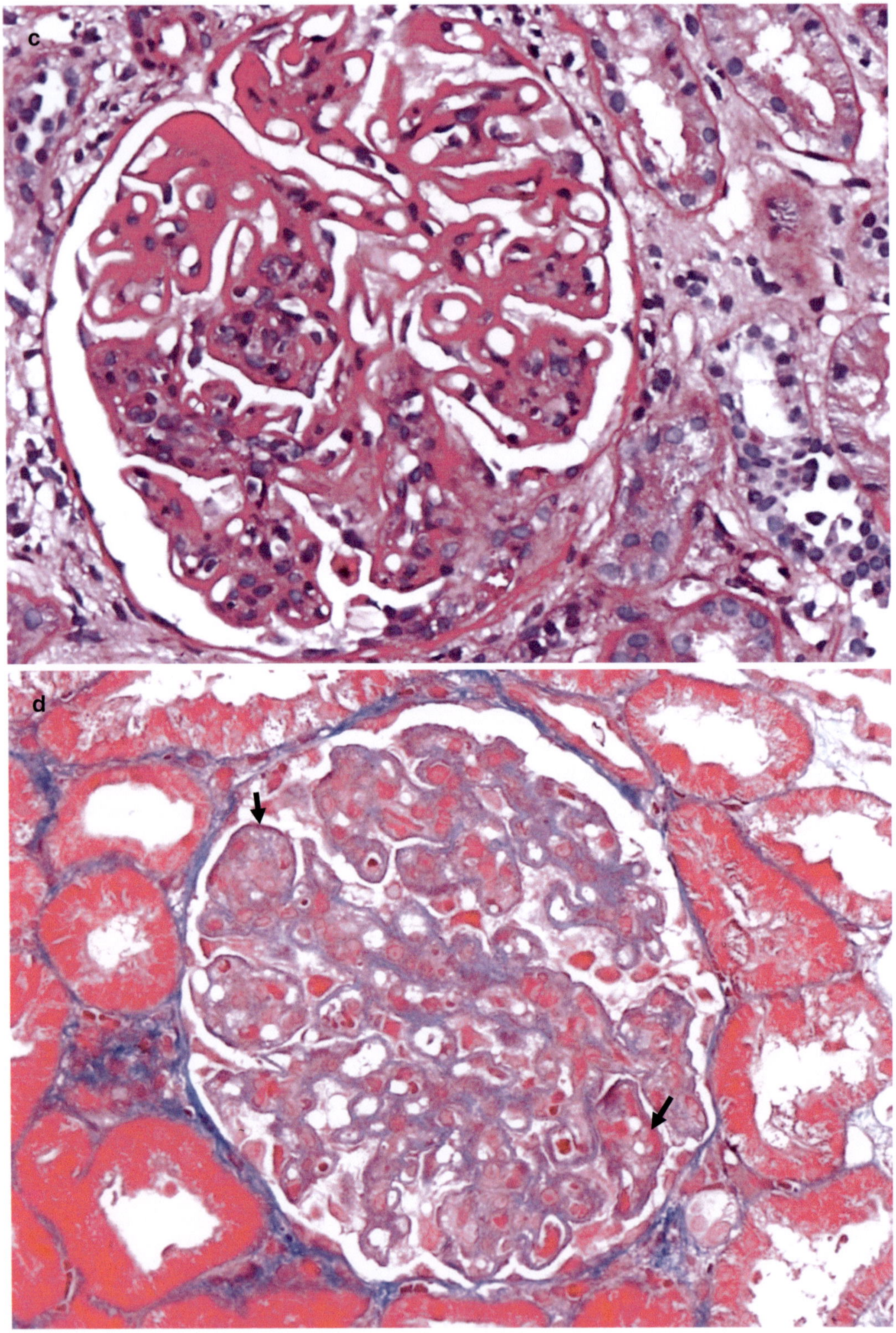

Fig. 11.8 (continued)

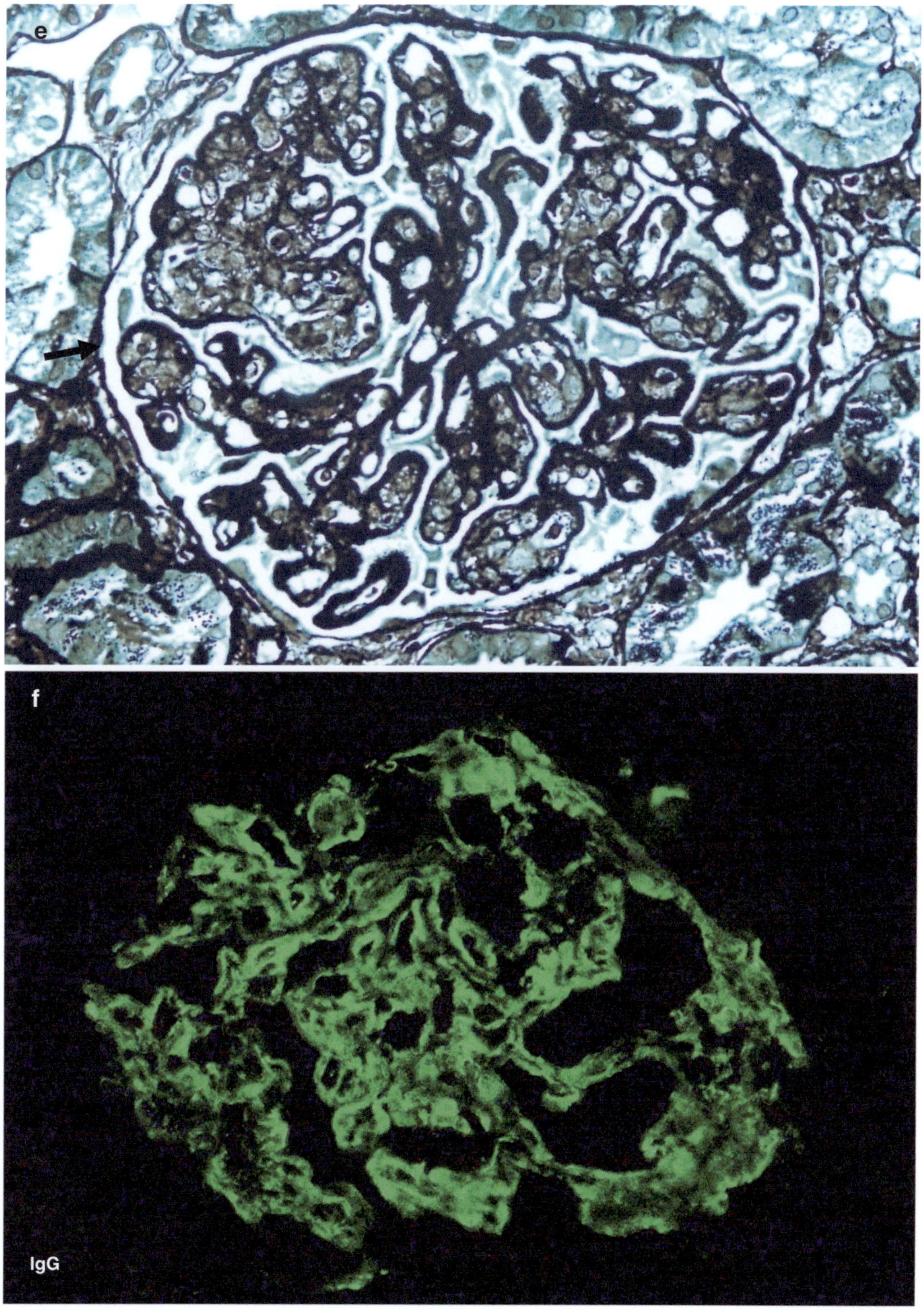

Fig. 11.8 (continued)

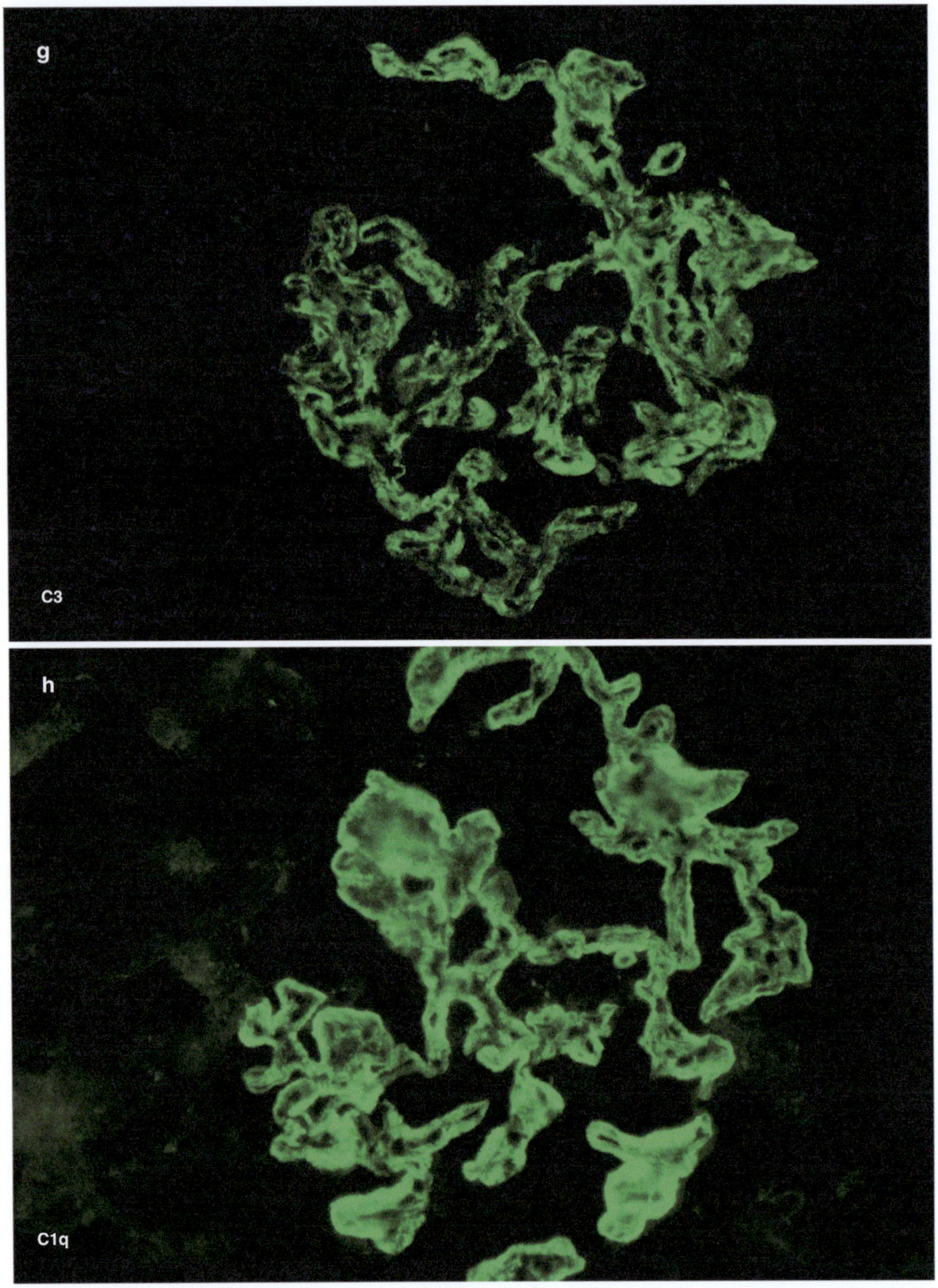

Fig. 11.8 (continued)

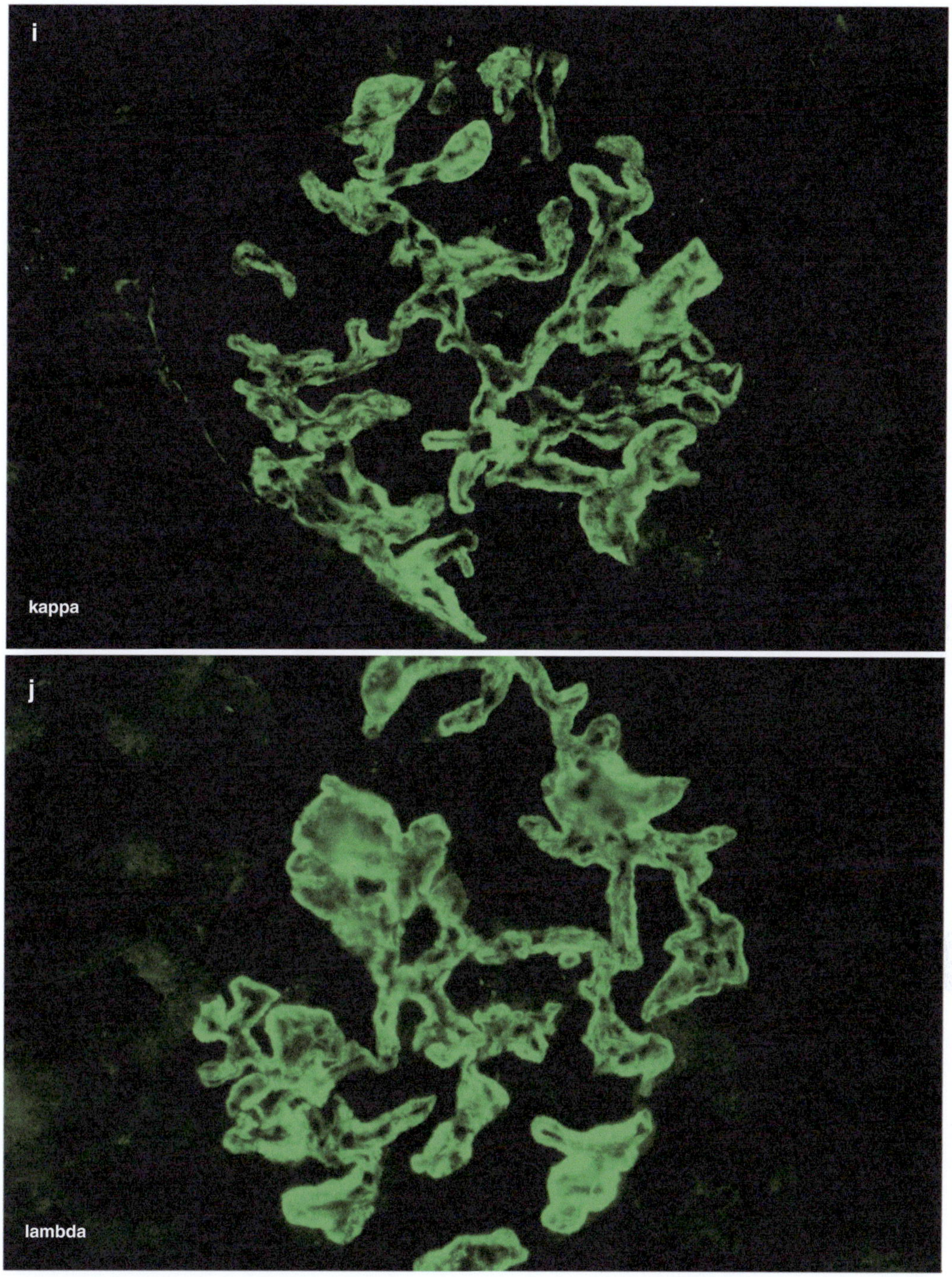

Fig. 11.8 (continued)

11.1.9 Lupus Nephritis Class V (Fig. 11.9)

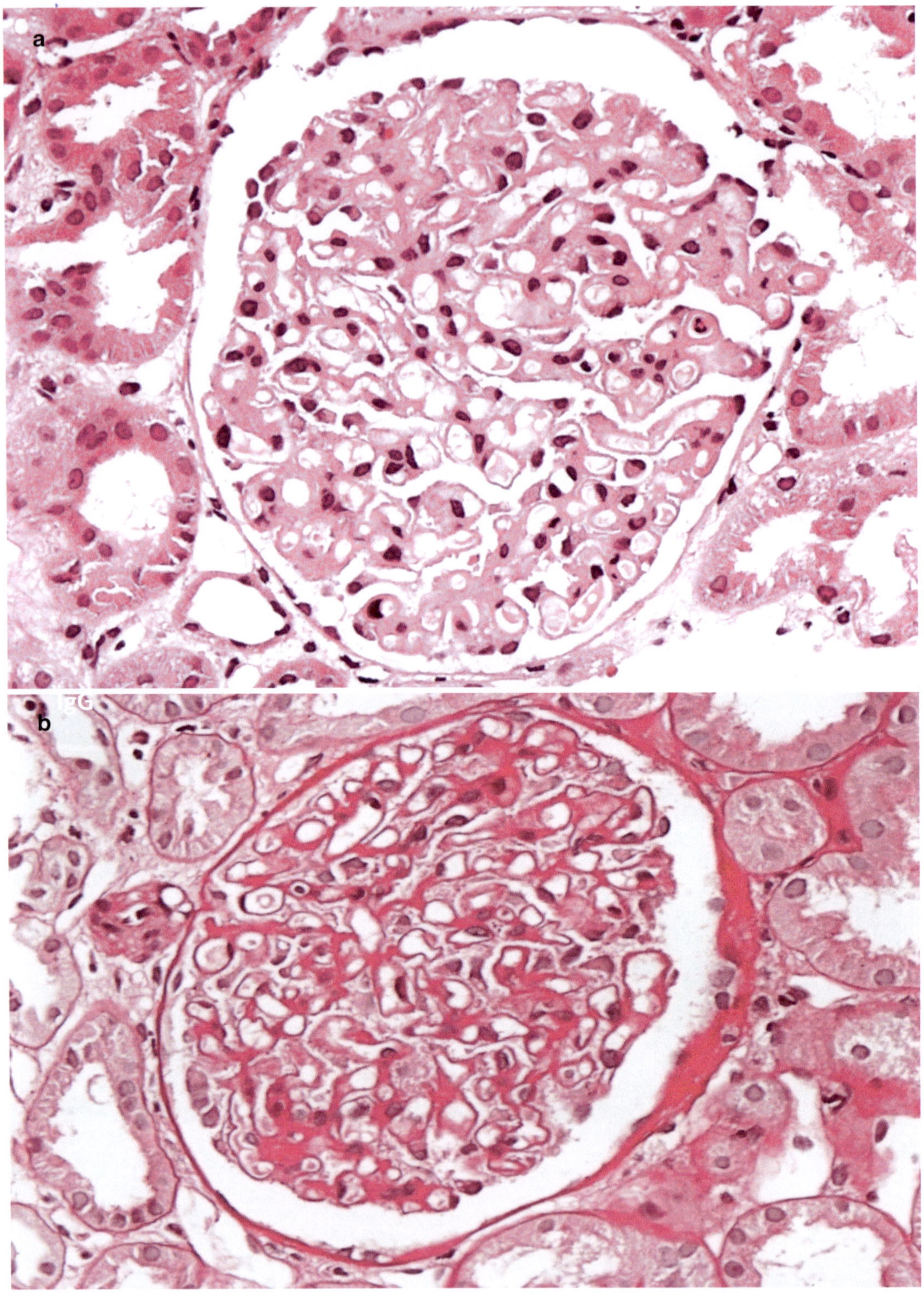

Fig. 11.9 Class V lupus nephritis. A 30-years female patient presented with fever off and on. She also complained of alopecia. On clinical examination, she was found to have bilateral pleural effusion. Laboratory workup revealed that the patient was anemic with Hb level of 8.9 g/dL. Her blood counts were wnl, platelets were 120,000 per cu mm. Direct Coombs test was positive. Urine examination revealed proteinuria of 5 g/day with the presence of 10–15 RBC /hpf. Her renal functions were within normal limits. Serum ANA was positive; ENA profile revealed that the antinucleosomal antibodies were present, Anti-ds-DNA was <10 IU/mL. Serum complement C3 and C4 were within normal limits. Renal biopsy showed enlarged glomeruli with thickened GBM and silver stain also showed thickened GBM with diffuse argyrophilic epimembranous spikes. IF showed full house pattern. EM showed several subepithelial electron-dense deposits and tubuloreticular inclusions within endothelial cell cytoplasm. (**a**) HE ×400, (**b**) PAS ×400, (**c**) PSM ×400, (**d**)–(**g**) IF ×400, (**h**) and (**i**) EM (identity of the patient has been concealed)

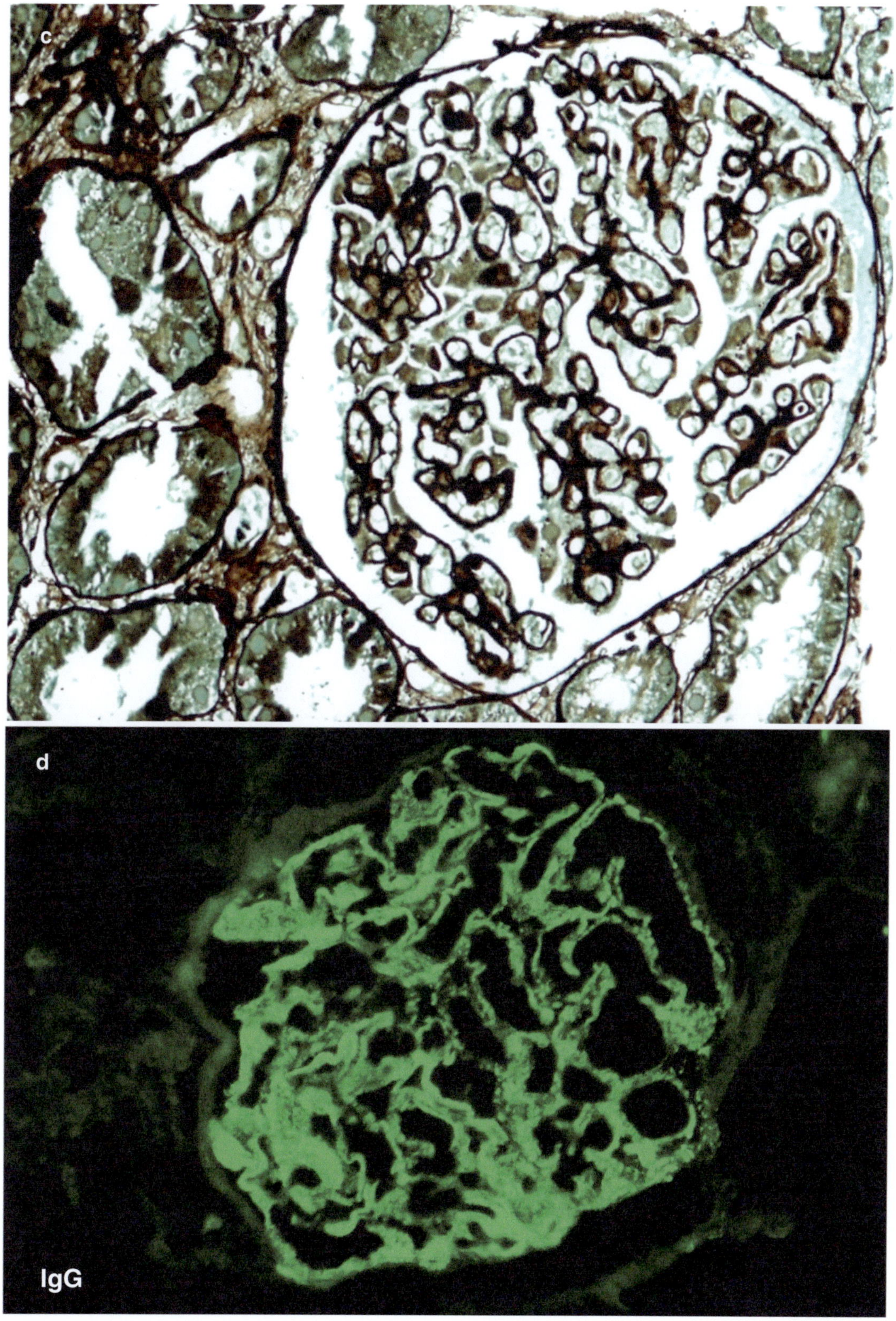

Fig. 11.9 (continued)

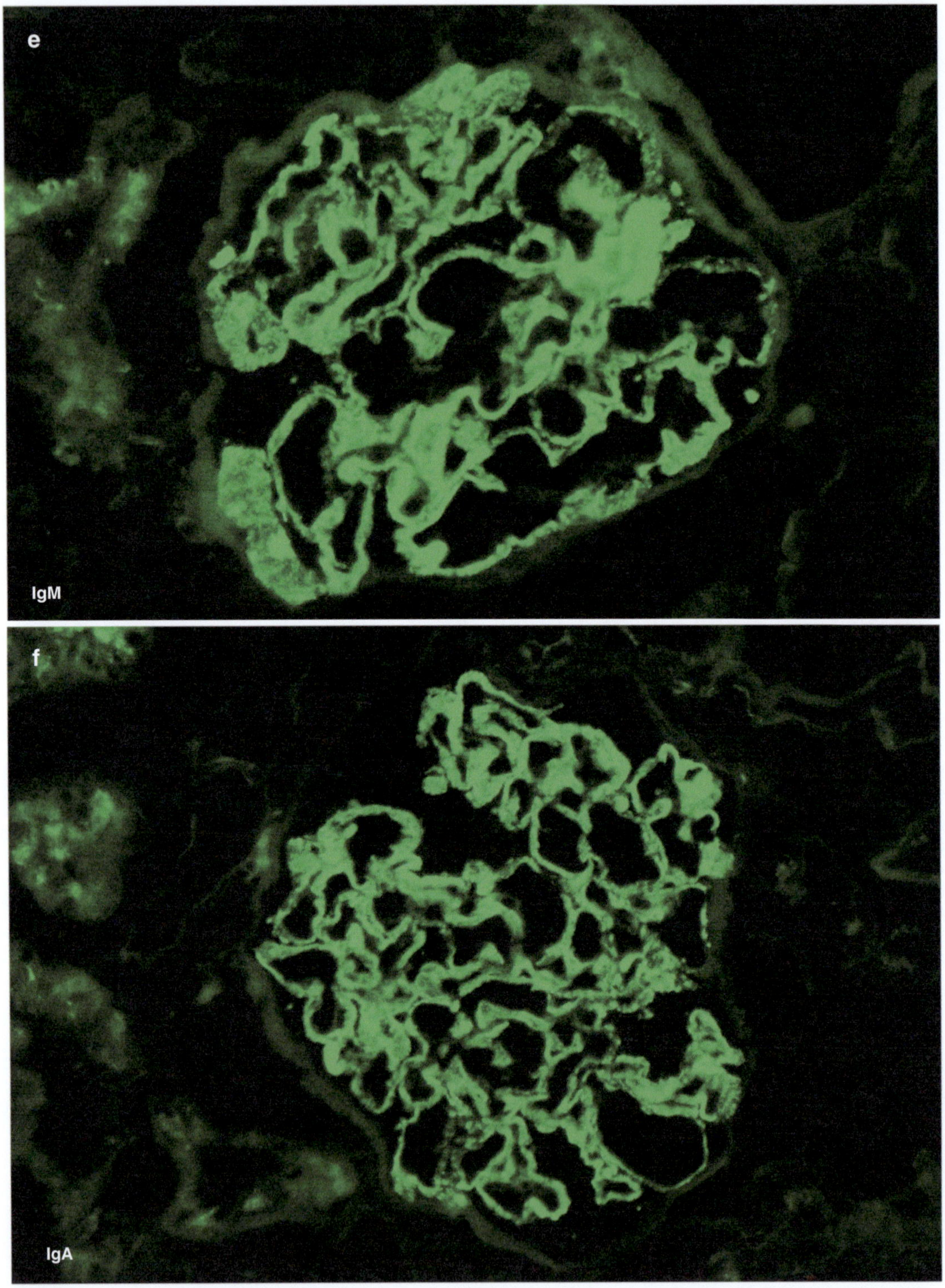

Fig. 11.9 (continued)

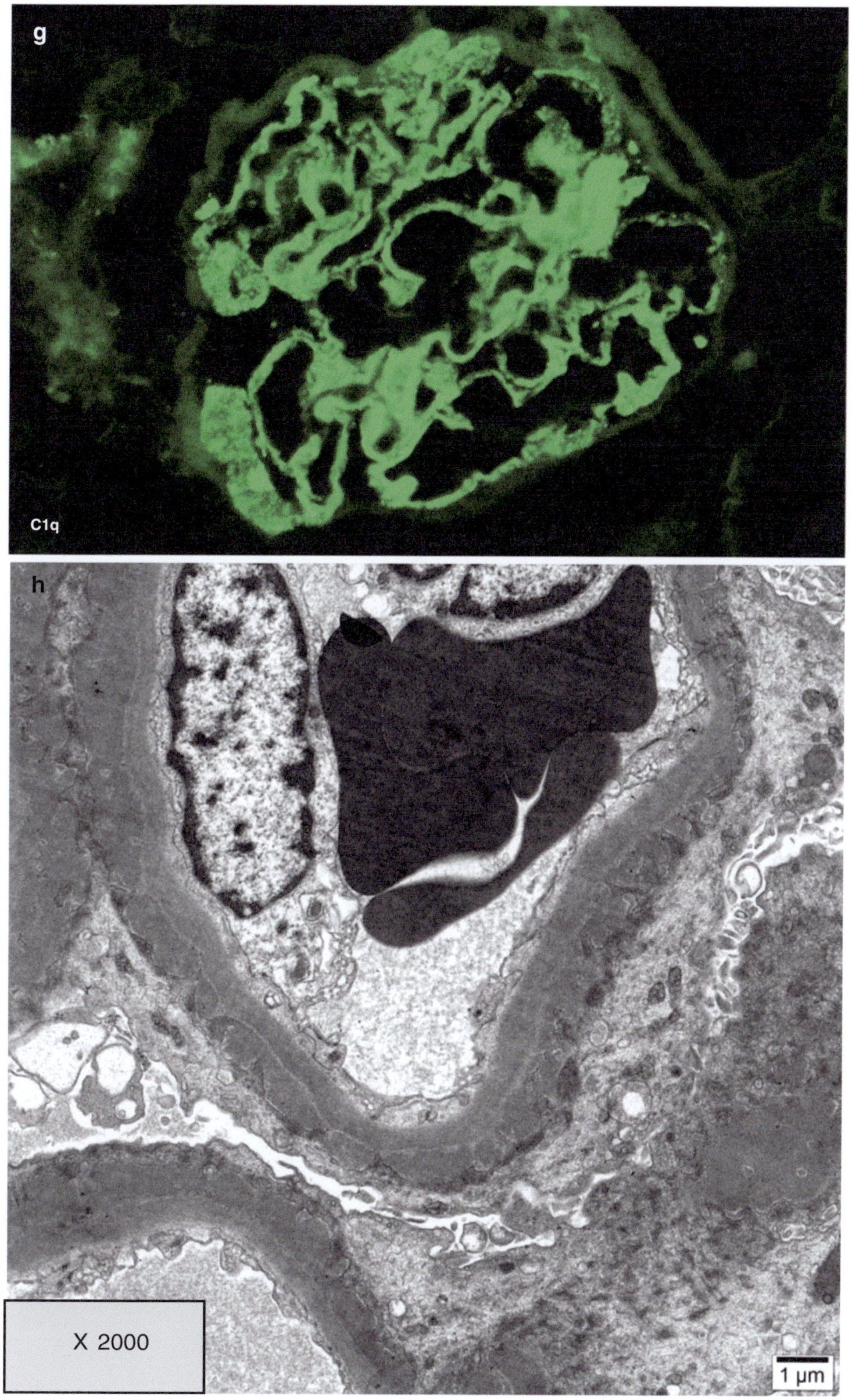

Fig. 11.9 (continued)

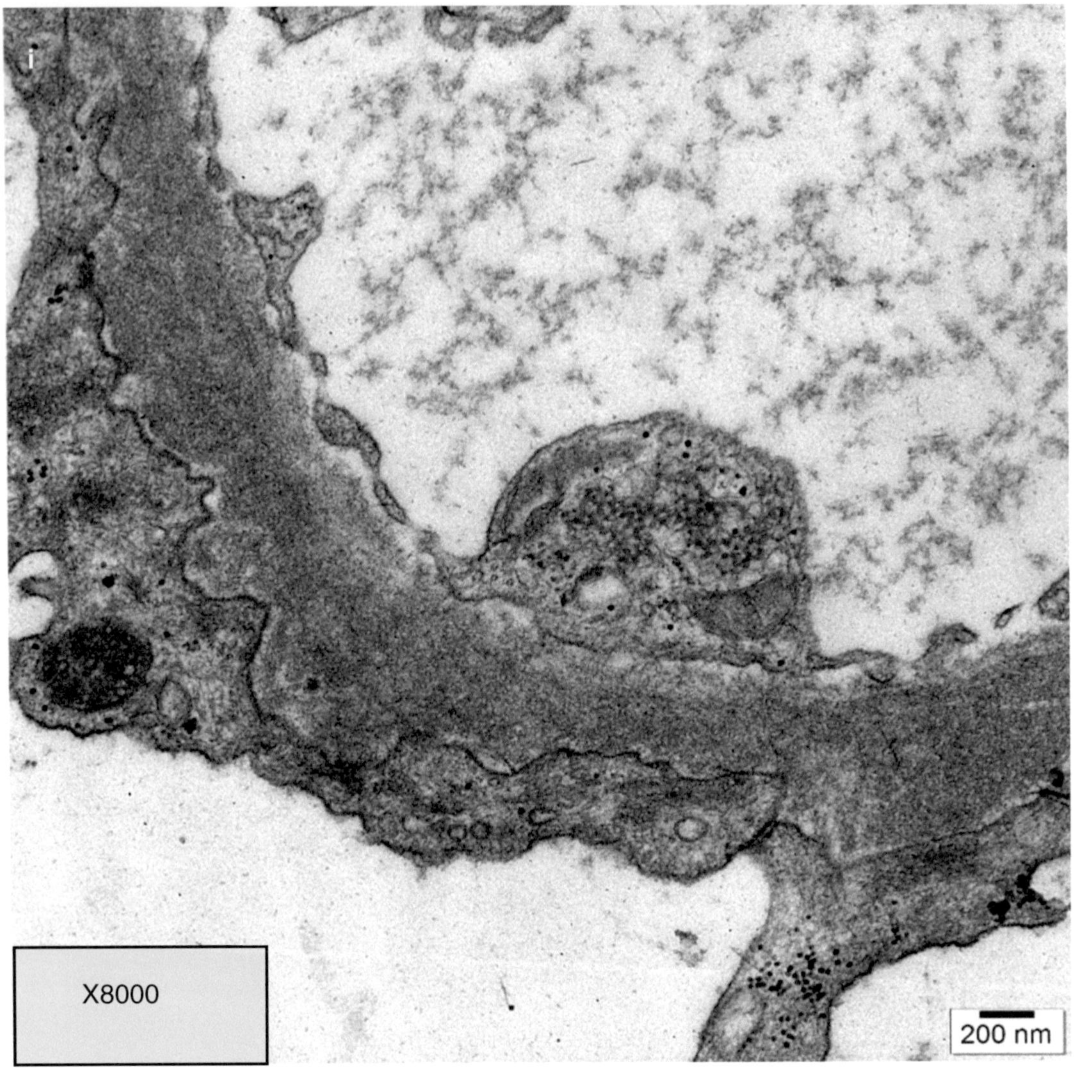

Fig. 11.9 (continued)

11.2 Lupus Podocytopathy

It is seen in patients with SLE presenting as nephrotic syndrome without hematuria or hypertension. It is more often seen in females than males. Patients can have thrombocytopenia, anemia or leucopenia and extrarenal manifestations like malar rash, arthritis, fever, and alopecia. ANA is positive in all patients. Patient with lupus podocytopathy can have morphological features of minimal change disease, focal segmental glomerulosclerosis or mesangioproliferative glomerulonephritis. On Immunofluorescence, no immune deposits or minimal mesangial deposits are seen. There are no capillary wall deposits. On electron microscopy, there is diffuse and widespread effacement of podocyte foot process without any subendothelial or subepithelial immune deposits. Mesangial deposits may be seen. Patients with FSGS like morphological appearance usually have a poor prognosis and are less likely to respond to immunosuppressive therapy. For other patients, steroids are the mainstay of treatment. A case of lupus podocytopathy is illustrated (Fig. 11.10).

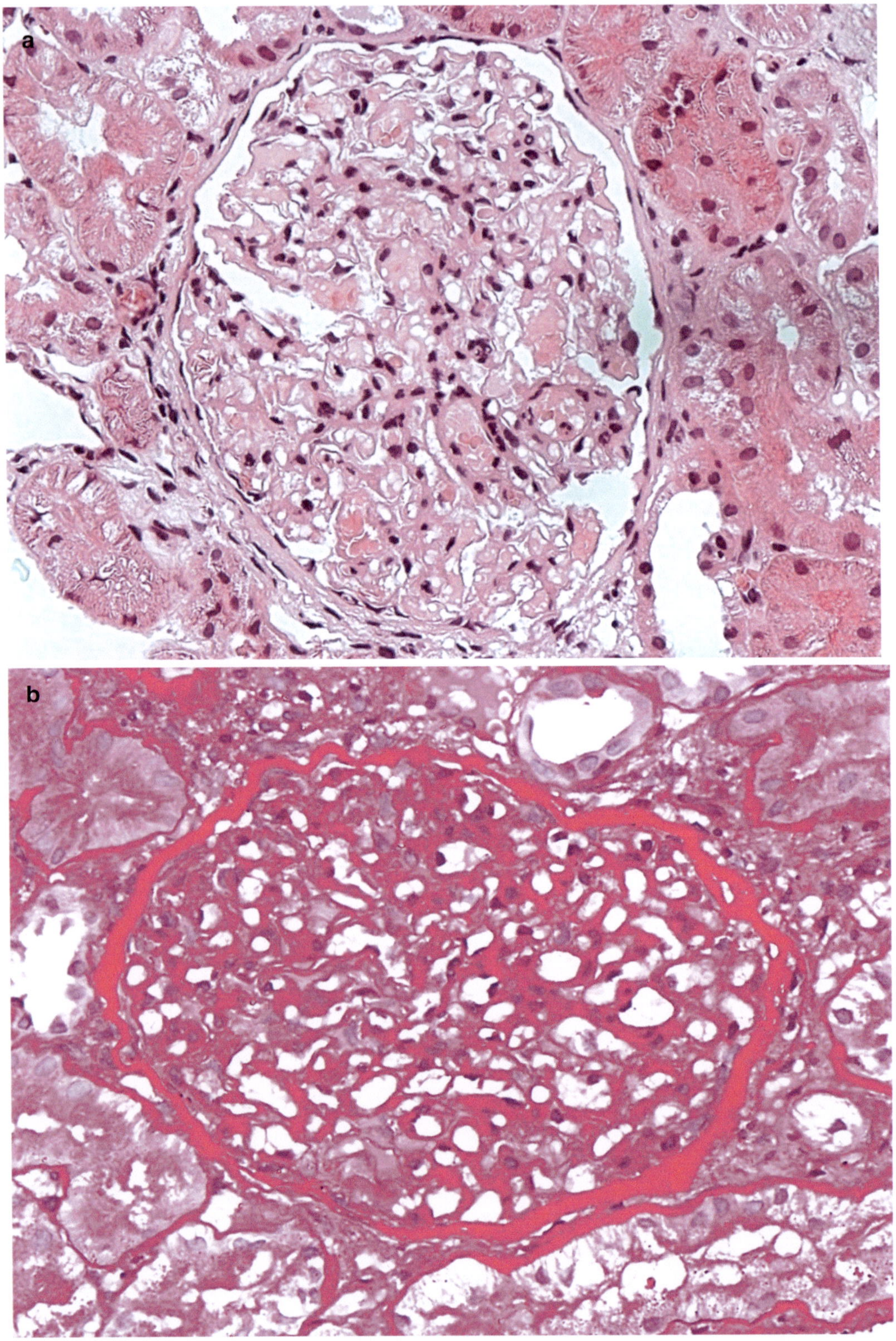

Fig. 11.10 Lupus Podocytopathy. A 46-years male patient, treated for SLE, presented with hypertension for 2 years and proteinuria for the last 5 months. His ESR was 44 mm for first hour (Westergren). Urinary protein was 3+ with bland sediment and urine PC ratio was 13.74. Renal function was within normal limits, serum ANA was positive and serum complement C3 was within normal limits. Kidney biopsy had 11 glomeruli, 1 of them was globally sclerosed and others were almost within normal limits except for mild increase of mesangial matrix. Patchy tubular atrophy was present and the interstitium showed mild lymphocytic infiltration, the blood vessels were unremarkable. IF for IgG, IgM, IgA, C3, C1q, kappa and lambda light chains was negative. EM revealed diffuse podocyte effacement/podocytopathy accompanied by scattered few mesangial electron-dense deposits. (**a**) HE ×400, (**b**) PAS ×400, (**c**) PSM ×400, (**d**) EM (identity of the patient has been concealed)

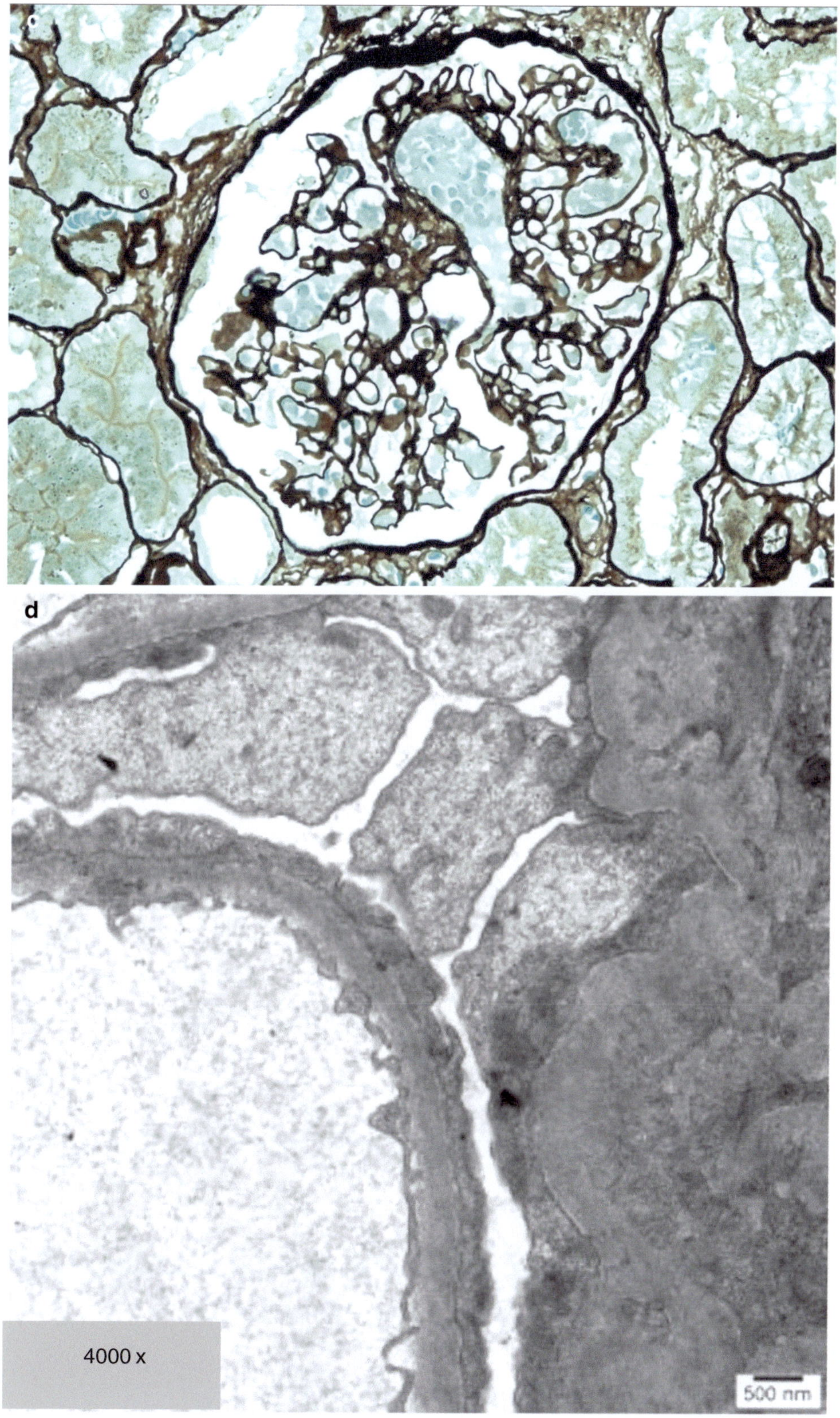

Fig. 11.10 (continued)

Further Reading

Almaani S, Meara A, Rovin BH. Update on lupus nephritis. Clin J Am Soc Nephrol. 2017;12:825–35.

Bajema IM, Wilhelmus S, Alpers CE, Bruijn JA, Colvin RB, Cook HT, D'Agati VD, Ferrario F, Haas M, Jennette JC, Joh K, Nast CC, Noël LH, Rijnink EC, Roberts ISD, Seshan SV, Sethi S, Fogo AB. Revision of the International Society of Nephrology/Renal Pathology Society classification for lupus nephritis: clarification of definitions, and modified National Institutes of Health activity and chronicity indices. Kidney Int. 2018;93:789–96.

Bomback AS, Markowitz GS. Lupus podocytopathy: a distinct entity. Clin J Am Soc Nephrol. 2016;11:547–8.

Chen D, Hu W. Lupus podocytopathy: a distinct entity of lupus nephritis. J Nephrol. 2018;31:629–34.

Hu W, Chen Y, Wang S, Chen H, Liu Z, Zeng C, Zhang H, Liu Z. Clinical-morphological features and outcomes of lupus podocytopathy. Clin J Am Soc Nephrol. 2016;11:585–92.

Oliva-Damaso N, Payan J, Oliva-Damaso E, Pereda T, Bomback AS. Lupus podocytopathy: an overview. Adv Chronic Kidney Dis. 2019;26:369–75.

Weening JJ, D'Agati VD, Schwartz MM, Seshan SV, Alpers CE, Appel GB, Balow JE, Bruijn JA, Cook T, Ferrario F, Fogo AB, Ginzler EM, Hebert L, Hill G, Hill P, Jennette JC, Kong NC, Lesavre P, Lockshin M, Looi LM, Makino H, Moura LA, Nagata M, International Society of Nephrology Working Group on the Classification of Lupus Nephritis, Renal Pathology Society Working Group on the Classification of Lupus Nephritis. The classification of glomerulonephritis in systemic lupus erythematosus revisited. Kidney Int. 2004;65:521–30.

Yu F, Haas M, Glassock R, Zhao MH. Redefining lupus nephritis: clinical implications of pathophysiologic subtypes. Nat Rev Nephrol. 2017;13:483–95.

12 Anti-GBM Disease

Anti-GBM glomerulonephritis or anti-glomerular basement membrane disease/Good Pasture disease is an autoimmune disorder affecting glomerular capillaries resulting in rapidly progressive glomerulonephritis and involvement of pulmonary capillaries manifesting as alveolar hemorrhage. It is considered an immune complex mediated small vessel vasculitis in the revised international Chapel Hill nomenclature and accounts for 10–15% cases of crescentic glomerulonephritis. It is caused by the binding of circulating IgG autoantibodies with the NC-1 domain of $\alpha 3$ chain of type IV collagen in the glomerular capillary basement membrane. On serological workup circulating anti-GBM antibodies can be identified in serum of affected patients by ELISA. Morphologically it is characterized by necrotizing and crescentic glomerulonephritis. Majority of patients will have crescents in >50% of glomeruli and crescents will be usually of uniform age, unlike the ANCA associated pauci-immune glomerulonephritis. Similar to pauci-immune crescentic glomerulonephritis rupture of Bowman's capsule and periglomerular granuloma can be appreciated. In the early phase of the disease segmental infiltration of polymorphs and mononuclear cells may be seen. On immunofluorescence linear deposit of IgG is seen along the glomerular capillary basement membrane. On electron microscopy, no electron-dense deposits are seen although rupture of glomerular capillary basement membrane and composition of crescent in the form of fibrin and proliferating cells are appreciated. Patients are treated with a combination of plasmapheresis, corticosteroids, and cyclophosphamide. Five years survival can be as low as 34%. A case of Anti-GBM disease is illustrated (Fig. 12.1).

P. Gupta, R. K. Gupta, *Pathology of Glomerular Diseases*, https://doi.org/10.1007/978-981-19-1430-0_12

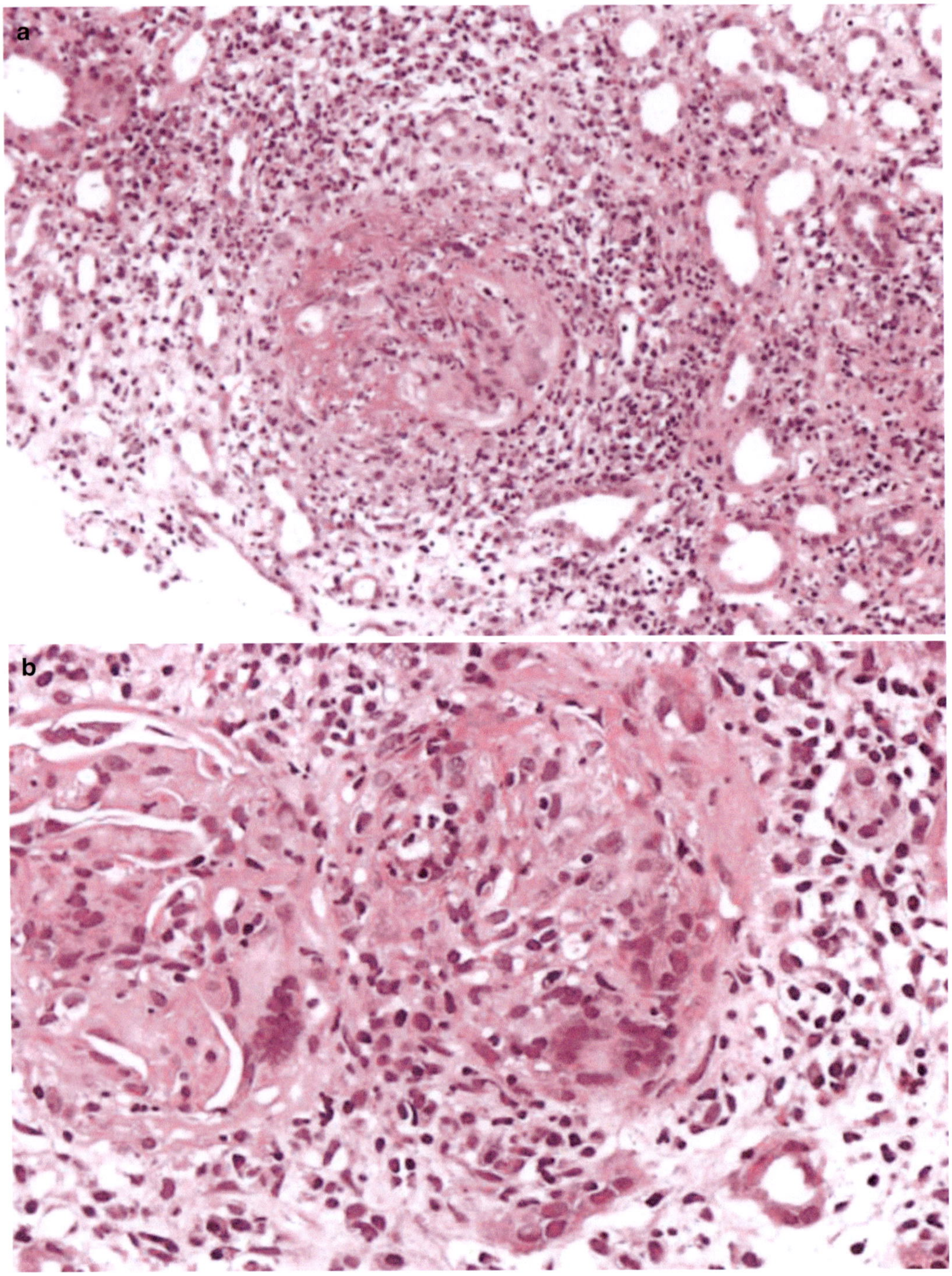

Fig. 12.1 **Anti-GBM disease** A 61-years female patient known to be hypothyroid, presented with cough and dyspnoea for 3 months and fever for 15 days. X-ray chest PA was wnl. Laboratory workup revealed hemoglobin 7.4 g/dL, TLC 16,690 per cu mL with 89% neutrophils, ESR 140 mm (Westergren) and the platelet count was 26.9 K/μL. Urine showed protein++ and plenty of RBC/hpf. Serum creatinine was 6.5 mg/dL. c-ANCA and p-ANCA were negative. Anti-GBM antibody titer was >100 AU. She was put on alternate day sessions of hemodialysis. Renal biopsy revealed 14 glomeruli, 1 of which was globally sclerosed and all other glomeruli showed circumferential cellular to fibrocellular crescents with fibrinoid necrosis and prolapse of the crescents into the tubular pole (PAS—short arrow). Glomeruli also showed granulomas with the presence of giant cells with breach of glomerular capillary basement membrane (PSM) and breach of Bowman's capsule (PAS—arrow heads) with periglomerulitis. Acute tubular injury and extensive interstitial inflammatory infiltrate, chiefly by polymorphonuclear leucocytes were apparent. Blood vessels were unremarkable. IF showed linear localization of IgG along GBM. IF for IgM, IgA, and complements was negative. (**a** and **b**) HE ×400, (**c** and **d**) PAS ×400, (**e**) PSM ×400, (**f**) IF ×400

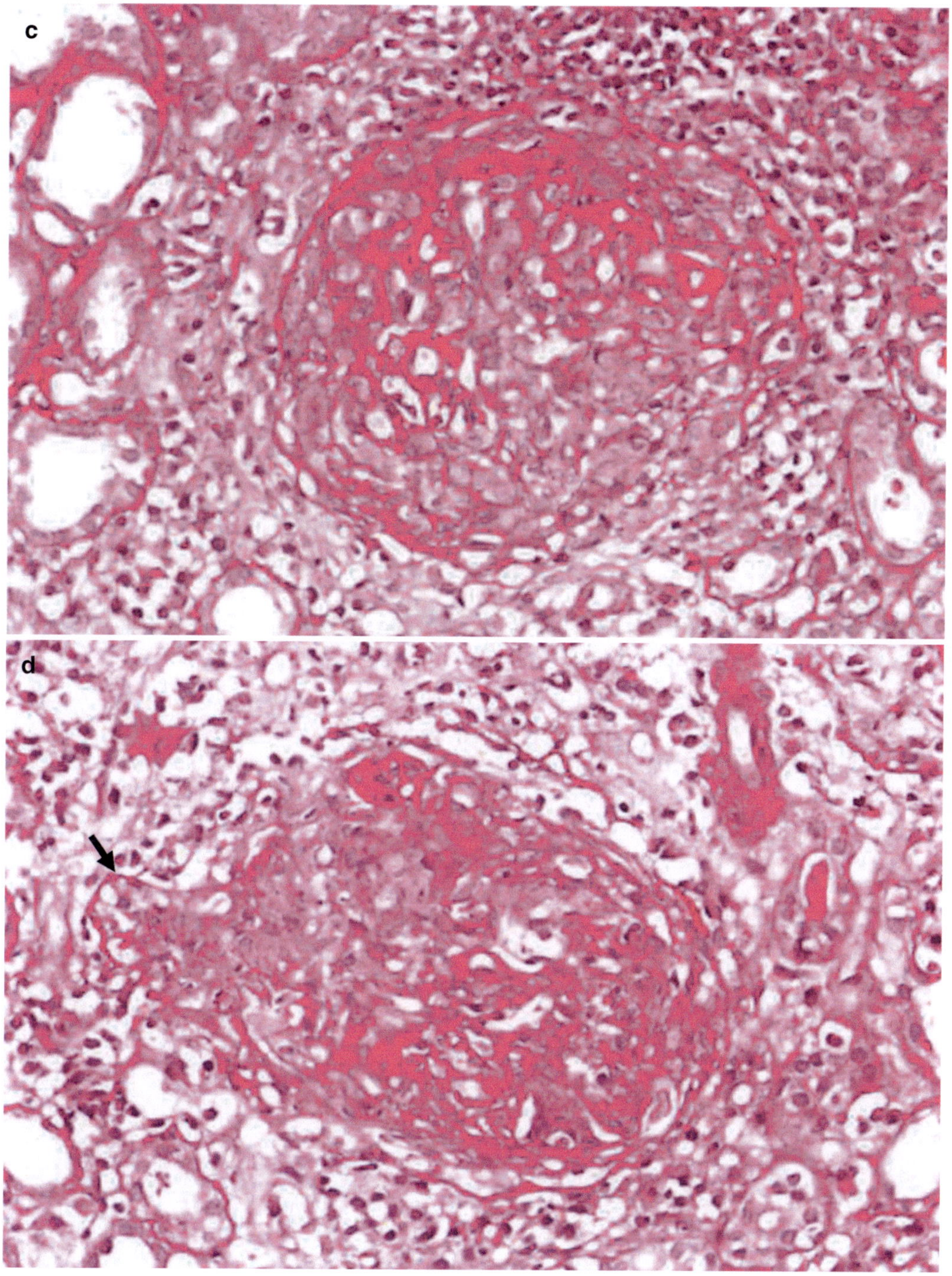

Fig. 12.1 (continued)

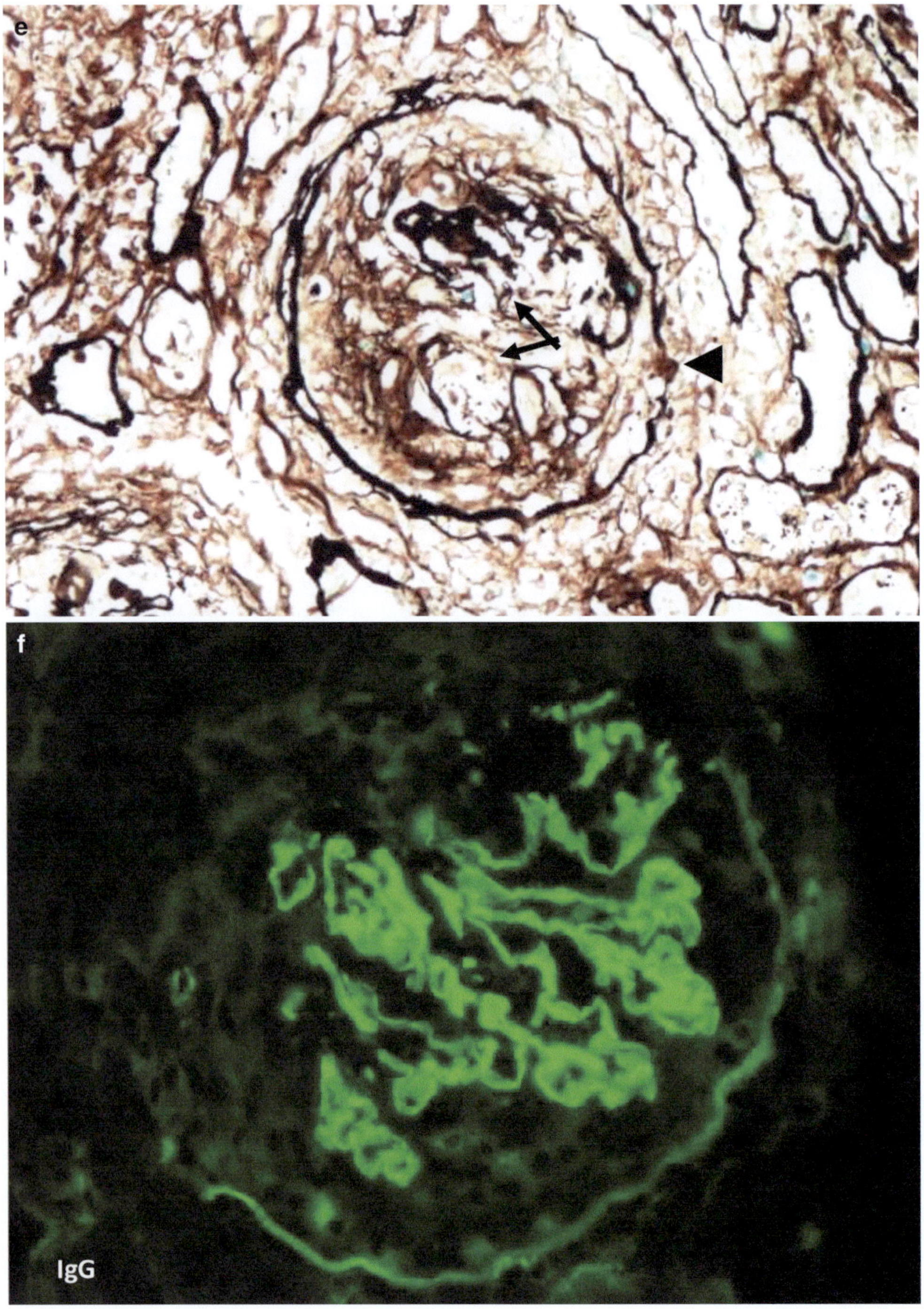

Fig. 12.1 (continued)

Further Reading

Gulati K, McAdoo SP. Anti-glomerular basement membrane disease. Rheum Dis Clin N Am. 2018;44:651–73.

Hellmark T, Segelmark M. Diagnosis and classification of Goodpasture's disease (anti-GBM). J Autoimmun. 2014;48–49:108–12.

McAdoo SP, Pusey CD. Anti-glomerular basement membrane disease. Clin J Am Soc Nephrol. 2017;12:1162–72.

van Daalen EE, Jennette JC, McAdoo SP, Pusey CD, Alba MA, Poulton CJ, Wolterbeek R, Nguyen TQ, Goldschmeding R, Alchi B, Griffiths M, de Zoysa JR, Vincent B, Bruijn JA, Bajema IM. Predicting outcome in patients with anti-GBM glomerulonephritis. Clin J Am Soc Nephrol. 2018;13:63–72.

13 Pauci-immune Crescentic Glomerulonephritis

Pauci-immune crescentic glomerulonephritis (PICGN) is the most important and common cause of rapidly progressive glomerulonephritis accounting for 80% of such cases. Patients present with rapidly progressive renal failure with a rapid rise in serum creatinine which may be accompanied by proteinuria and hematuria. On serology patients have c-ANCA or p-ANCA positivity; however, 30% or more of these patients can have ANCA-negative serology. The patients may have clinical evidence of granulomatosis with polyangiitis (Wegener's granulomatosis), Eosinophilic granulomatosis with polyangiitis (Churg–Strauss syndrome), or microscopic polyangiitis. Sometimes the condition can be renal limited. On light microscopy, patients have necrotizing crescentic glomerulonephritis with crescents in 50% or more glomeruli. Usually, cellular crescents are the predominant type. At times rupture of glomerular capillary basement membrane and fibrinoid necrosis of glomerular capillary tuft may be seen. Periglomerular and interstitial granulomas may be present. Evidence of vasculitis is seen in <10% of cases. On Immunofluorescence either no immunoglobulin deposits are seen or the intensity of deposits is <2+. On electron microscopy, crescents are seen to be composed of fibrin tactoids, macrophages, and epithelial cells. Endothelial cell swelling can be seen in glomerular capillaries. Rupture of glomerular capillary basement membrane and Bowman's capsule can also be seen. No electron-dense deposits are identified in glomerular, tubular, or vascular compartment in classic cases.

Granulomatosis with polyangiitis, GPA (Wegener's granulomatosis) will show granulomatous vasculitis. Renal biopsy may show periglomerular granuloma and rupture of Bowman's capsule. Necrotizing small vessel vasculitis with granulomatous inflammation can be seen in the respiratory tract also. In majority of cases in these patients, c-ANCA is positive (Figs. 13.1 and 13.2).

Eosinophilic granulomatosis with polyangiitis, EGPA (Churg–Strauss disease) will have a history of asthma, peripheral blood eosinophilia, and pulmonary granuloma with renal involvement in 45% of patients in the form of necrotizing crescentic glomerulonephritis. More than 50% of these patients can be ANCA-negative. Of those who are ANCA positive, predominantly MPO ANCA has been found positive although few cases can show PR3 ANCA as well (Fig. 13.3).

Microscopic polyangiitis, MPA will show renal involvement in 90% of cases. They are frequently p-ANCA positive; some may have c-ANCA positivity. They will have systemic vasculitis without evidence of asthma or granulomatous inflammation (Fig. 13.4).

P. Gupta, R. K. Gupta, *Pathology of Glomerular Diseases*, https://doi.org/10.1007/978-981-19-1430-0_13

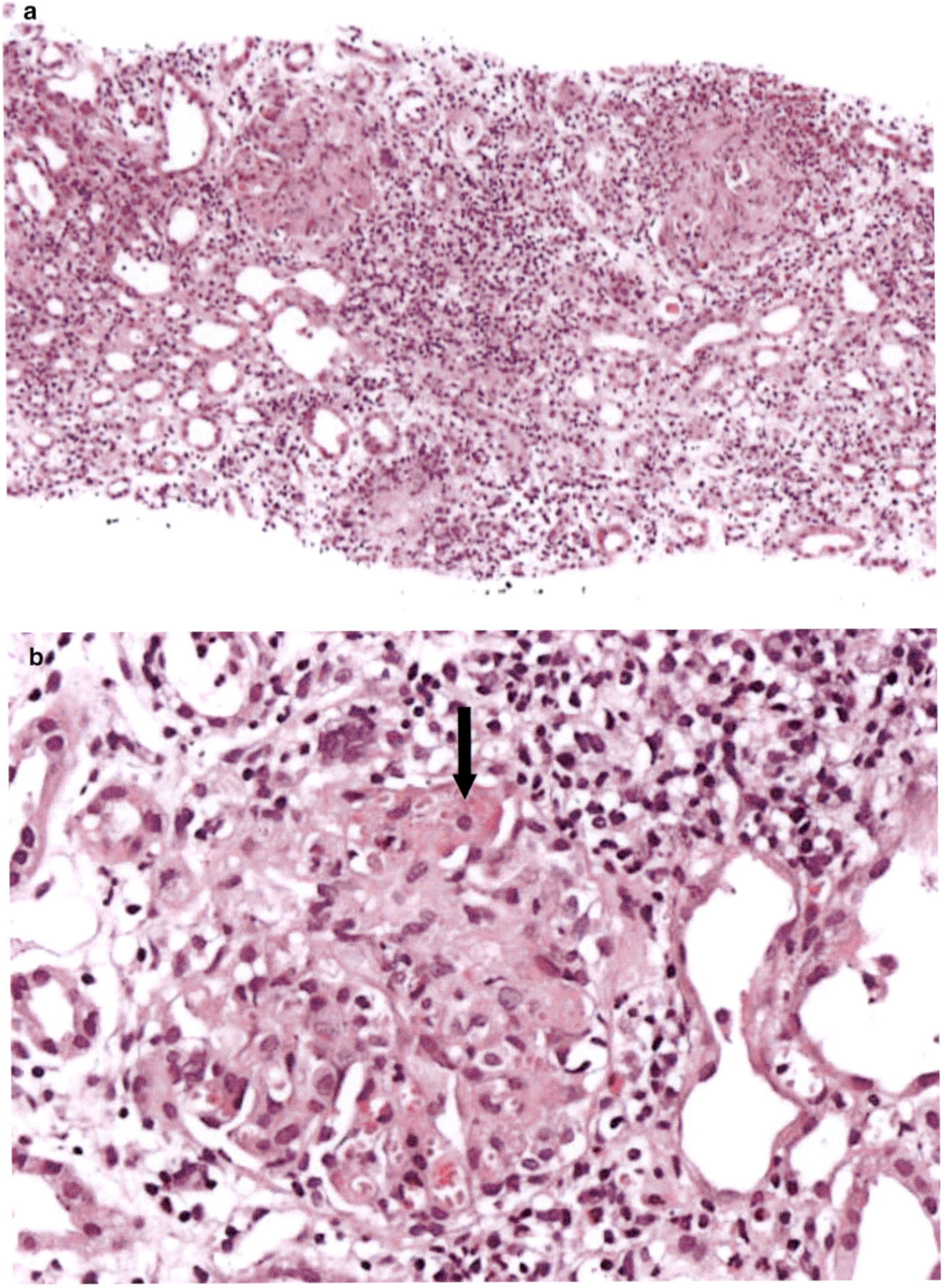

Fig. 13.1 **GPA** A 69-years male patient presented with rapidly progressive renal failure. Patient had history of flu-like symptoms with fever and myalgia, epistaxis, and hemoptysis. CT thorax revealed intra-alveolar hemorrhage. Routine hematological workup revealed Hb 8.7 g/dL, ESR was 135 mm for the first hour (Westergren); blood counts were wnl. Urine examination showed proteinuria (+) with active sediment: WBC 5–10/hpf and RBC 10–20/hpf. Serum creatinine increased from 1.2 mg/dL to 6.5 mg/dL during last 6 weeks. Serological workup revealed that c-ANCA was positive (581 AU/mL) and p-ANCA and ANA were negative. Serum complement C3 and C4 were wnl. Renal biopsy revealed 17 glomeruli, all of them had cellular crescents; some of the glomeruli also had loop necrosis (arrow); there was associated periglomerulitis with breach of the Bowman's capsule. Blood vessels showed arteriosclerosis accompanied with acute tubular injury. Interstitium showed periglomerular epithelioid cell granulomas. IF was negative for IgG, IgM, IgA, C3, C1q, kappa and lambda light chains. (**a**) HE ×100, (**b–d**) HE ×400, (**e**) PAS ×400, (**f**) PSM ×400

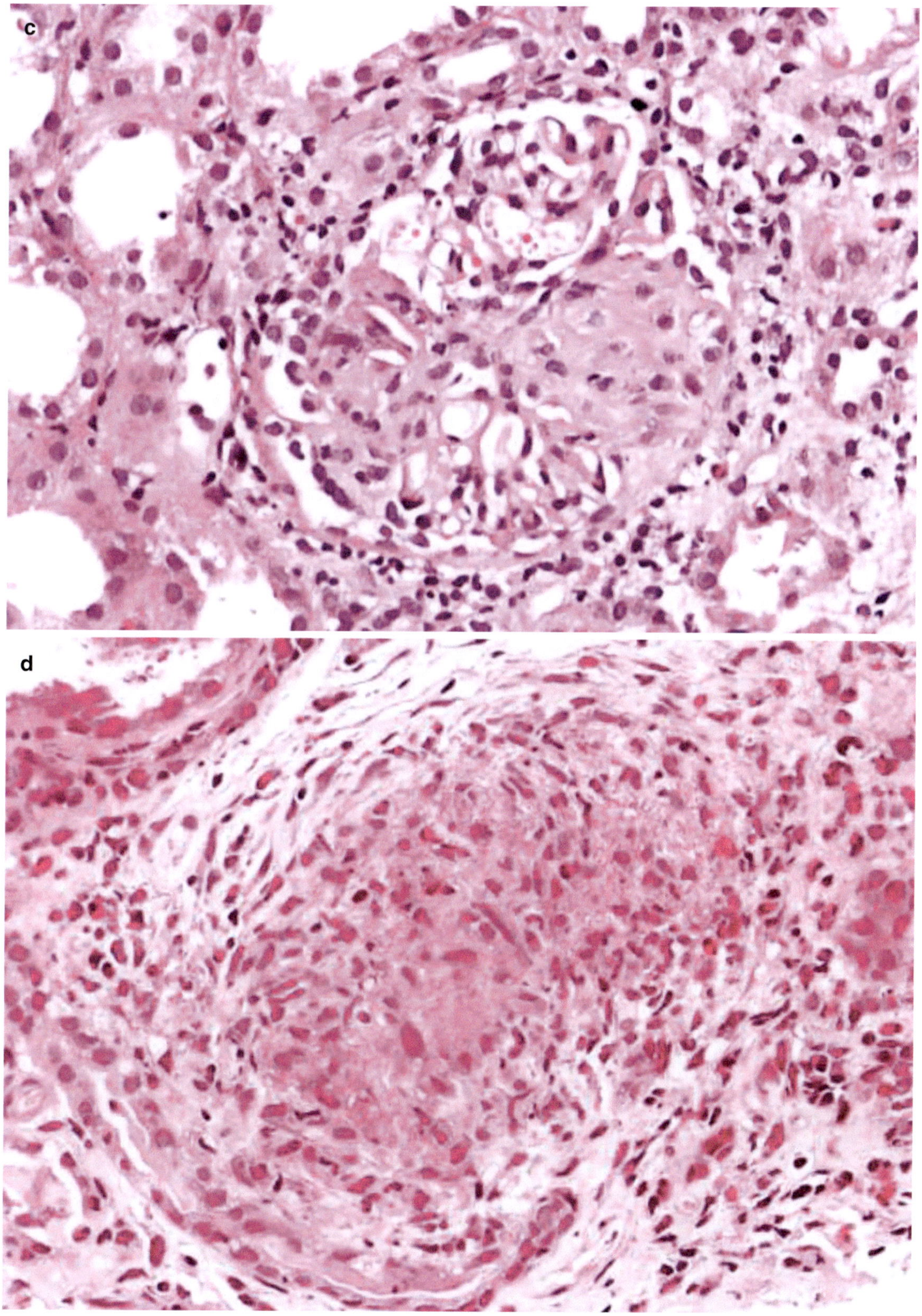

Fig. 13.1 (continued)

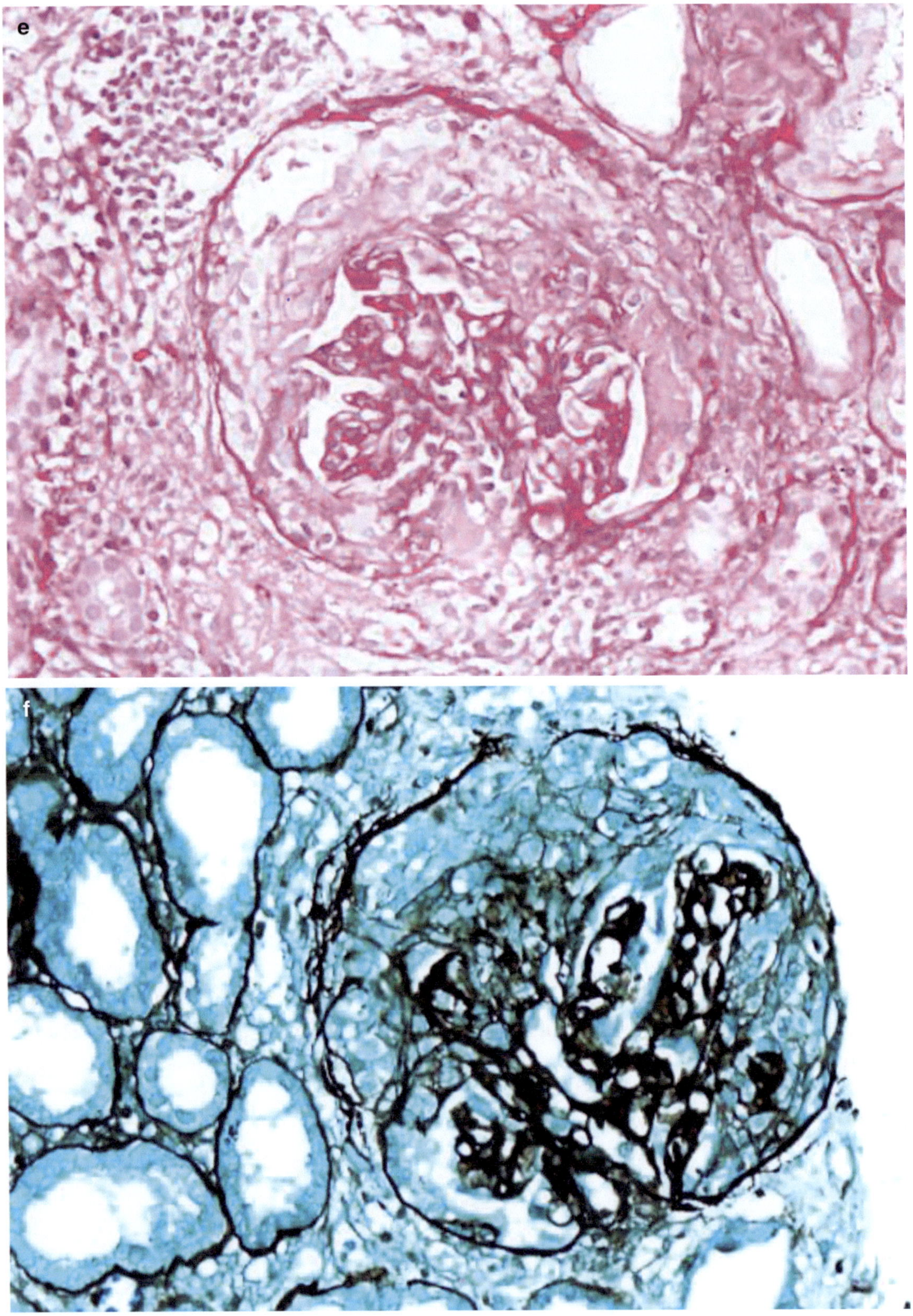

Fig. 13.1 (continued)

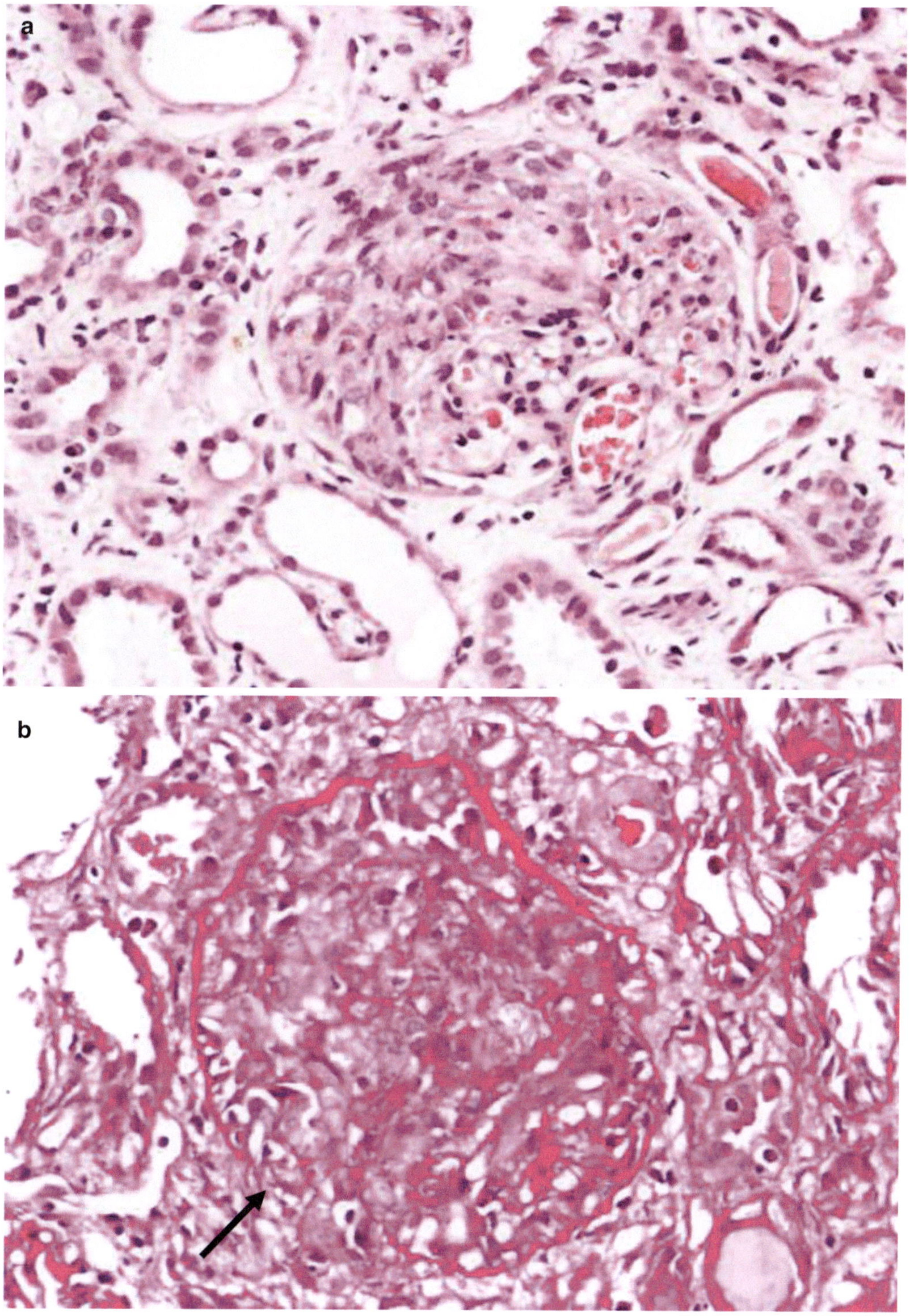

Fig. 13.2 **GPA in a child** A 12-years male patient presented with joint pain and body ache for 3 months, subsequently for the past 2 weeks he had fever with rashes over knuckles and swelling of body for 10 days. He passed cola-colored urine for the past 9 days. On physical examination, the child had swelling over face and legs and he was hypertensive. On USG both kidneys showed raised cortical echogenicity. Urine analysis revealed protein 2+ with 5–10 WBC/hpf and numerous RBC/hpf. Serum total protein was 6.6 g/dL with serum albumin of 2.7 g/dL. Serial serum creatinine estimation showed rising trend from 1.6 to 3.3 mg/dL over 3 days. ASO titer was <200 IU/mL and ANA was negative by IIF. c-ANCA was markedly raised being >1000 AU/mL while p-ANCA was <3 AU/mL. Serum C3 was 1863 mg/L. Renal biopsy had 12 glomeruli, 8 glomeruli had cellular crescents; breach of the Bowman's capsule was seen (arrow), areas of acute tubular injury were also evident with interstitial inflammation and edema and focal tubular atrophy. (**a**) HE ×400, (**b**) PAS ×400, (**c**) PAS ×200

c

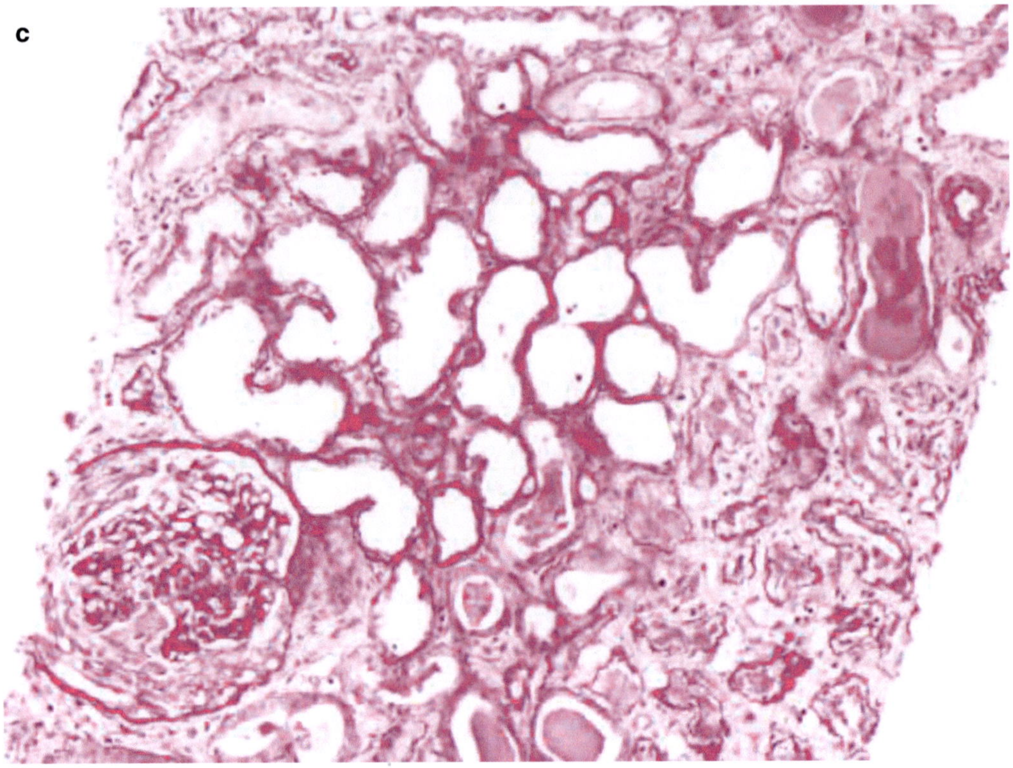

Fig. 13.2 (continued)

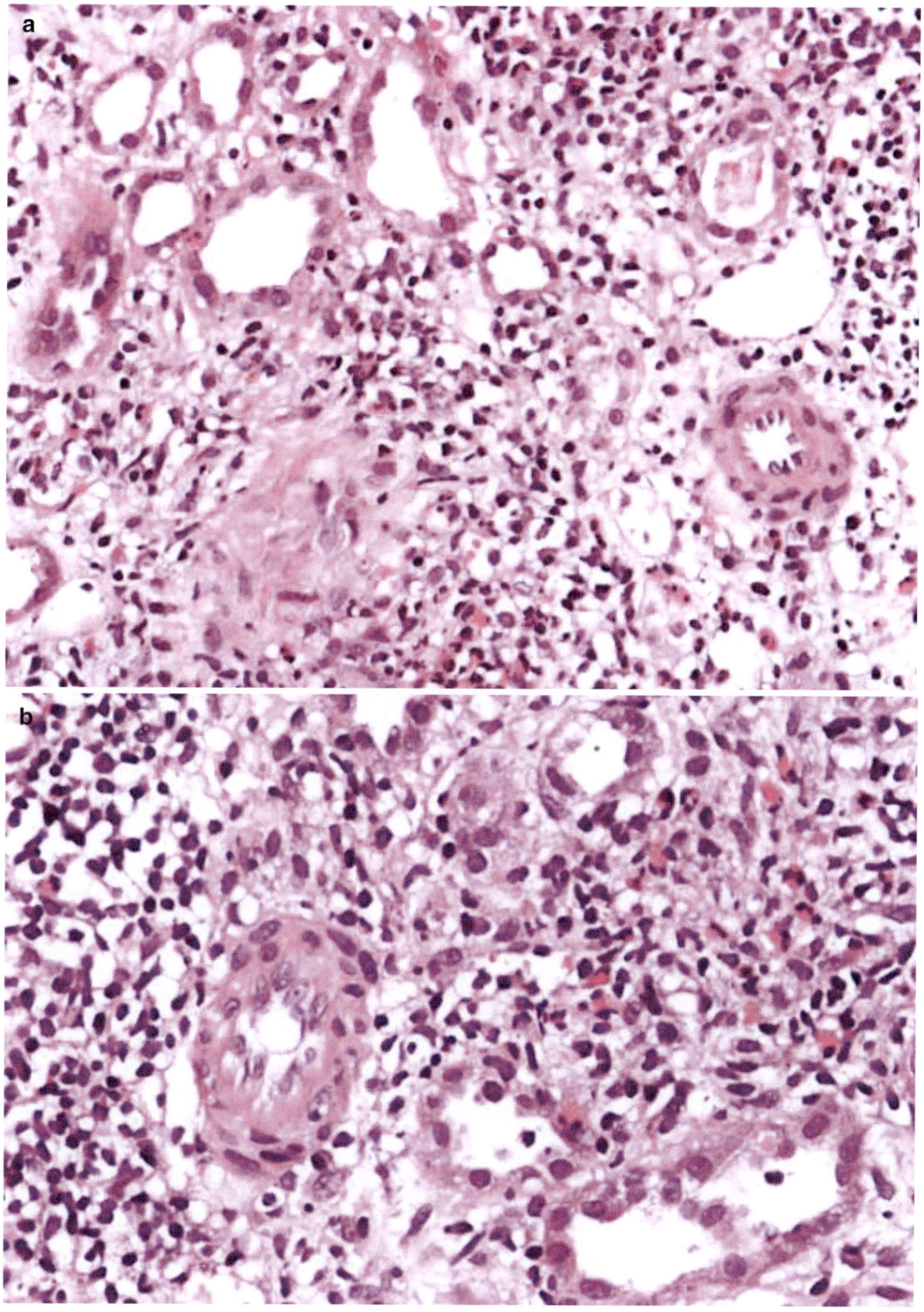

Fig. 13.3 **EGPA** A 45-years asthmatic male patient presented with fever and breathlessness along with rapidly progressive renal failure. PFT showed reversible airway obstruction. Urine analysis revealed proteinuria 2+ with 80–100 RBC/hpf and 0–2 WBC/hpf. Patient had peripheral blood eosinophilia, total WBC count was 15,600 per cu mm with 23% eosinophils and absolute eosinophil count of 3588 per cu mm. He had mild anemia with Hb of 11 g%; ESR was 72 mm for the first hour (Westergren). Serum creatinine was 8.1 mg/dL. p-ANCA was positive; anti-MPO ELISA was78 RU/mL. Renal biopsy had 12 glomeruli, 8 having cellular, 3 with fibrocellular, and 1 showing fibrous crescent. Focal tubular atrophy was seen and the interstitium showed moderate eosinophilic infiltrate. Blood vessels were unremarkable. (**a** and **b**) HE ×200, (**c**) PAS ×400, (**d**) PSM ×400

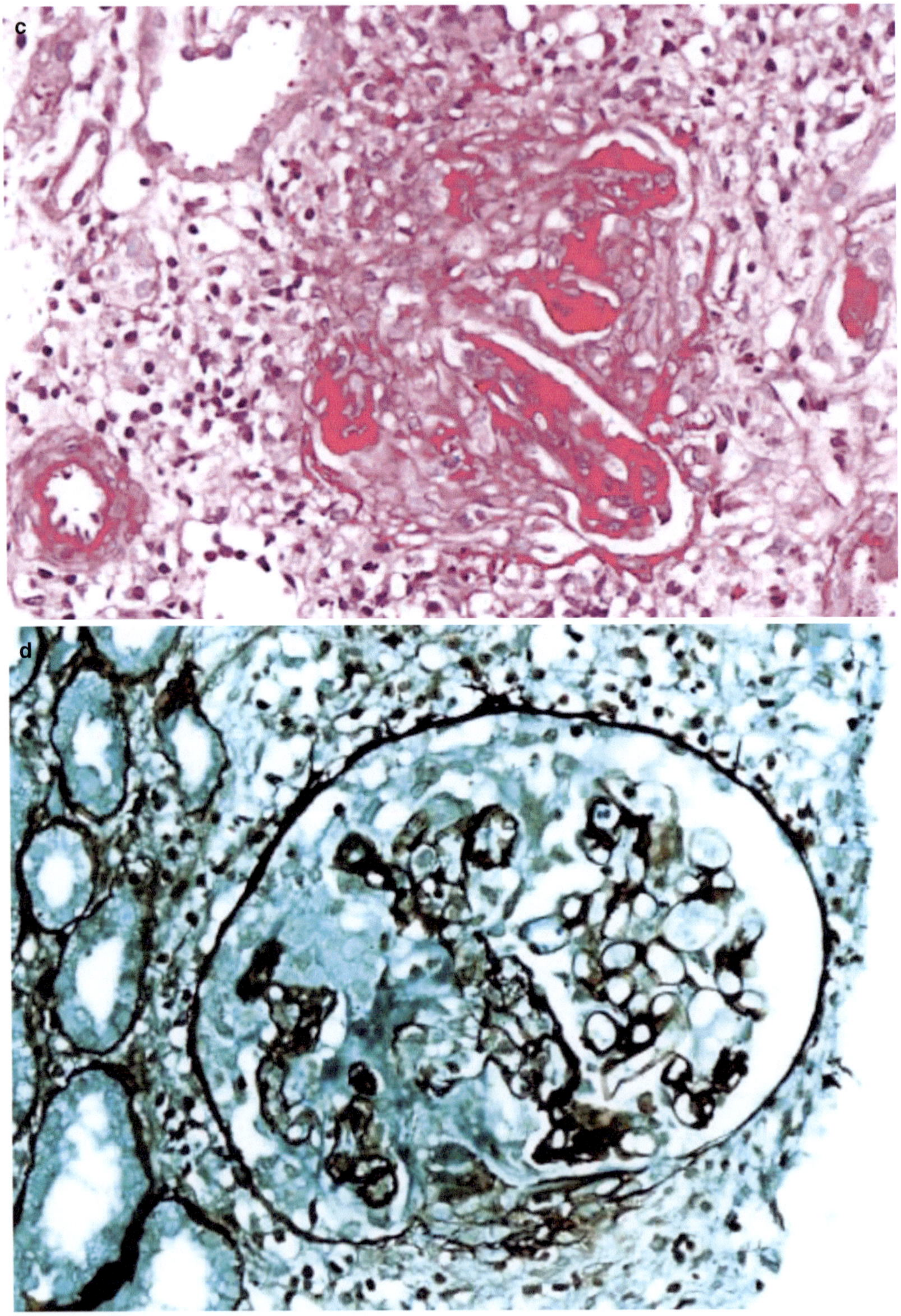

Fig. 13.3 (continued)

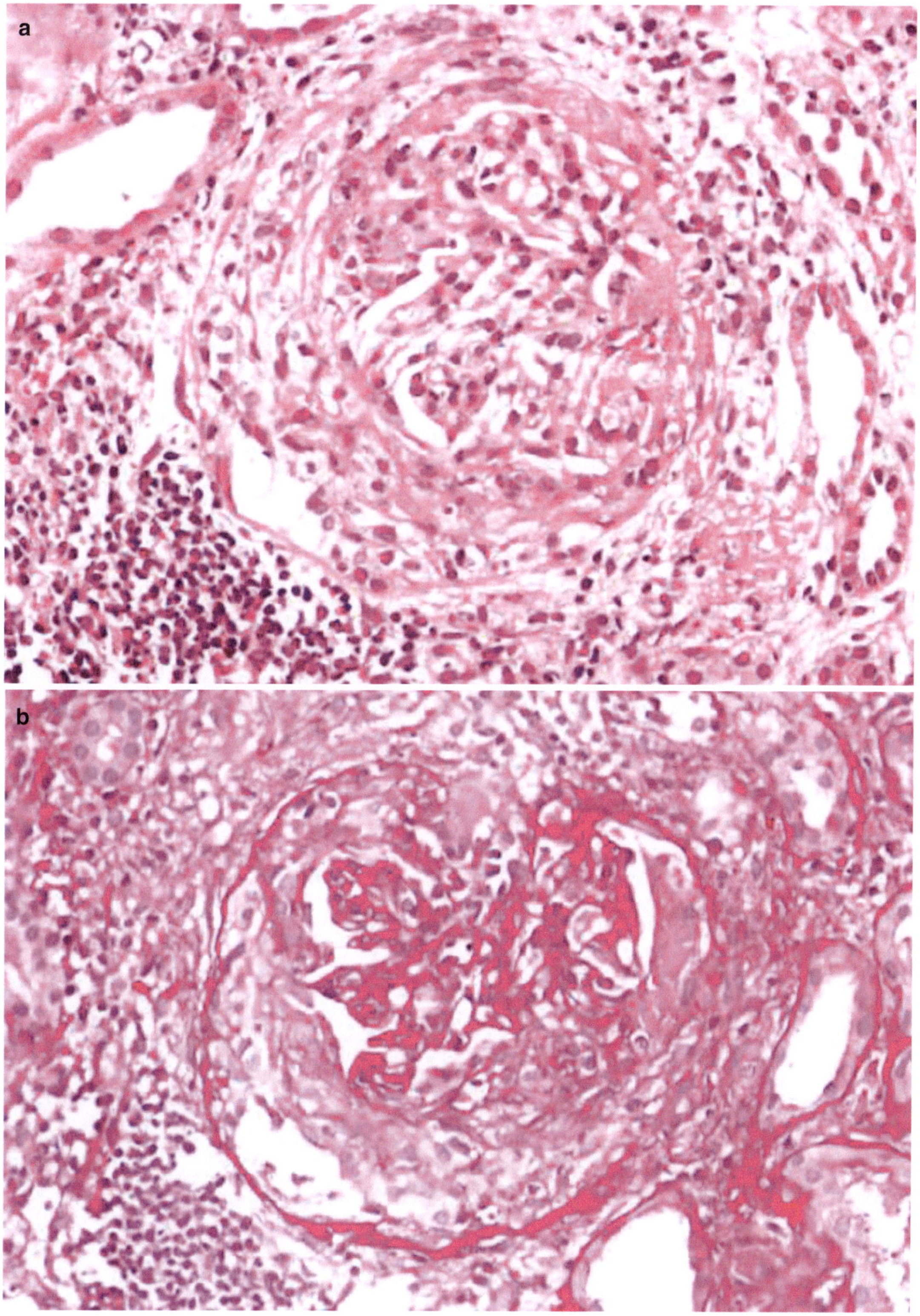

Fig. 13.4 **MPA** A 44-years female patient presented with rapidly progressive renal failure. Urine analysis revealed protein (+) with 20–30 RBC/phf, 24 h protein being 0.4 g. Routine CBC revealed hemoglobin of 11 g/dL with total WBC count of 11,200 per cu mm and platelets 1.6 lakh per cu mm; she had an ESR of 140 mm for first hour (Westergren). Her serum complement C3 and C4 were wnl. ANA was negative. Serum p-ANCA was >1000 AU/mL. Renal biopsy had nine glomeruli, seven of them showed cellular to fibrocellular crescents with breach of Bowman's capsule, while two glomeruli were unremarkable. Some of the tubules showed hyaline casts and presence of WBC, occasional foci of tubular atrophy were present. Interstitium had moderate lymphocytic infiltrate. One of the blood vessels showed vasculitis with fibrinoid necrosis of the wall. IF for IgG, IgM, IgA, C3, C1q, kappa and lambda light chains was negative. (**a**) HE ×400, (**b** and **c**) PAS ×400 and (**d**) Masson's trichrome (MT) ×400

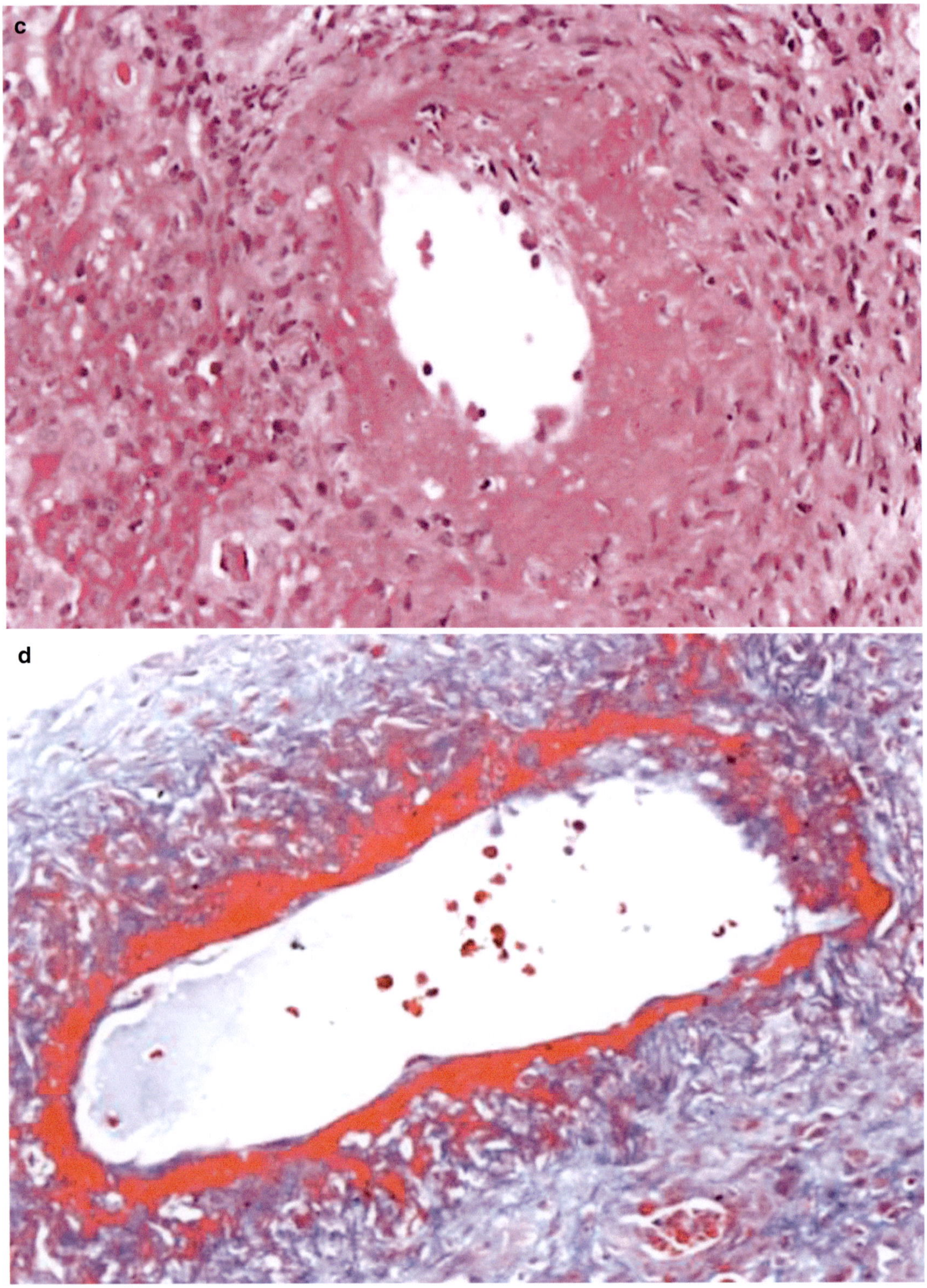

Fig. 13.4 (continued)

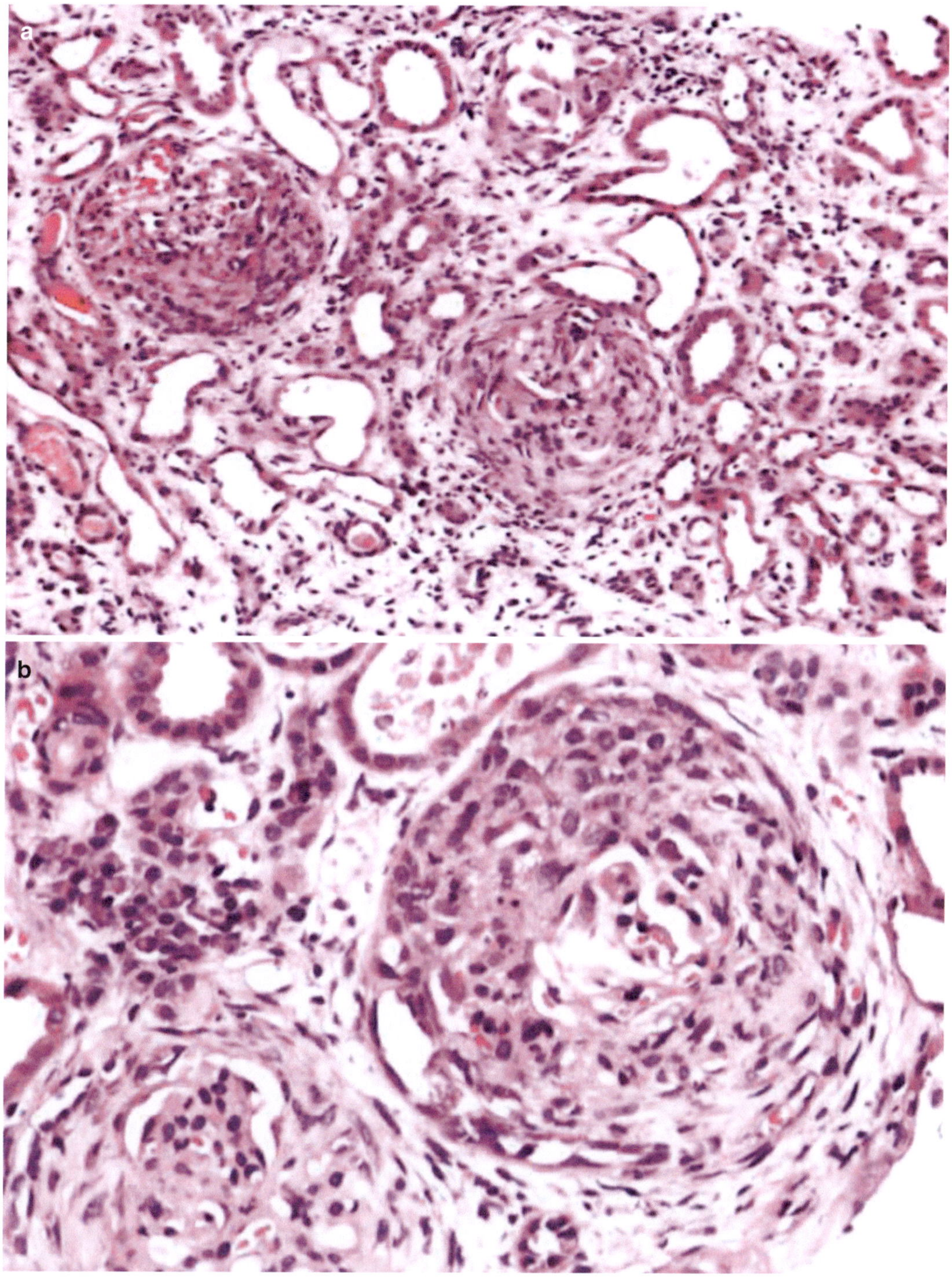

Fig. 13.5 **ANCA -ve PICGN** A 56-years female patient having hypertension for the past 10 years, was admitted to the hospital with multiple joint pains for which she had been taking NSAID. During her reproductive life, she had two episodes of spontaneous abortion. She had no history of DM, rashes, oral ulceration or hair loss. On laboratory workup she was found to have moderate anemia with hemoglobin of 8.7 g/dL, total WBC count was raised 16.18 × 10^3 per cu mm and the ESR was 79 mm for first hour (Westergren). Urine analysis revealed the presence of albumin (+++) with active sediment (RBC 20–30/phf); P:C ratio was 10.7. Serum biochemistry revealed hypoalbuminemia with serum albumin being 2.2 g/dL; serum creatinine was 13 mg/dL. Complement C3 and C4 were wnl. Both c-ANCA and p-ANCA were negative. Anti dsDNA was also negative. Renal biopsy showed 14 glomeruli and all of them had circumferential cellular or fibrocellular crescents with marked tubulointerstitial changes; breach of the Bowman's capsule was seen. IF for IgG, IgM, IgA, C3, and C1q was negative. EM showed prominent subendothelial rarefaction of glomerular capillaries, expansion of endothelial cell cytoplasm and few fibrin tactoids both within capillary lumina and in extra capillary location. (**a**) HE ×200, (**b**) HE ×400, (**c**) PAS ×400, (**d**) PSM ×400, (**e**) EM (identity of the patient has been concealed)

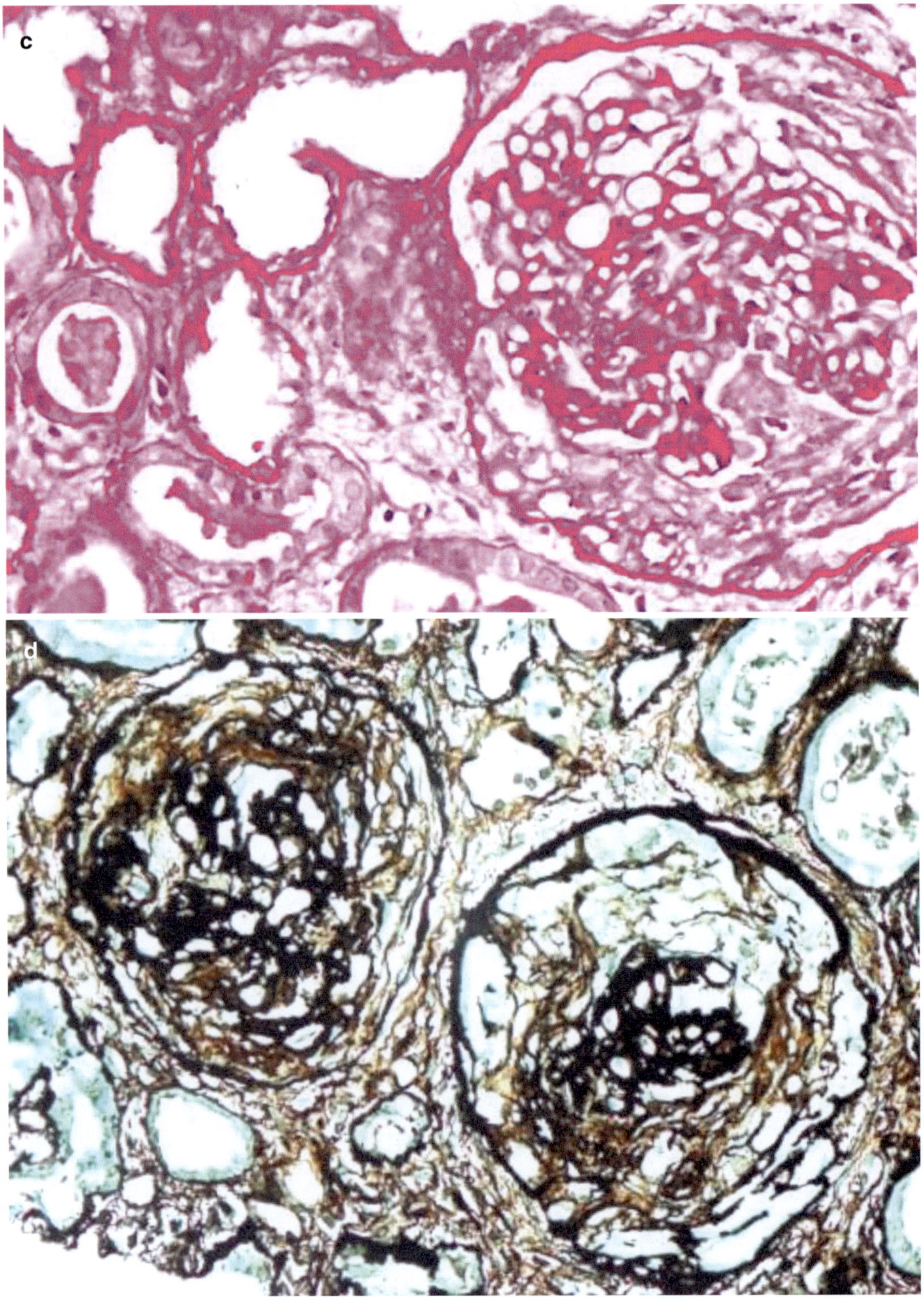

Fig. 13.5 (continued)

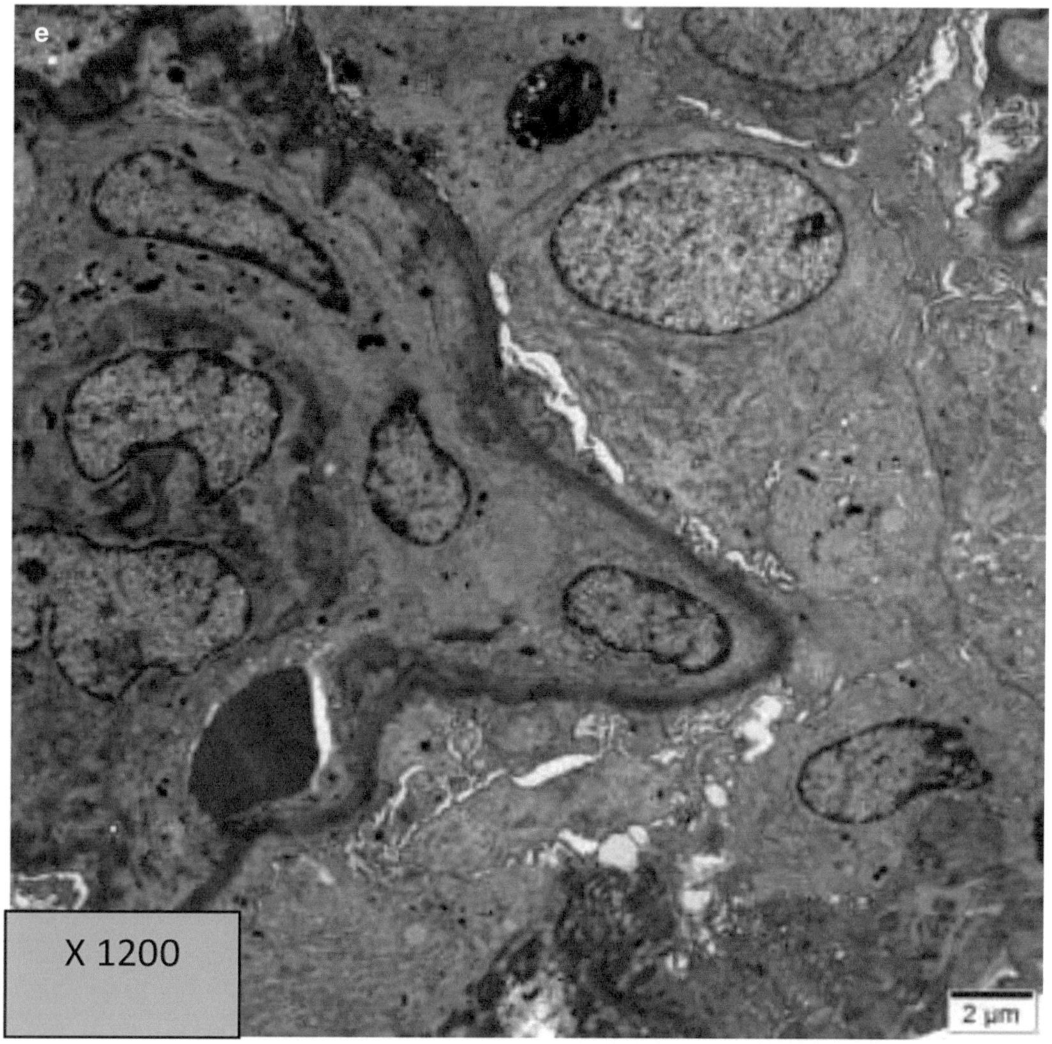

Fig. 13.5 (continued)

Further Reading

Andreiana I, Stancu S, Avram A, Taran L, Mircescu G. ANCA positive crescentic glomerulonephritis outcome in a Central East European cohort: a retrospective study. BMC Nephrol. 2015;16:90.

Booth AD, Almond MK, Burns A, Ellis P, Gaskin G, Neild GH, et al. Outcome of ANCA-associated renal vasculitis: a 5-year retrospective study. Am J Kidney Dis. 2003;41:776–84.

Brix SR, Noriega M, Tennstedt P, Vettorazzi E, Busch M, Nitschke M, et al. Development and validation of a renal risk score in ANCA-associated glomerulonephritis. Kidney Int. 2018;94:1177–88.

Gupta P, Dharamdasani S, Gupta A, Bhalla AK, Gupta A, Malik M, Bhargava V, Tiwari V, Rana DS, Sapra RL. Evaluation of factors influencing outcomes in pauci-immune crescentic glomerulonephritis: single centre experience of 51 cases. Indian J Nephrol. 2021;31:503–6.

Tanna A, Guarino L, Tam FW, Rodriquez-Cubillo B, Levy JB, Cairns TD, et al. Long-term outcome of anti-neutrophil cytoplasm antibody-associated glomerulonephritis: evaluation of the international histological classification and other prognostic factors. Nephrol Dial Transplant. 2015;30:1185–92.

14 Postpartum Thrombotic Microangiopathy

Postpartum or pregnancy-associated thrombotic microangiopathy can be seen in the setting of pre-eclampsia/HELLP syndrome, thrombotic thrombocytopenic purpura, and atypical hemolytic uremic syndrome (complement-mediated TMA). Patients have microangiopathic hemolytic anemia, thrombocytopenia, and renal dysfunction.

Glomeruli are enlarged and show endothelial cell swelling. Solid bloodless appearance of glomeruli with luminal narrowing and endothelial cell swelling (endotheliosis) can be seen in cases with pre-eclampsia. Fibrillary or bubbly appearance of mesangium may be seen. Fibrin thrombi may be seen within the glomerular capillary lumen.

Renal cortical necrosis may be seen which can be patchy or diffuse in severe cases. Blood vessels may show evidence of arteriosclerosis or the presence of fibrin thrombi. Artery and arteriolar changes in the form of endothelial cell swelling, narrowing of lumen, fragmented red blood cells in arteriolar wall and fibrinoid necrosis can be seen and are more common in the setting of atypical HUS and TTP.

On immunofluorescence, fibrinogen deposits can be seen in the glomeruli along glomerular capillary loops and blood vessels.

On electron microscopy endothelial cell swelling, widening of subendothelial space, widening of lamina rara interna with electron-lucent appearance can be seen. Thickening of glomerular capillary wall and intracapillary thrombi (amorphous osmiophilic) may also be seen. Mesangial matrix may appear swollen (Fig. 14.1).

P. Gupta, R. K. Gupta, *Pathology of Glomerular Diseases*, https://doi.org/10.1007/978-981-19-1430-0_14

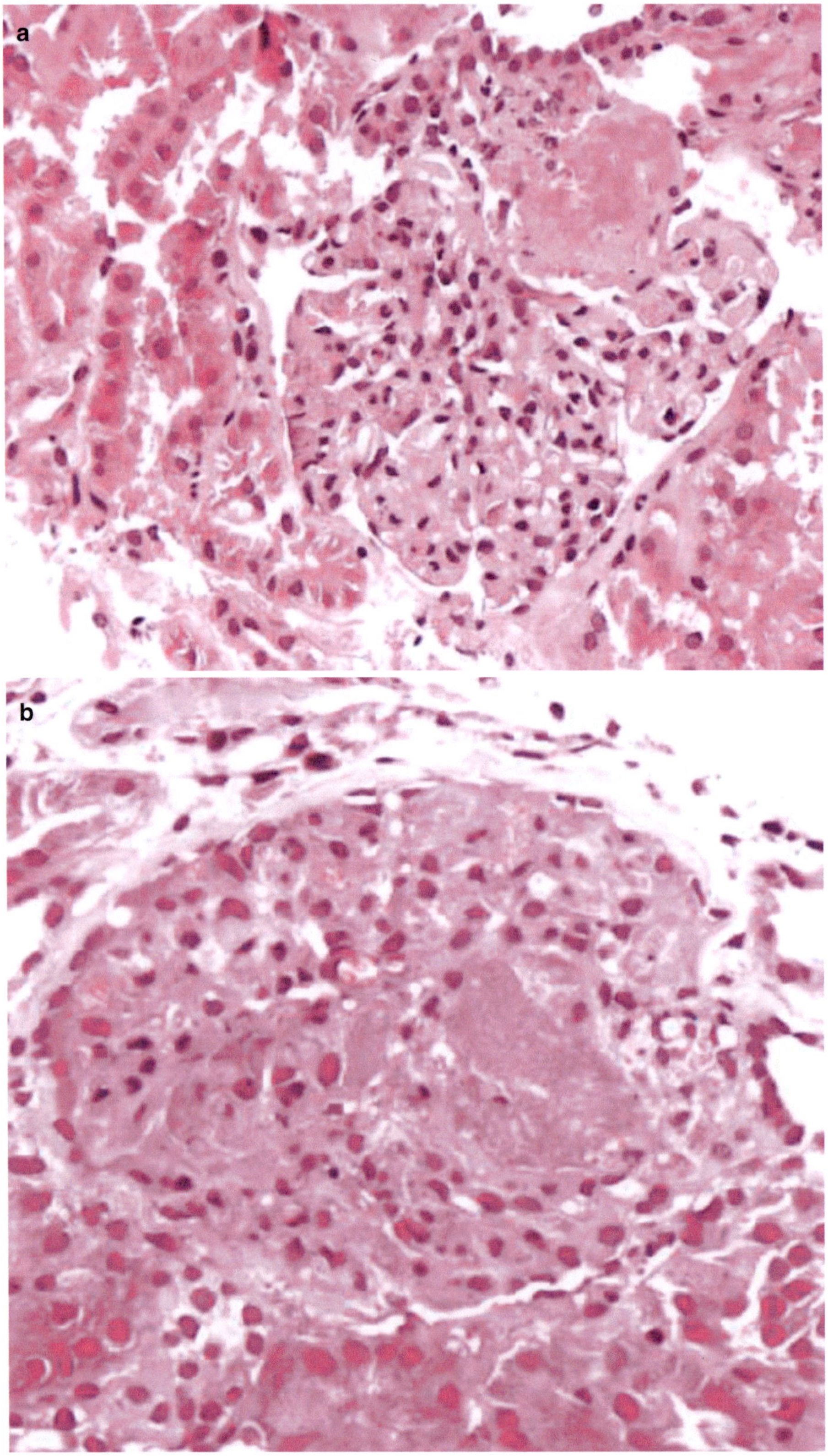

Fig. 14.1 **Post Partum TMA** A 24-years female patient with h/o pre-eclampsia presented with acute kidney injury during postpartum period. Patient had undergone LSCS and also had postpartum hemorrhage. On routine investigations her Hb was 8.2 g/dl, Platelet count was 1.2 million; peripheral smear showed presence of schistocytes. Serum creatinine was 5.8 mg/dl and LDH was 521 IU/L. Renal biopsy showed 8 glomeruli which were enlarged and appeared solid blood less; endotheliosis and endothelial cell swelling were evident. Some of the glomeruli showed fibrillary appearance of mesangium. Fibrin thrombi were seen in capillary loops. Part of the renal cortex showed cortical necrosis with ghost outlines of glomeruli and tubules. (**a**, **b**) HE × 400, (**c**) HE × 200, and (**d**) MT × 400

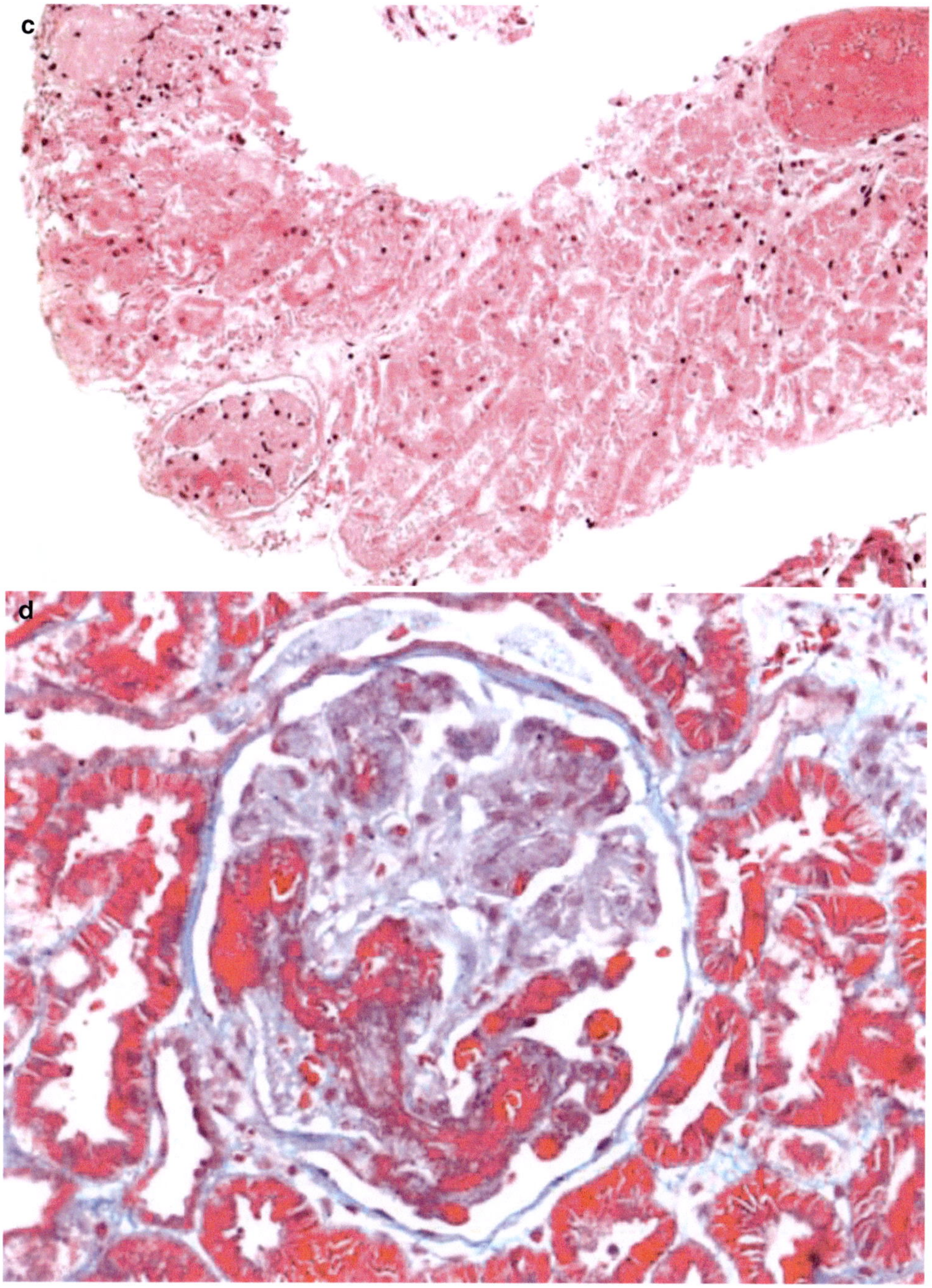

Fig. 14.1 (continued)

Further Reading

Bruel A, Kavanagh D, Noris M, Delmas Y, Wong EKS, Bresin E, Provôt F, Brocklebank V, Mele C, Remuzzi G, Loirat C, Frémeaux-Bacchi V, Fakhouri F. Hemolytic uremic syndrome in pregnancy and postpartum. Clin J Am Soc Nephrol. 2017;12:1237–47.

George JN, Nester CM, McIntosh JJ. Syndromes of thrombotic microangiopathy associated with pregnancy. Hematology Am Soc Hematol Educ Program. 2015;2015:644–8.

Gupta M, Govindappagari S, Burwick RM. Pregnancy associated atypical hemolytic uremic syndrome: a systematic review. Obstet Gynecol. 2020;135:46–58.

Sibai BM. Imitators of severe preeclampsia. Obstet Gynecol. 2007;109:956–66.

15 Hemolytic Uremic Syndrome (HUS)

Hemolytic uremic syndrome is characterized by acute kidney injury along with microangiopathic hemolytic anemia and thrombocytopenia. HUS can be typical Shiga toxin-associated (diarrhea associated) or atypical HUS which is commonly seen due to defects in the alternate complement pathway. Many other causes of atypical HUS are known including influenza, streptococcal pneumonia, HIV infection, autoimmune disorders, cobalamin C disorder, idiopathic and familial.

Shiga toxin-associated HUS (following *E. coli* diarrhea) accounts for majority of cases of childhood hemolytic uremic syndrome. Clinical presentation includes diarrhea, nausea, vomiting, decreased urine output, pallor along with microangiopathic hemolytic anemia, thrombocytopenia and acute renal dysfunction. Proteinuria and hematuria can be seen.

Atypical HUS can occur both in children and adults with hypertension and proteinuria as common presenting features. Microangiopathic hemolytic anemia, thrombocytopenia, and acute renal dysfunction are seen in most patients. These patients can show reduced serum C3 levels. In addition serum factor H and I levels can be altered and anti-factor H antibodies can be detected.

On light microscopy, features of thrombotic microangiopathy are seen comprising thickened glomerular capillaries, endothelial cell swelling; fibrin and platelet-rich thrombi can also be seen in lumen of glomerular capillaries and in arterioles. In addition, fragmented red blood cells in mesangium, bloodless appearance of glomeruli, fibrinoid necrosis of blood vessels, or mucoid intimal hyperplasia in arteries can be seen. Chronic changes include mesangiolysis, double contour of glomerular capillary basement membranes, glomerulosclerosis, and arterial intimal fibrosis. A case of typical hemolytic uremic syndrome is illustrated in (Fig. 15.1). Atypical hemolytic uremic syndrome shows more pronounced vascular changes in the form of endothelial cell swelling, widening of subendothelial space, luminal narrowing, fibrinoid necrosis, and fragmented red blood cells in vessel wall. Immunofluorescence shows fibrin and non-specific IgM deposits within glomeruli and arterioles. Electron microscopy will show endothelial cell swelling, subendothelial expansion by electron-lucent material, fibrils in mesangium, capillary wall, and subendothelium (Fig 15.2).

P. Gupta, R. K. Gupta, *Pathology of Glomerular Diseases*, https://doi.org/10.1007/978-981-19-1430-0_15

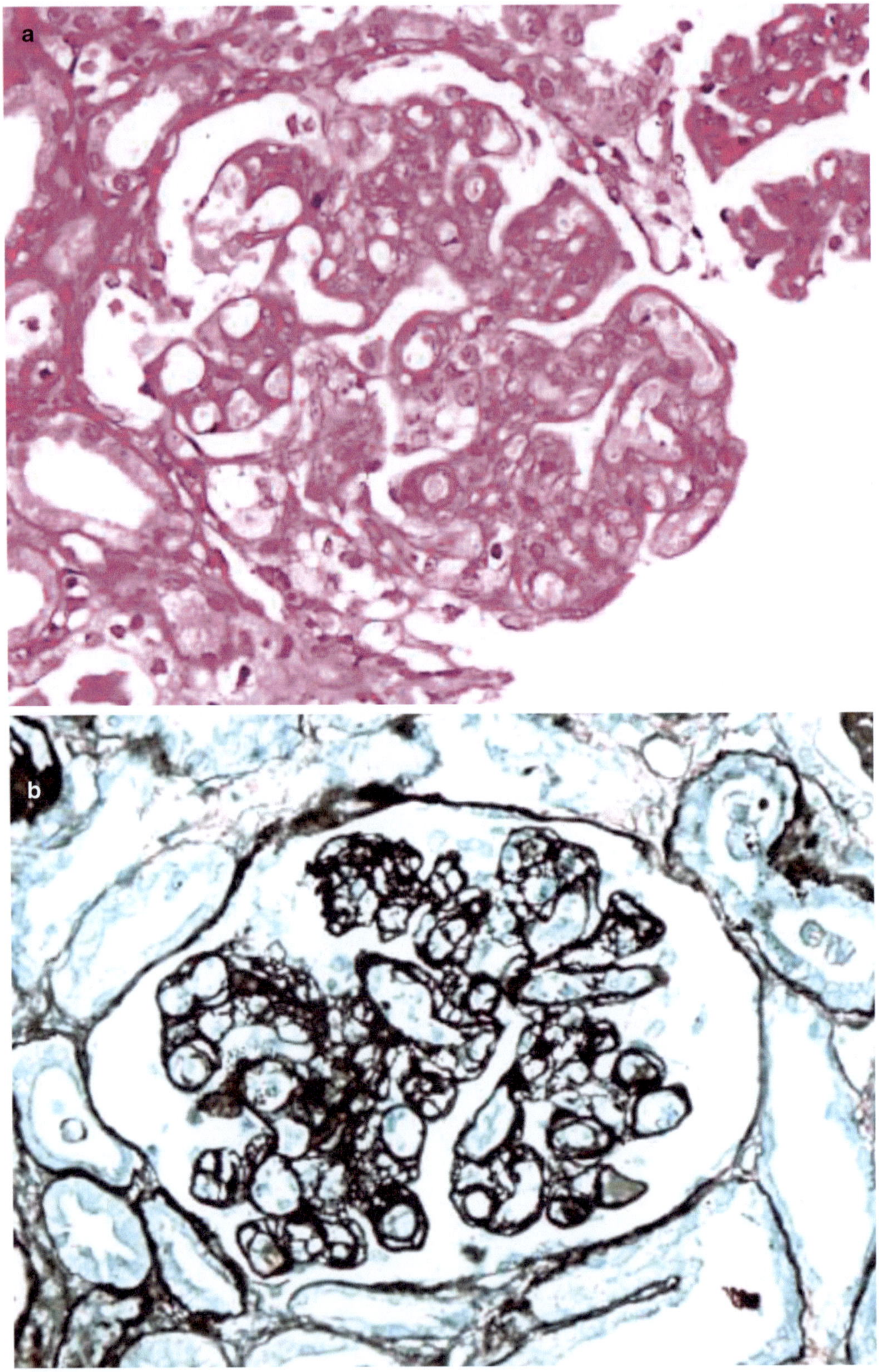

Fig. 15.1 **Typical HUS** A 21-years male patient with no co-morbidities, presented with decreased appetite and nausea associated with vomiting for 3 days. He also had h/o bloody diarrhea, 5–6 episodes/day for 3–4 days, 7 days back. USG KUB showed B/L unremarkable kidneys. On laboratory workup, he was found to have serum creatinine of 7.3 mg/dl and serum LDH was 1604, his hemoglobin was 7 g/dl and the platelet count was 85,000/cu mm. Peripheral blood smear showed bicytopenia with schitocyte index of 8.2%. Urine examination revealed 1+ proteinuria with numerous rbc and 10–15 wbc/hpf. Two core renal biopsy was obtained which revealed 42 glomeruli, some of the glomeruli showed congested capillary loops along with endothelial cell swelling, occasional fibrin thrombi in capillary loops and few had fibrillary appearance of mesangium; focal duplication of GBM was observed. Tubules showed flattening and distalization of lining epithelium along with RBC casts. Blood vessels showed mucoid intimal hyperplasia with luminal narrowing. Interstitium was edematous. IF for IgG, IgM, IgA, C3, C1q, kappa and lambda was uniformly negative. (**a**) HE × 400, (**b**) PSM × 400, and (**c**) HE × 400

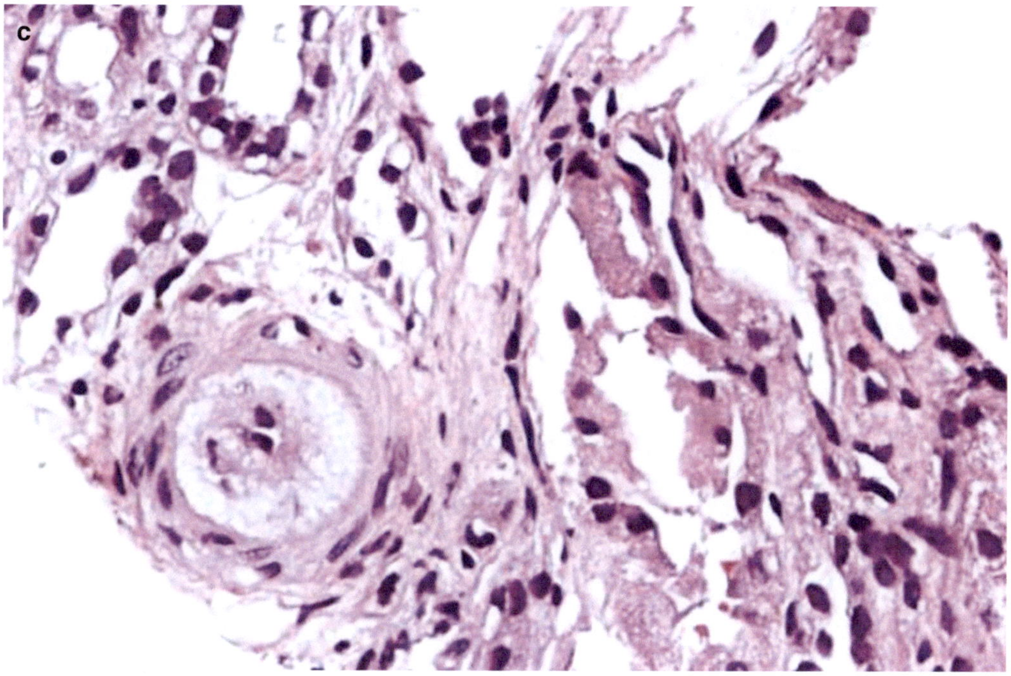

Fig. 15.1 (continued)

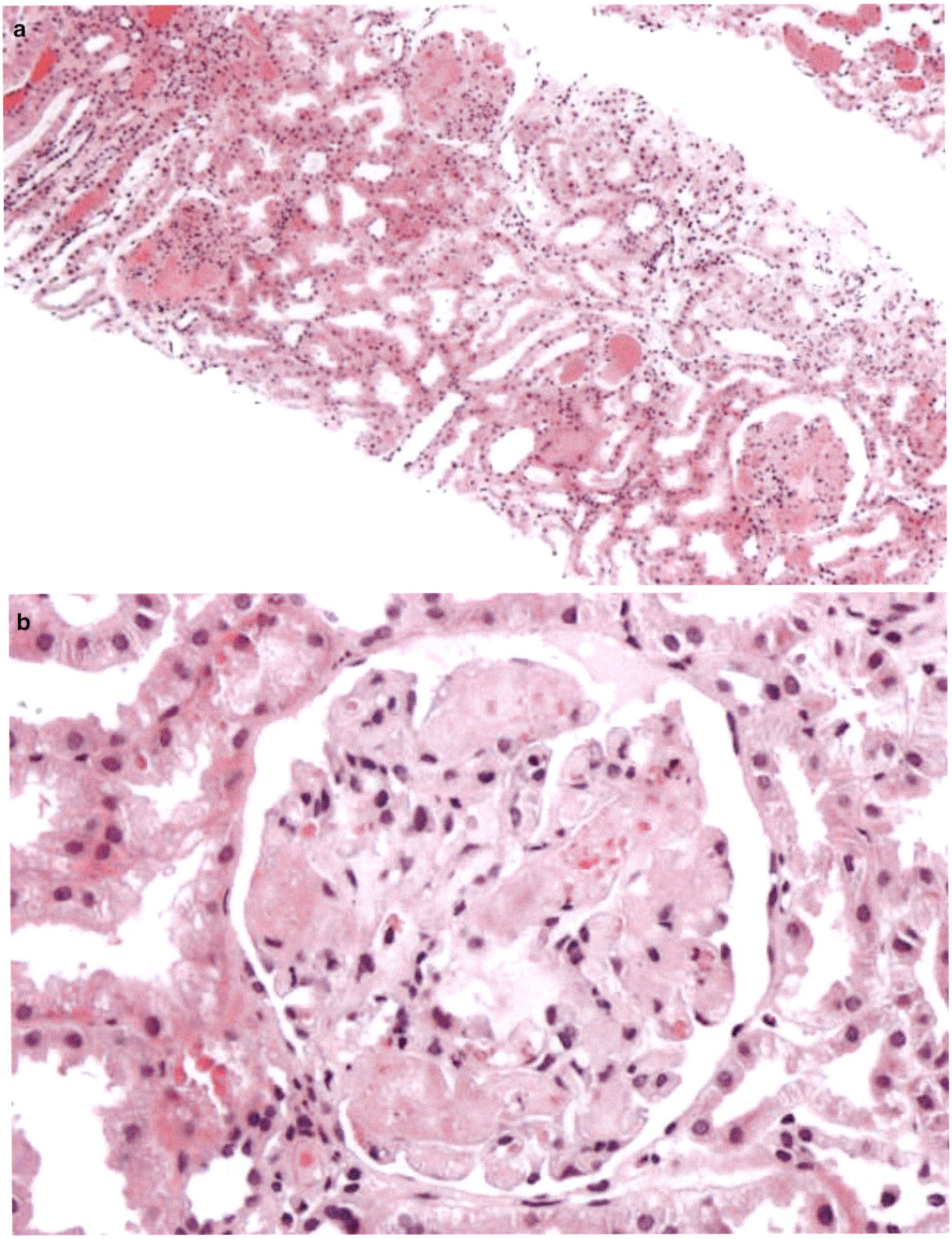

Fig. 15.2 Atypical HUS A 40-years male patient presented with nausea, lethargy, and reduced urine output; his blood pressure was 190/100 mm Hg. Urine analysis showed 1+ proteinuria and 8–10 RBC/hpf . His hemoglobin was 9.6 gm/dl and the platelet count was 1.2 lakhs/ cu mm; peripheral blood smear showed the presence of schistocytes (schistocyte index 2%). Serum creatinine was 5.5 mg/dl, BUN 32 mg/dl; serum C 3 was reduced to 950 mg/L and serum LDH was 530 IU/L. Two core renal biopsy was obtained which had 28 glomeruli of which four were globally sclerosed and one showed collapse of glomerular tuft; one of the glomerulus was enlarged and had loop necrosis. Fibrin thrombi were seen in glomerular capillary loops and arteriole at hilar pole. Remaining glomeruli showed thickening and wrinkling of glomerular capillary basement membrane; some of these glomeruli also showed fibrillary appearance of the mesangium. Focal tubular atrophy with interstitial mononuclear inflammatory infiltrate was also observed. Interlobular arteries and arterioles showed intimal mucoid edema, luminal narrowing along with onion peal appearance. IF showed mesangial positivity for IgM (+) and C3 (2+) and along the GBM. IgG, IgA, C1q, kappa and lambda were negative. EM showed focal effacement of foot processes of visceral epithelial cells. Basement membrane of few capillary loops showed prominent subendothelial rarefaction and accumulation of granular material in the widened subendothelial spaces. Endothelial swelling, focal neo-basement membrane formation was discernible. No electron dense/organized deposits were observed in glomerular capillaries or mesangial areas. (**a**) HE × 100, (**b–d**) HE × 400, (**e**) MT × 400, (**f**) PSM × 400, (**g**) HE × 200, (**h**) PAS × 200, (**i**) MT × 200 and (**j**, **k**) EM (identity of the patient has been concealed)

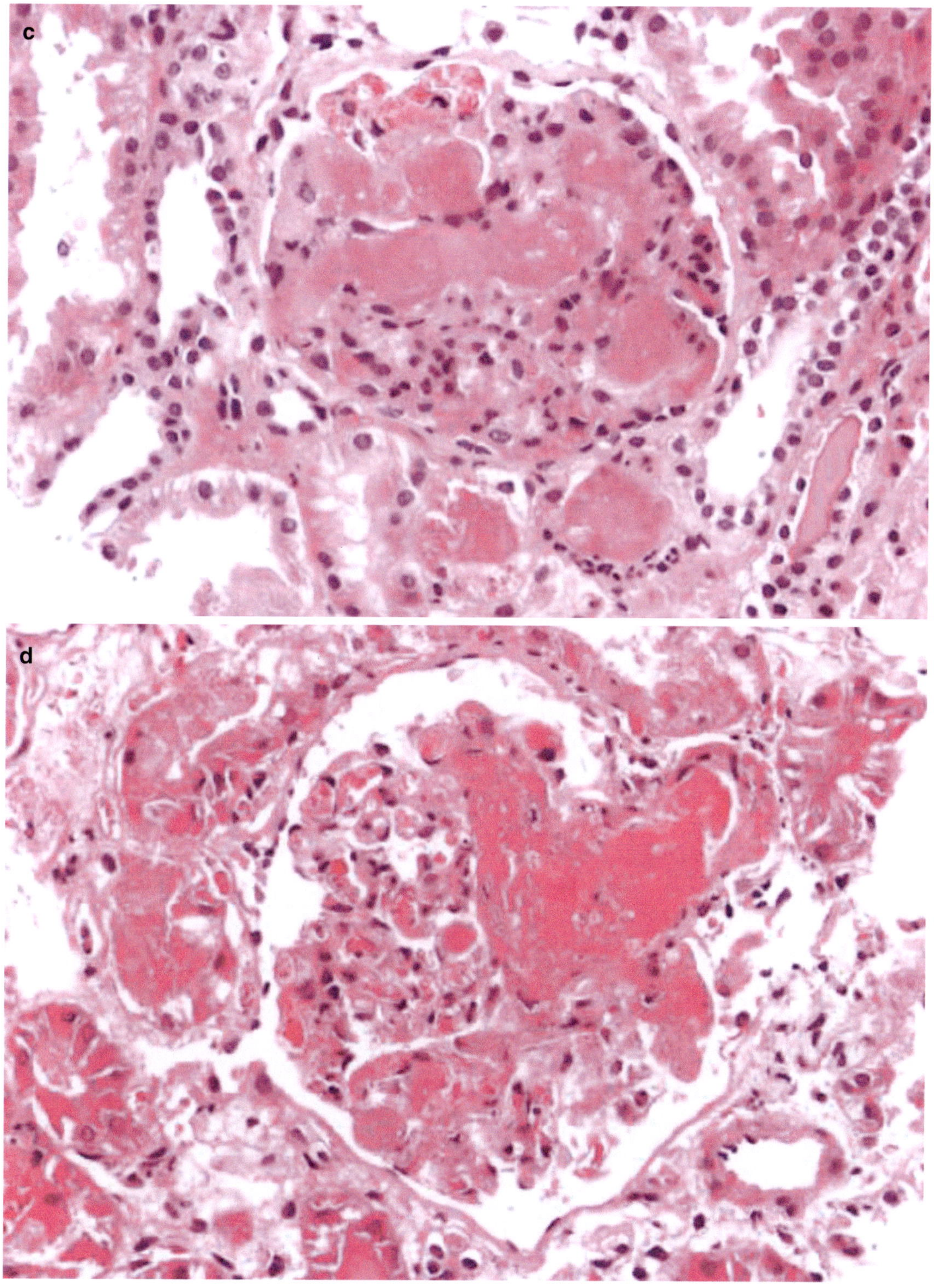

Fig. 15.2 (continued)

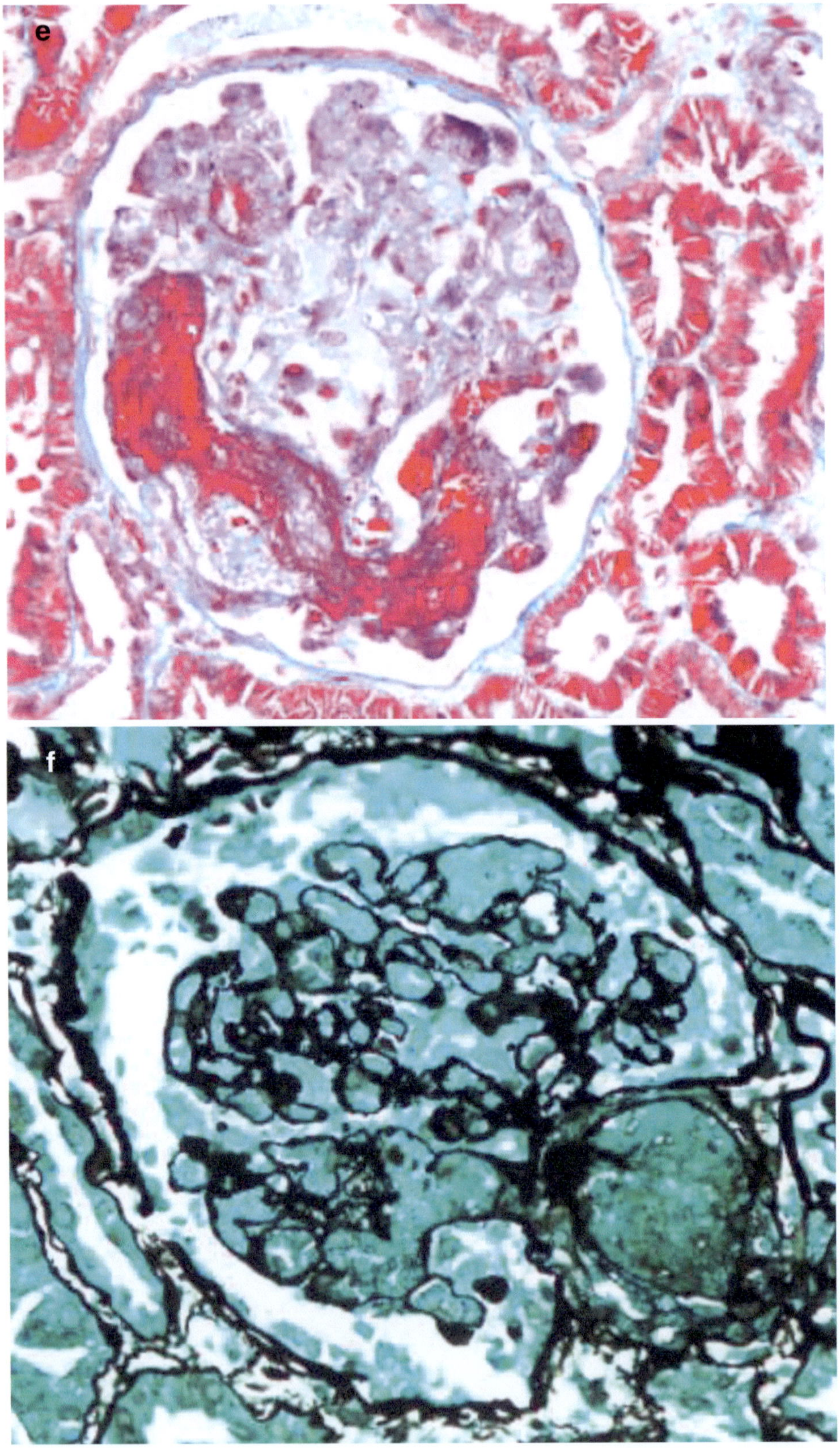

Fig. 15.2 (continued)

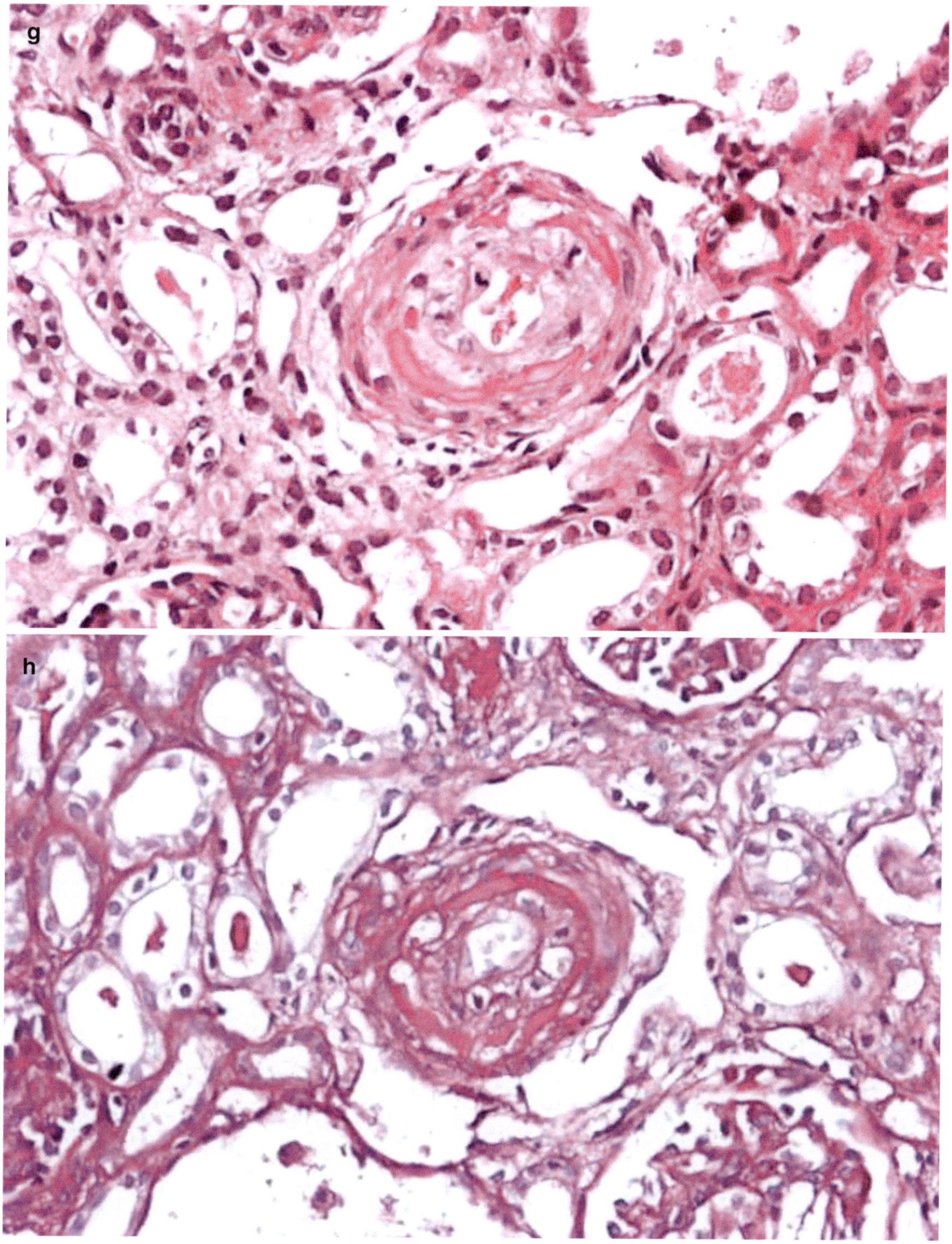

Fig. 15.2 (continued)

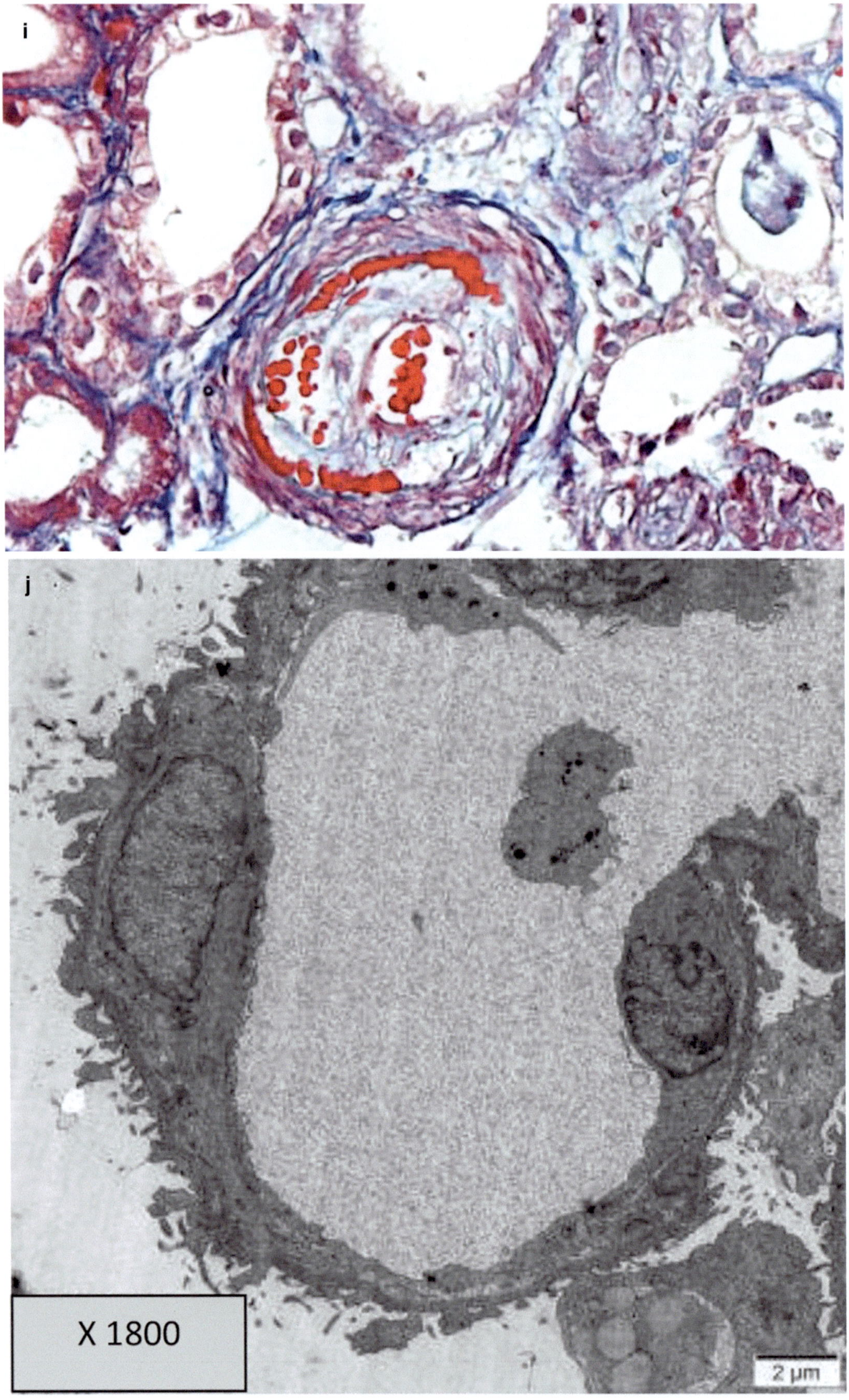

Fig. 15.2 (continued)

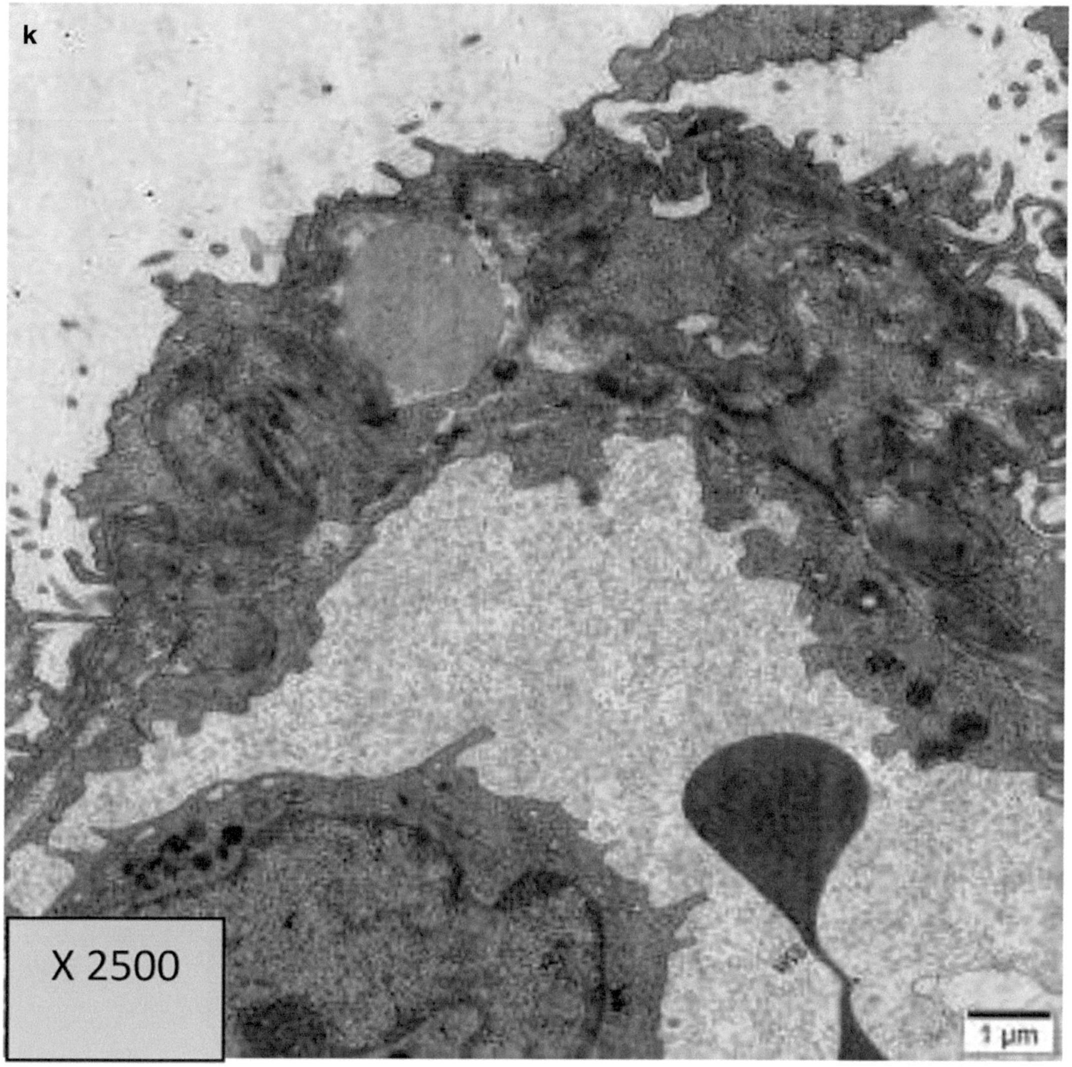

Fig. 15.2 (continued)

Further Reading

Bitzan M, Lapeyraque AL. Postinfectious hemolytic uremic syndrome. Pediatr Kidney Dis. 2016;2016:653–731.

Canpolat N. Hemolytic uremic syndrome. Turk Pediatri Ars. 2015;50:73–82.

Joseph A, Cointe A, Mariani Kurkdjian P, Rafat C, Hertig A. Shiga toxin-associated hemolytic uremic syndrome: a narrative review. Toxins (Basel). 2020;12:67.

Lee H, Kang E, Kang HG, et al. Consensus regarding diagnosis and management of atypical hemolytic uremic syndrome. Korean J Intern Med. 2020;35:25–40.

Yoshida Y, Kato H, Ikeda Y, Nangaku M. Pathogenesis of atypical hemolytic uremic syndrome. J Atheroscler Thromb. 2019;26:99–110.5.

Zhang K, Lu Y, Harley KT, Tran MH. Atypical hemolytic uremic syndrome: a brief review. Hematol Rep. 2017;9:7053.

16 Diabetic Nephropathy

Diabetic nephropathy is one of the important complications of diabetes mellitus and is an important cause of end-stage renal disease worldwide. Clinically patients with diabetic nephropathy initially have microalbuminuria (30–300 mg/day) and later develop frank proteinuria (>300 mg/day). There can be accompanying microscopic hematuria in a few patients. With the progression of renal disease, rise in serum creatinine and deteriorating GFR are evident. Renal biopsy changes are characterized into four different classes by Tervaert. Class I shows features of early diabetic nephropathy with normal-appearing glomeruli or with mild thickening of glomerular capillary basement membrane demonstrated by electron microscopy (GBM thickness more than 430 nm in patients 9 years and older and >395 nm in females). Class II diabetic nephropathy is also called diffuse diabetic glomerulosclerosis and is characterized by mesangial expansion (Fig 16.1). Class III diabetic nephropathy (nodular sclerosis) shows Kimmelstiel-Wilson lesions (Fig 16.2). Class IV shows global glomerulosclerosis involving >50% glomeruli and is also called advanced diabetic glomerulosclerosis. Other glomerular lesions seen in diabetic nephropathy include fibrin cap and capsular drop. Thickening of tubular basement membrane, varying degrees of interstitial fibrosis and tubular atrophy, afferent arteriolar hyalinosis, and arteriosclerosis can also be seen. On Immunofluorescence, sometimes linear staining of IgG can be observed along glomerular capillary basement membrane. On electron microscopy thickening of glomerular capillary basement membrane, mesangial widening and varying degrees of podocyte foot process effacement can be seen. Nonspecific mesangial fibrils can be observed in few patients with nodular glomerulosclerosis and this is referred as Diabetic Fibrillosis (Fig 16.3). These changes were first described in the 1970s and are seen secondary to chronic injury to mesangium. At times they need to be differentiated from amyloid fibrils (congored positive) and fibrillary glomerulonephritis (DNAJB9-positive and larger fibril size of 12–20 nm in diameter and also positive immunofluorescence for immunoglobulin IgG) Non diabetic glomerular diseases can be observed in patients with type 2 diabetes either alone or on a background of diabetic nephropathy and include membranous nephropathy, FSGS, amyloidosis, IgA nephropathy and post infectious glomerulonephritis. A case of post infectious glomerulonephritis on background of diabetic nephropathy is illustrated (Fig. 16.4).

P. Gupta, R. K. Gupta, *Pathology of Glomerular Diseases*, https://doi.org/10.1007/978-981-19-1430-0_16

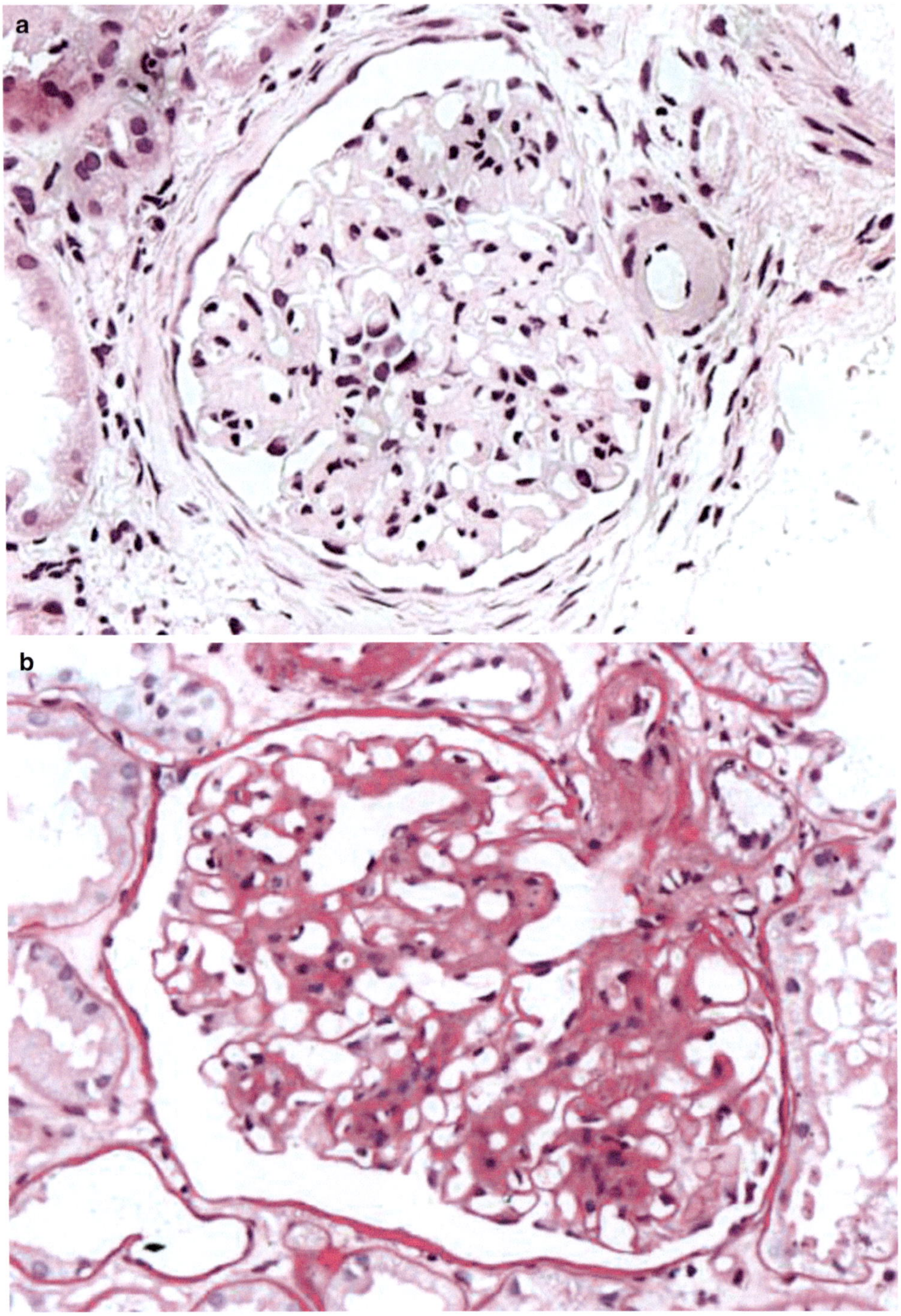

Fig. 16.1 **Class II DN** A 43-years male patient, known to have hypertension and type II DM for 10 years, presented with anasarca. Urine analysis revealed protein 3+ with bland sediment, urinary P/C ratio was 8. Serum creatinine was 1.1 mg/dL. Fasting blood glucose was 168 mg/dl with HbA1c of 7.2%. Renal biopsy showed 11 glomeruli, all showed diffuse increase in mesangial matrix with focal increase in its cellularity. GBM showed diffuse thickening; some of the glomeruli showed solidification of glomerular tuft. Hyalinosis of afferent arteriole with moderate hyaline arteriosclerosis was also observed. Interstitium showed moderate mixed inflammatory cell infiltrate and mild tubular atrophy with thickened tubular basement membrane. (**a**) HE × 400, (**b–e**) PAS × 400

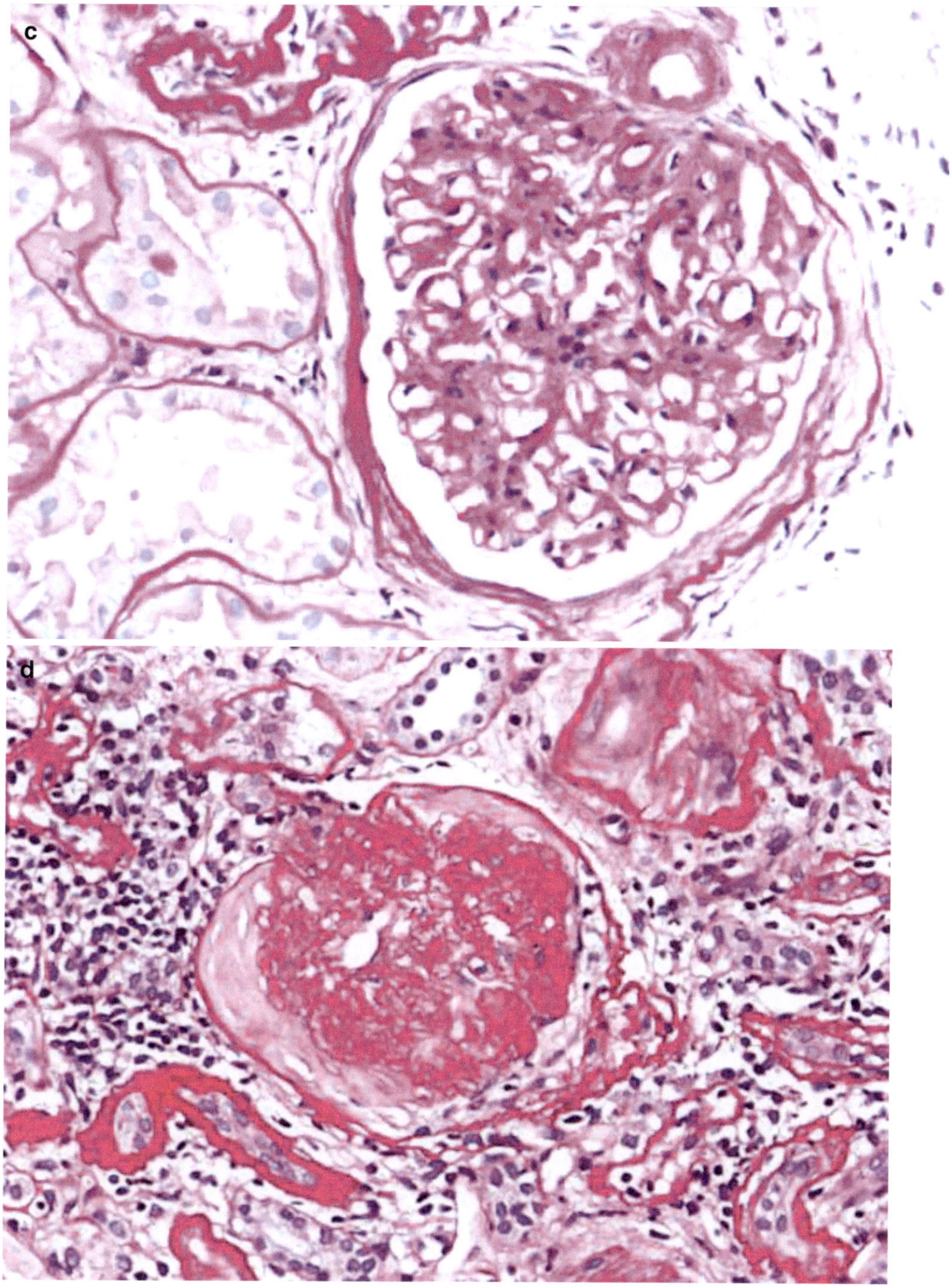

Fig. 16.1 (continued)

e

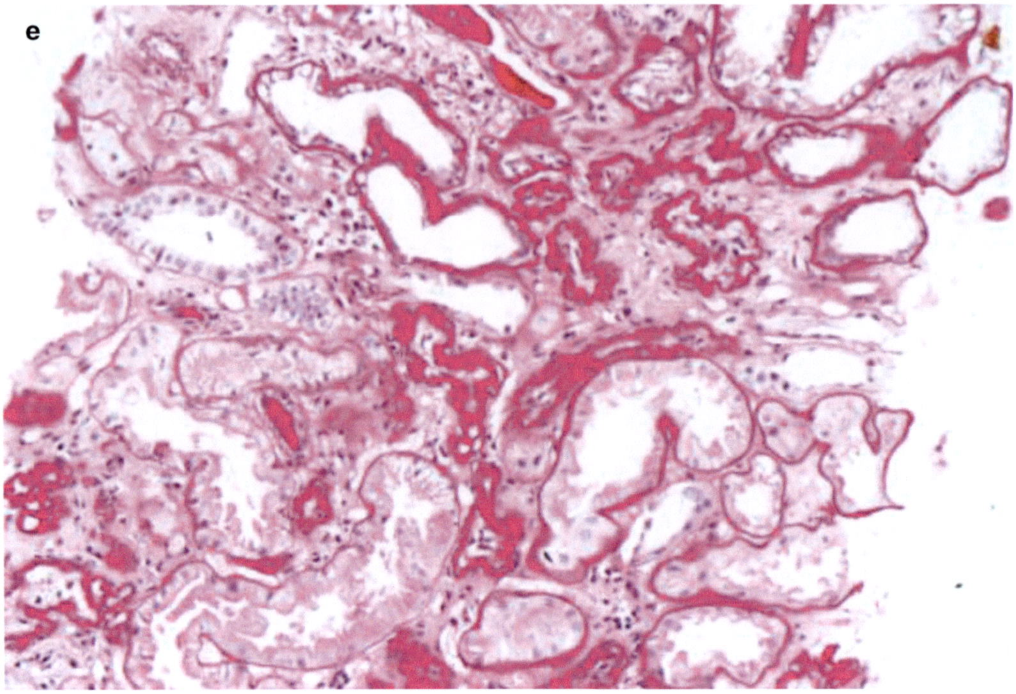

Fig. 16.1 (continued)

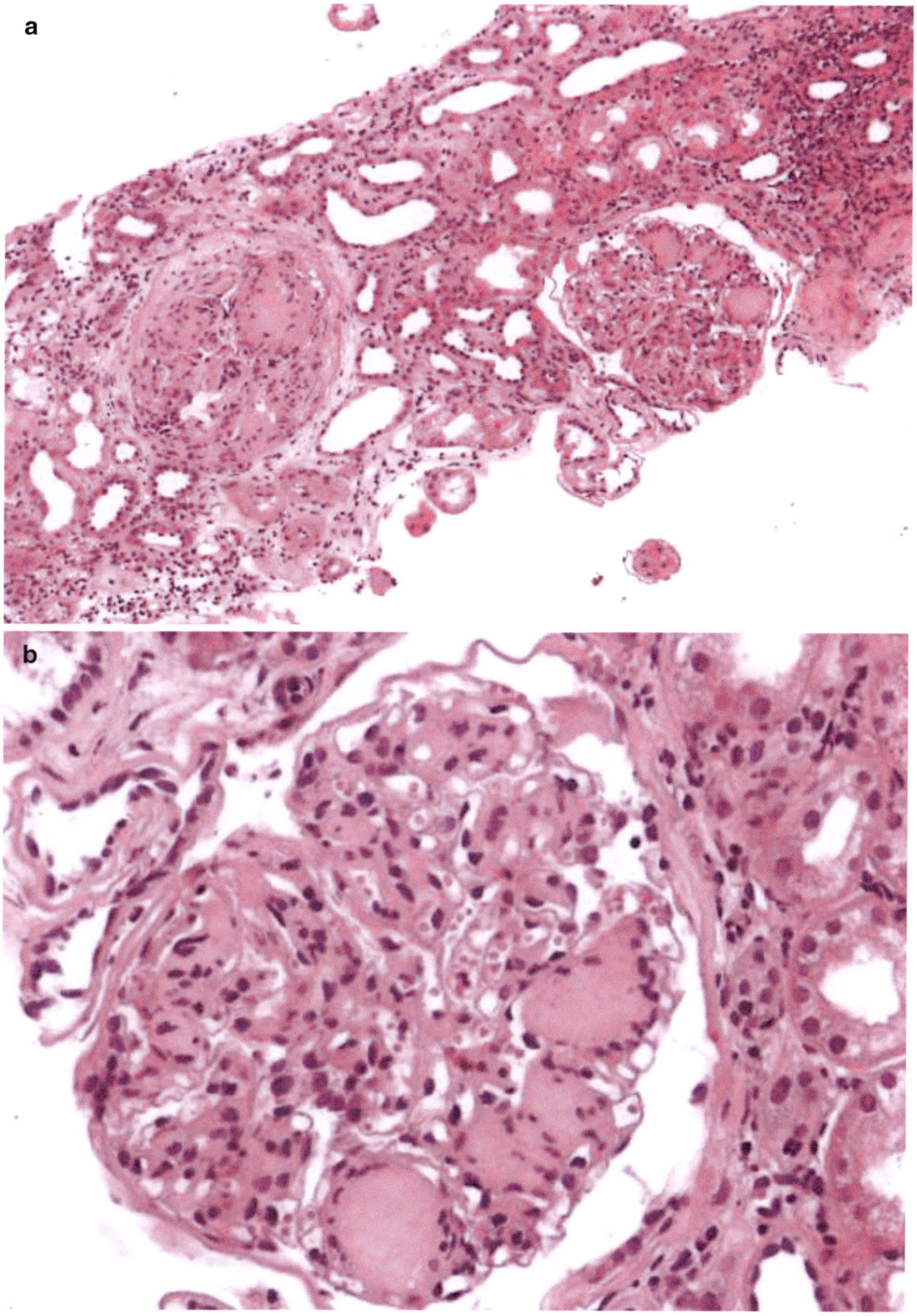

Fig. 16.2 **Class III DN** A 56-years male patient known to have type II DM and hypertension, presented with pedal edema and nephrotic range proteinuria. Urine analysis revealed 3+ proteinuria with P/C ratio of 3.1 and serum creatinine was 7.5 mg/dl. Renal biopsy had 10 glomeruli, six were globally sclerosed and four showed mesangial expansion with the formation of mesangial nodules (KW lesion), periglomerular fibrosis was also present. Moderate tubular atrophy with mild interstitial lymphocytic infiltration was evident. The blood vessels showed hyaline arteriosclerosis. Immunofluorescence for IgG, IgM, IgA, C3, C1q, kappa and lambda light chains was negative. EM showed glomerular capillary basement membrane thickening with marked mesangial expansion and effacement of podocyte foot processes. (**a**) HE × 100, (**b**) HE × 400, (**c**) PAS × 100, (**d**) PAS × 400, (**e**) PSM × 400, (**f** and **g**) EM (identity of the patient has been concealed)

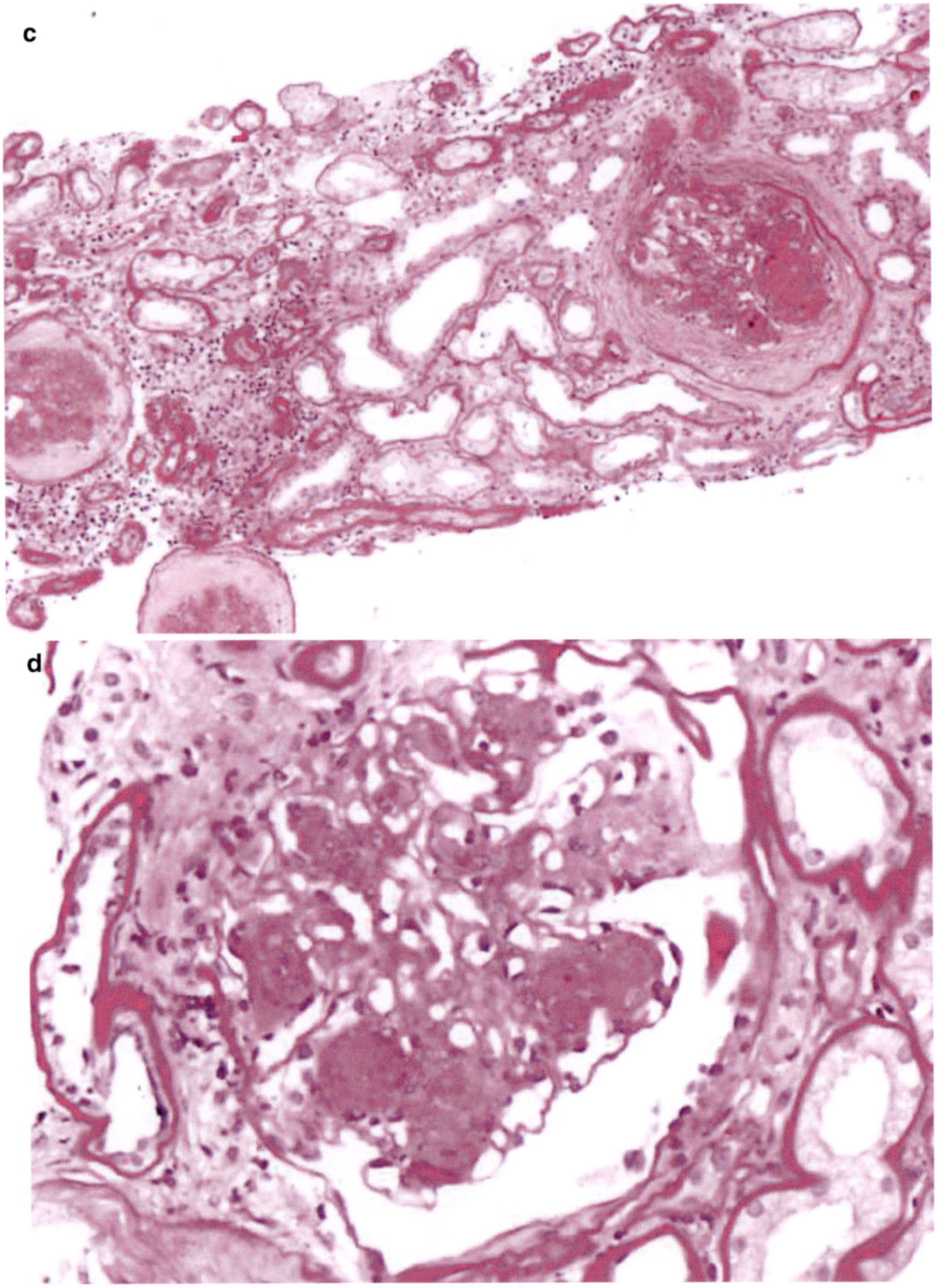

Fig. 16.2 (continued)

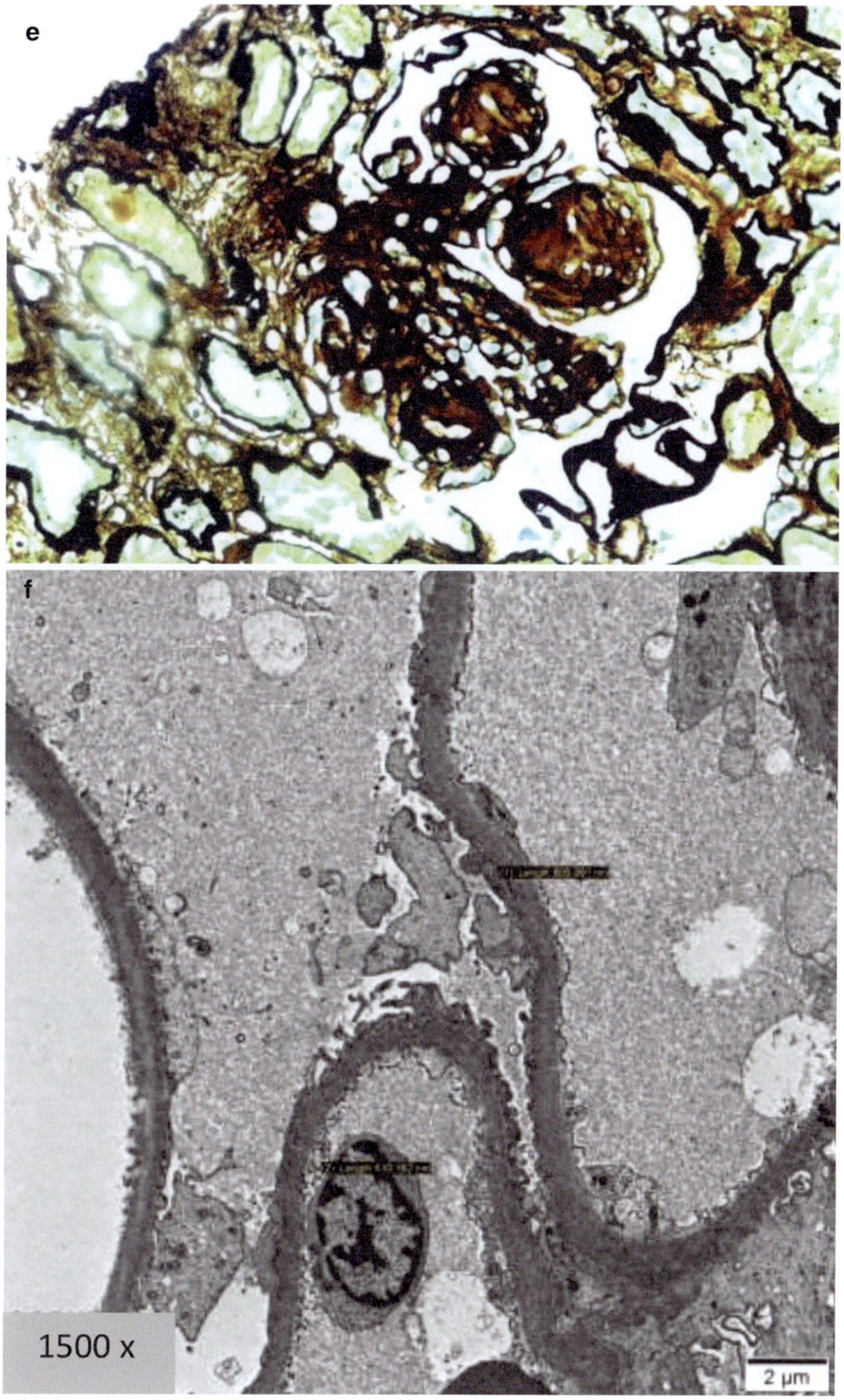

Fig. 16.2 (continued)

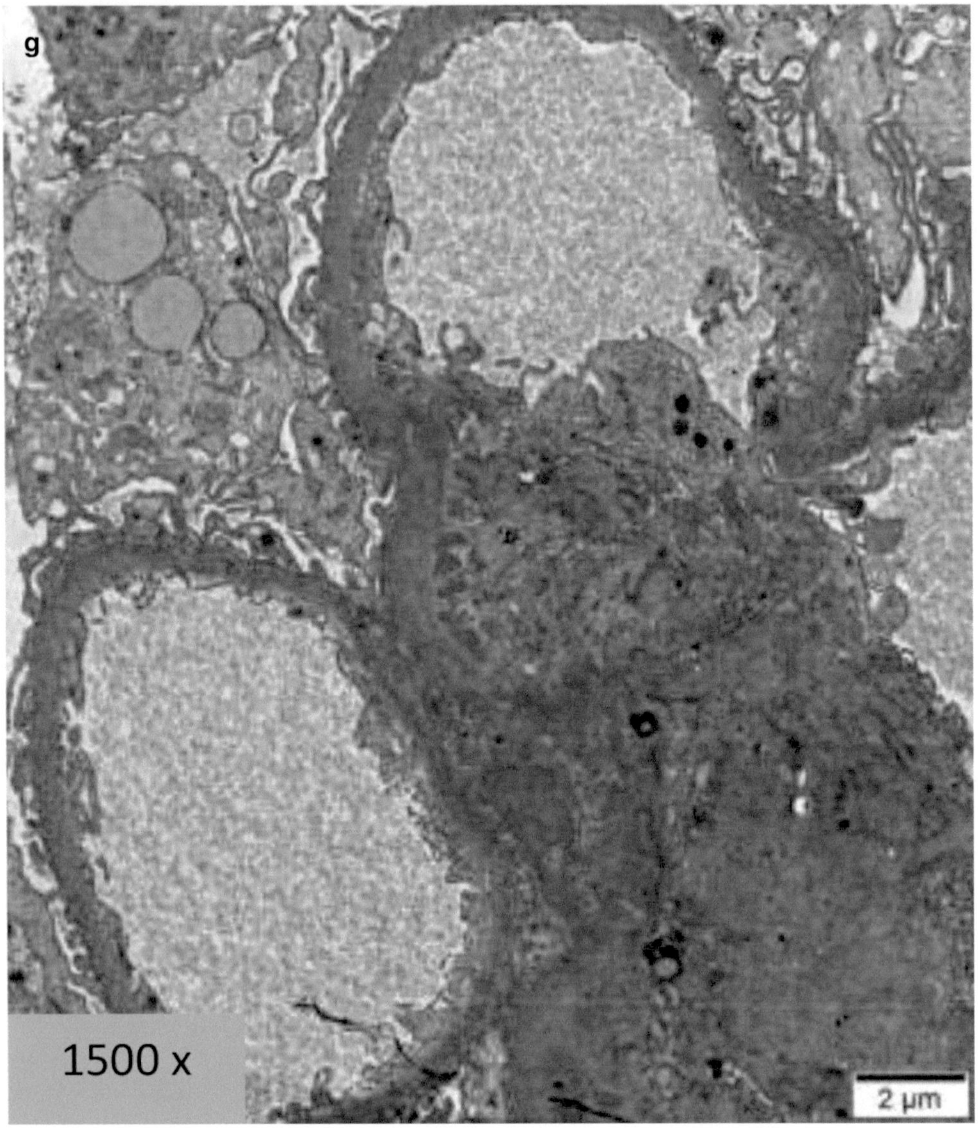

Fig. 16.2 (continued)

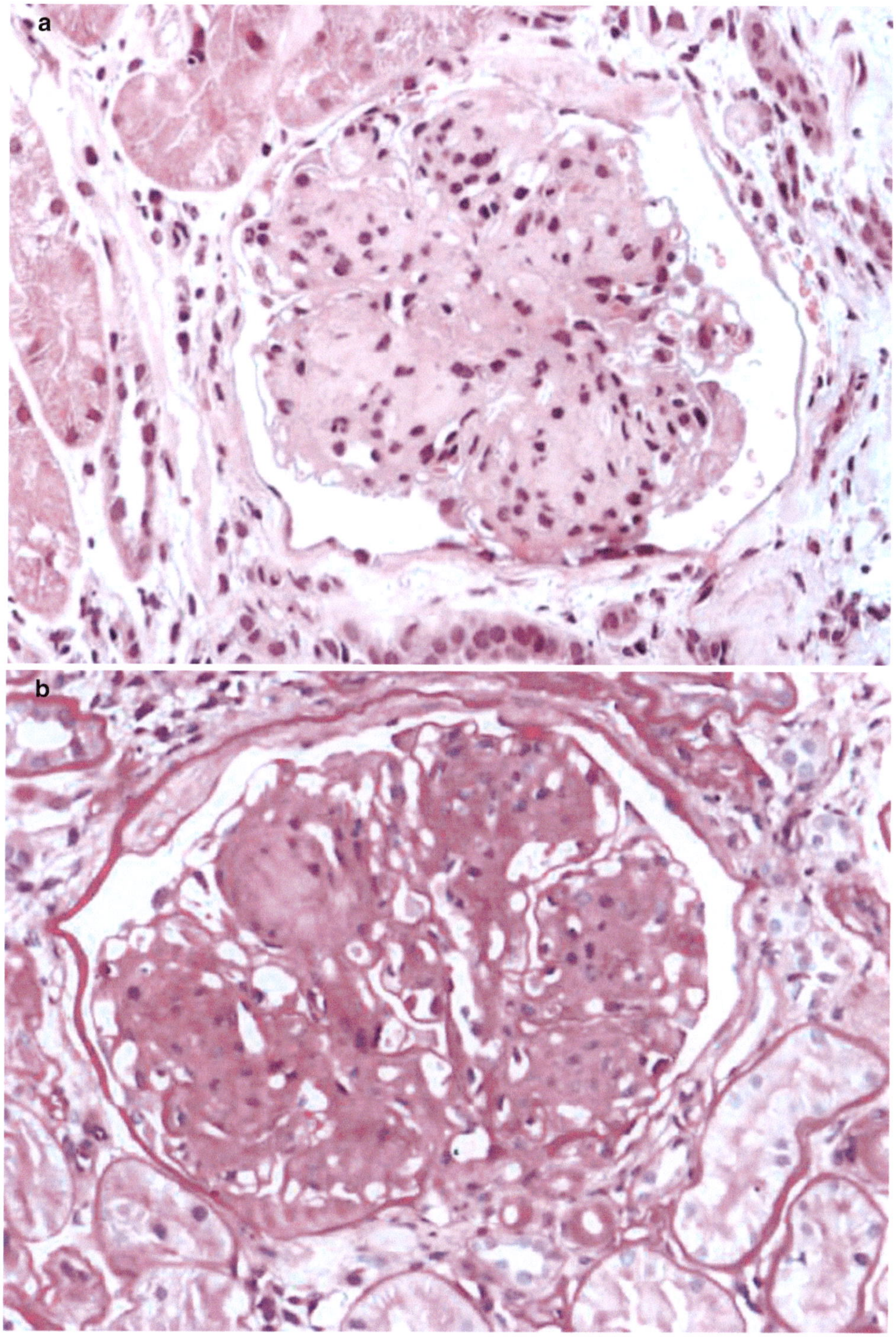

Fig. 16.3 Diabetic Fibrillosis A 34-years male patient with h/o diabetes mellitus for the past nine years presented with nephrotic range proteinuria and mild renal dysfunction. Patient had bilateral pedal edema. There was no history of hematuria. On fundus examination, there was no evidence of diabetic retinopathy. Patient also had history of tuberculosis 5 years back. Blood pressure was within normal limits. Lab investigations revealed 24 h urine protein of 16 g, Serum creatinine of 2.1 mg/dl, urine analysis showed proteins 3+, no active sediments. Hb was 12.2 gm% with total WBC count of 6800/cu mm. Renal Biopsy showed 16 glomeruli, 6 were globally sclerosed. Remaining glomeruli showed mesangial nodules of varying sizes with patent capillary loops at periphery in a few of them. These nodules were weakly PAS-positive and also weak PSM-positive. Glomerular capillary basement membrane appeared thickened. Periglomerular fibrosis was seen. Tubular atrophy, interstitial fibrosis, and arteriolar hyalinosis were seen. Congored for amyloid was negative. IHC for type III collagen was also negative. Immunofluorescence microscopy did not show any immunoglobulin, complement or light chain deposits. On electron microscopy GBM appeared diffusely thickened (mean 678 nm), mesangium appeared markedly expanded. Nonbanded, nonbranching fibrillary structures (9–16 nm) were seen with focal streaming pattern. No electron-dense deposits were seen. (**a**) H E × 400, (**b**) PAS × 400, (**c**) PAS × 200, (**d**) PSM × 400, (**e**–**g**) EM (identity of the patient has been concealed)

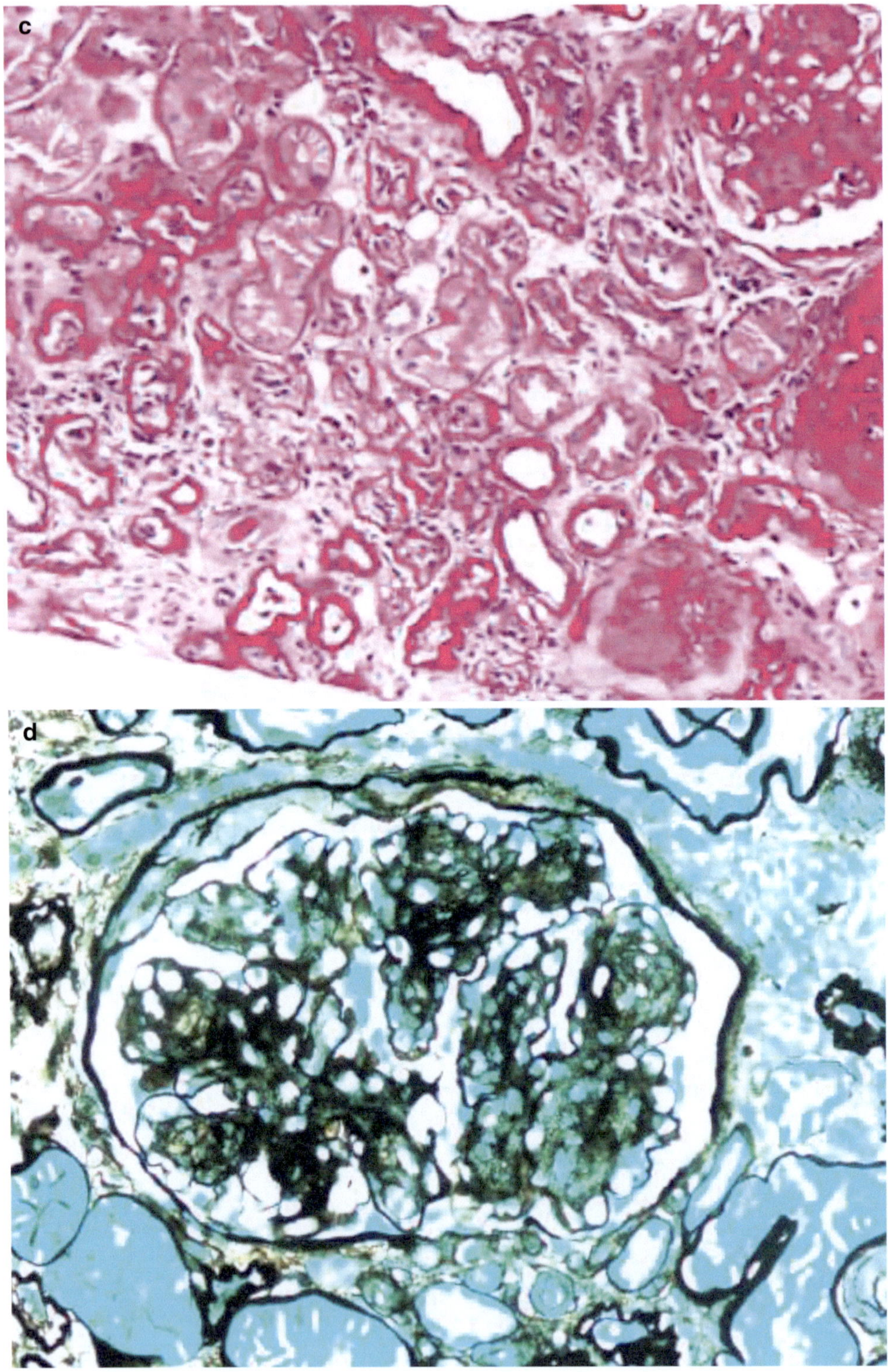

Fig. 16.3 (continued)

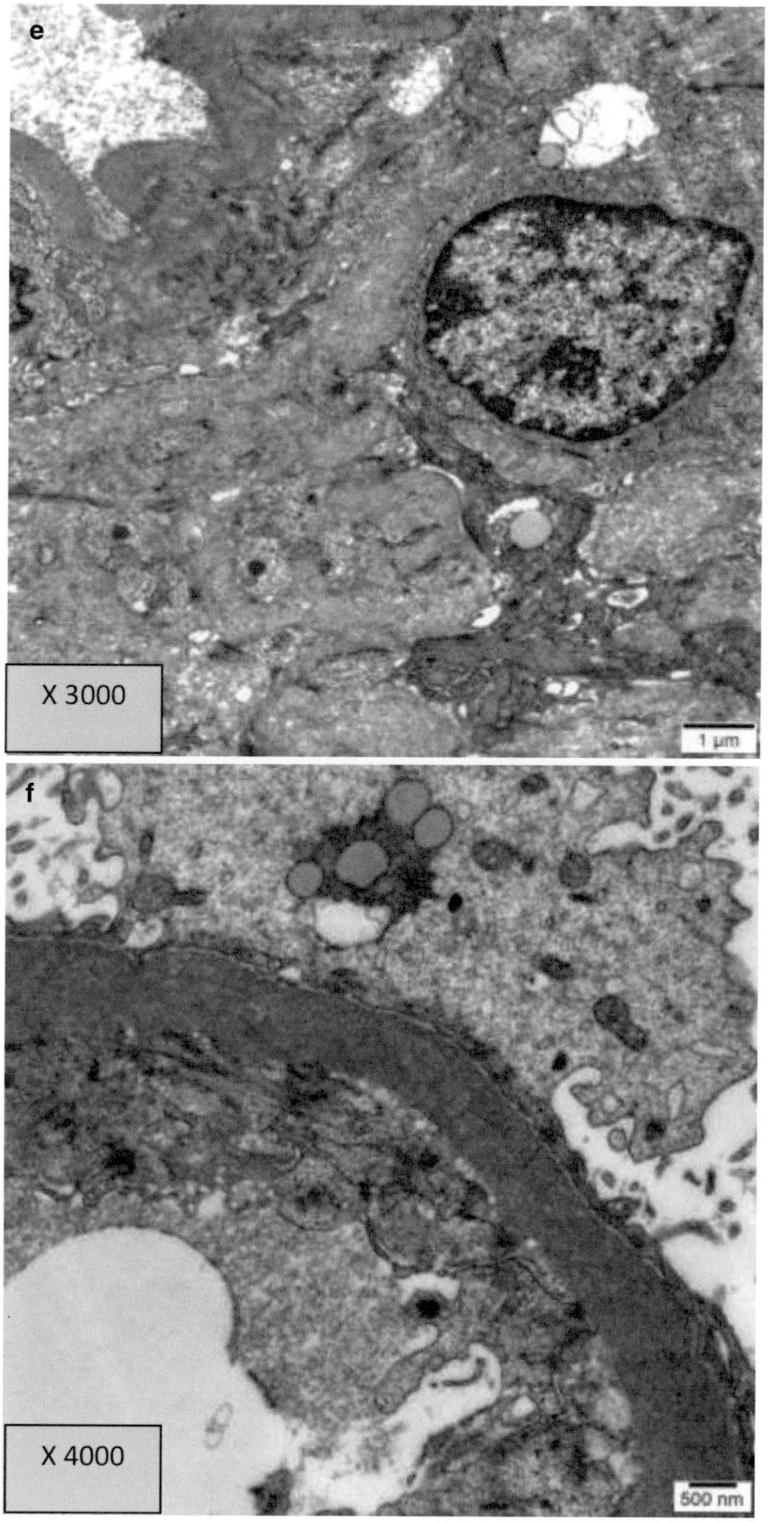

Fig. 16.3 (continued)

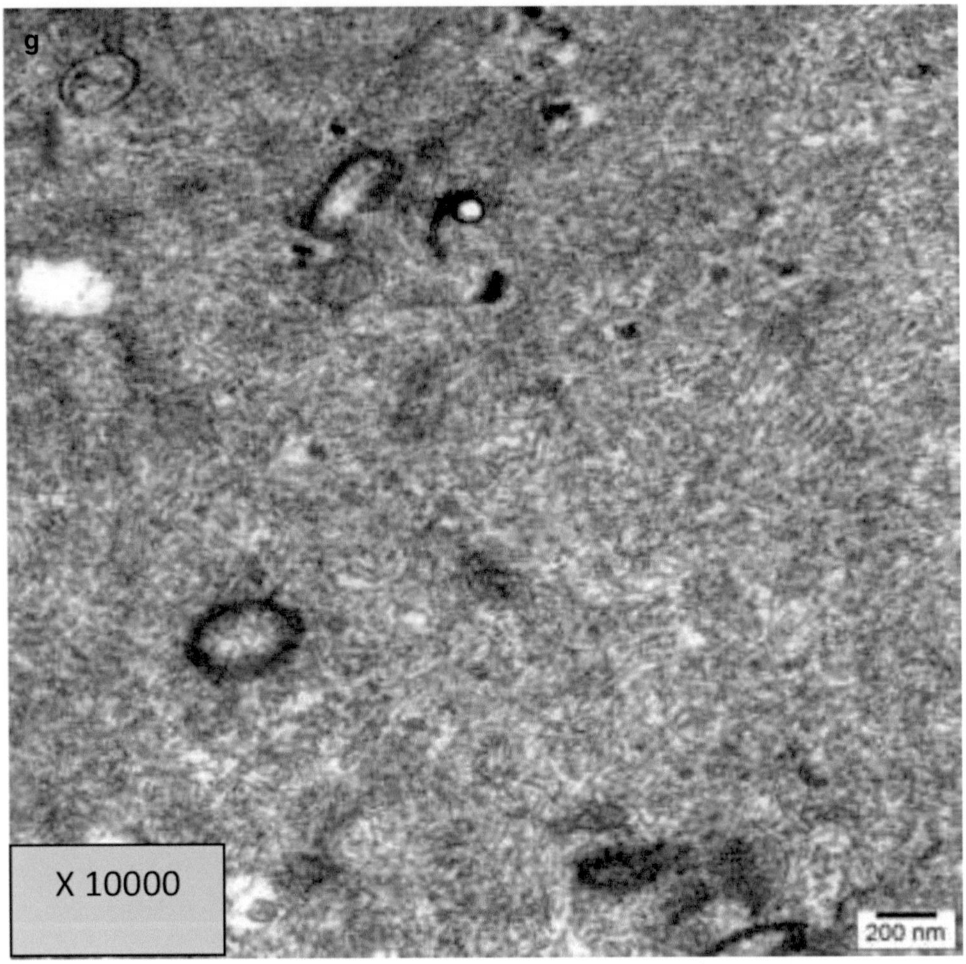

Fig. 16.3 (continued)

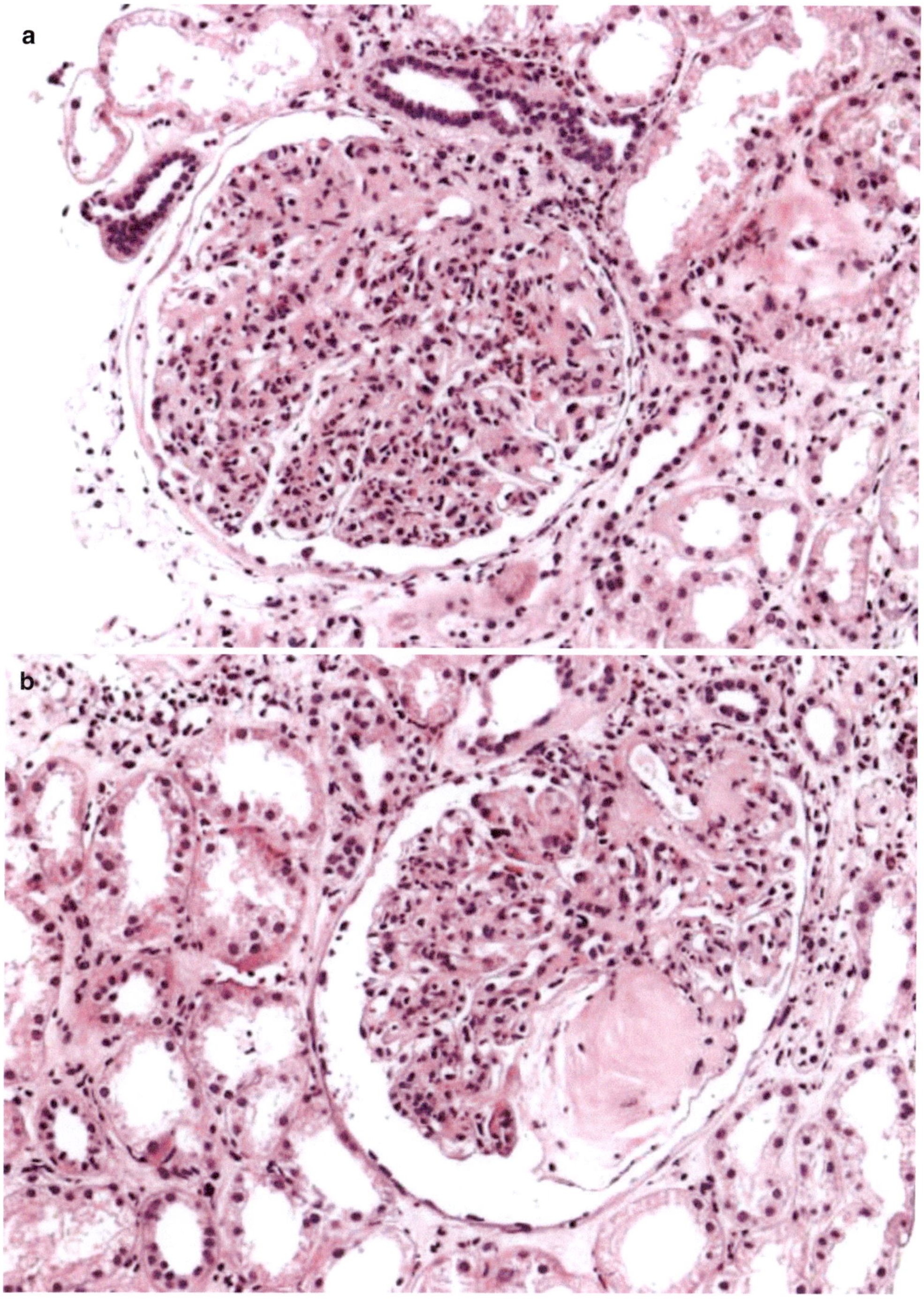

Fig. 16.4 PIGN on background of DN A 53-years male patient, known to have type II diabetes mellitus for the last 14 years, presented with pedal edema. He suffered URTI 3 weeks back. Urine examination revealed nephrotic range proteinuria (+++) with microscopic hematuria (30–40 RBC/hpf); P/C ratio was 3.2. His HbA1C level was 7.8% and serum creatinine was 3.5 mg/dl. ASO titer was >200 U. Serum complement C3 was low being 762 mg/L and C4 was wnl; ANCA was negative. Renal biopsy showed 14 glomeruli and all were enlarged with an accentuated lobular pattern, endocapillary hyperplasia with neutrophilic infiltration. The glomeruli also had associated nodular diabetic glomerulosclerosis. Silver stain also showed mild thickening of GBM with segmental GBM double contour, the diabetic KW nodule was also silver positive. IF for IgG, C3 and C1q showed glomerular capillary wall and mesangial immune deposits. EM Showed subepithelial hump with scattered subendothelial and mesangial electron-dense deposits. (**a**) HE × 200, (**b**) HE × 400, (**c**) PSM × 200, (**d–f**) IF × 400. (**g**) EM (identity of the patient has been concealed)

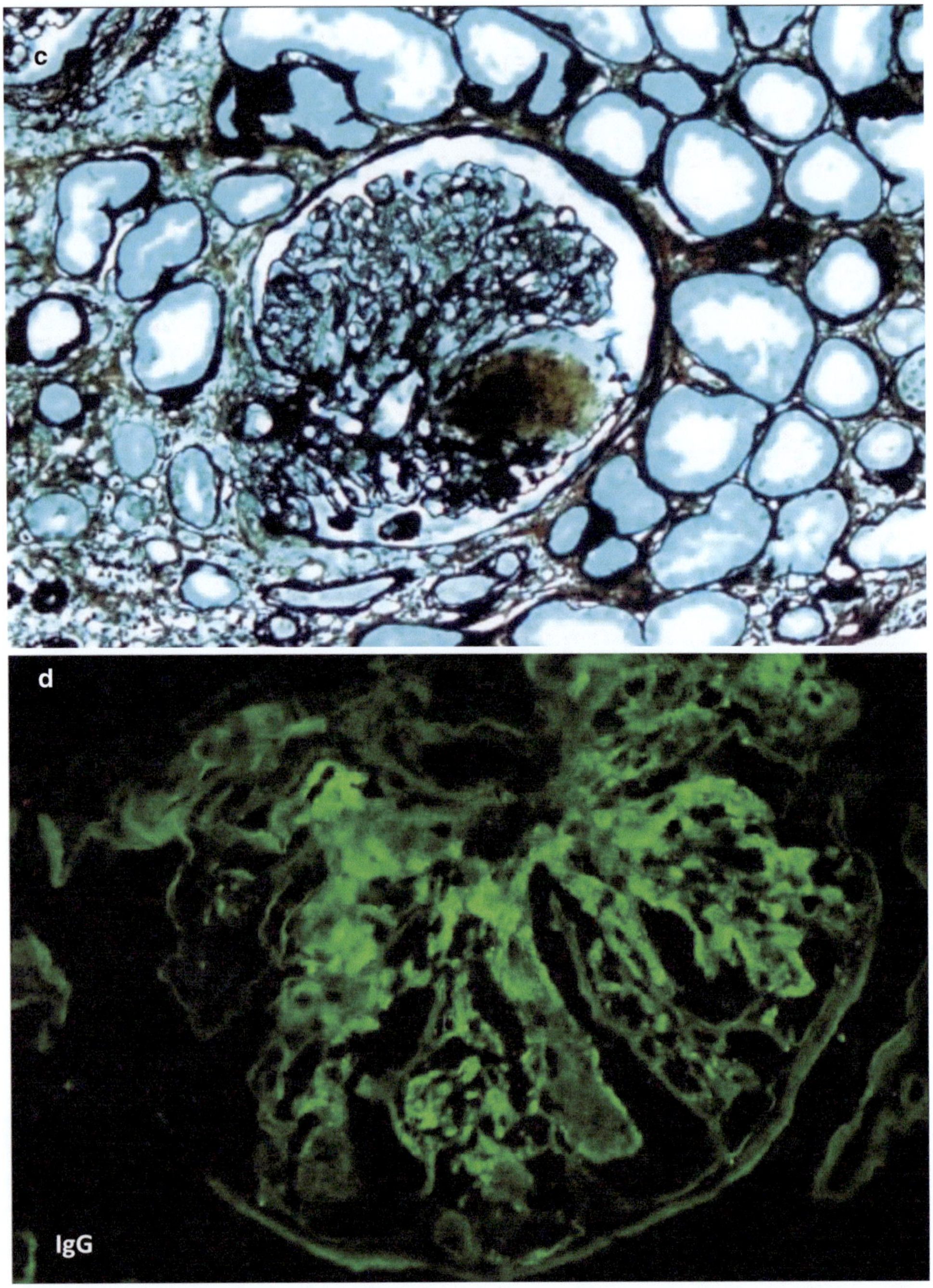

Fig. 16.4 (continued)

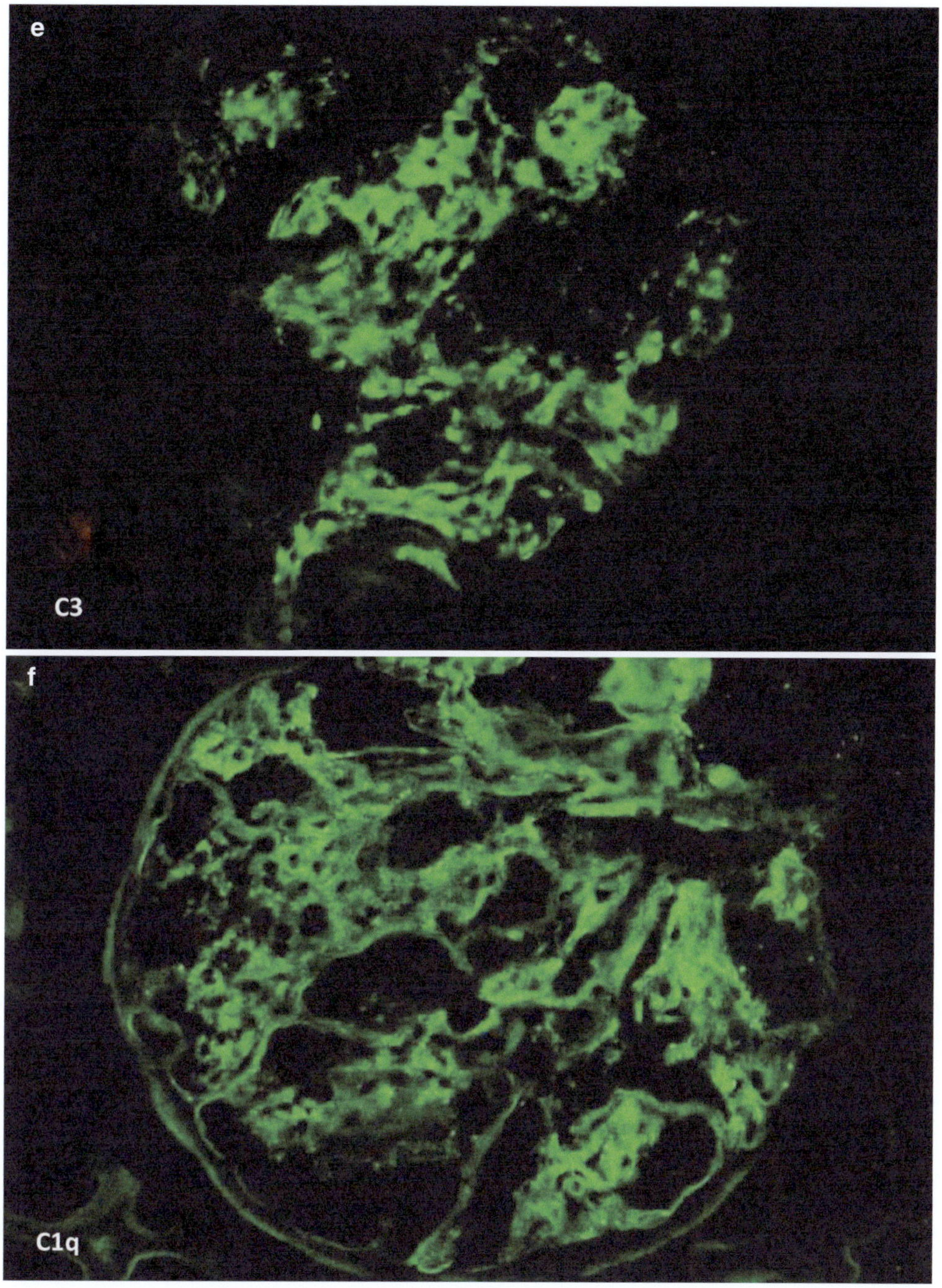

Fig. 16.4 (continued)

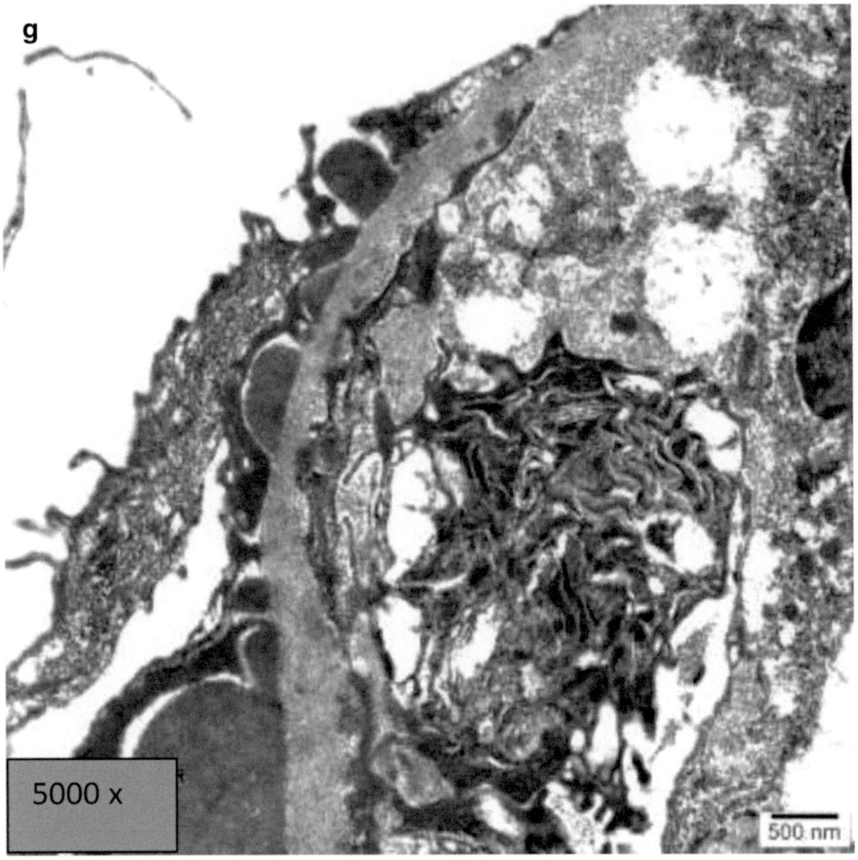

Fig. 16.4 (continued)

Further Reading

Alsaad KO, Herzenberg AM. Distinguishing diabetic nephropathy from other causes of glomerulosclerosis: an update. J Clin Pathol. 2007;60:18–26.

Qi C, Mao X, Zhang Z, Wu H. Classification and differential diagnosis of diabetic nephropathy. J Diabetes Res. 2017;2017:8637138.

Sohar E, Ravid M, Ben-Shaul Y, Reshef T, Gafni J. Diabetic fibrillosis. A report of three cases. Am J Med. 1970;1970(49):64–9.

Tervaert TW, Mooyaart AL, Amann K, Cohen AH, Cook HT, Drachenberg CB, Ferrario F, Fogo AB, Haas M, de Heer E, Joh K, Noël LH, Radhakrishnan J, Seshan SV, Bajema IM, Bruijn JA, Renal Pathology Society. Pathologic classification of diabetic nephropathy. J Am Soc Nephrol. 2010;21:556–63.

Tung CW, Hsu YC, Shih YH, Chang PJ, Lin CL. Glomerular mesangial cell and podocyte injuries in diabetic nephropathy. Nephrology (Carlton). 2018;23(Suppl 4):32–7.

Valk EJ, Bruijn JA, Bajema IM. Diabetic nephropathy in humans: pathologic diversity. Curr Opin Nephrol Hypertens. 2011;20:285–9.

17 Renal Amyloidosis

Amyloidosis is a systemic disorder characterized by the extracellular deposition of amorphous acellular fibrillary material in organs. The amyloidosis can be a result of deposition of abnormal protein like AL as seen in patients with myeloma, mutant thyretin as in cases of familial Mediterranean fever, or as a result of deposition of excess of normal protein as in cases of AA amyloidosis (chronic inflammatory disorder like rheumatoid arthritis), Aβ2M as in patients on long term dialysis. More than 30 amyloid proteins have been described.

Renal amyloidosis presents as massive proteinuria which can be in the form of nephrotic syndrome. Renal dysfunction may also be seen.

On light microscopy, glomerular deposition of the amyloid begins in the mesangium with later involvement of peripheral glomerular capillary walls. Mesangial deposits may be diffuse or have nodular configuration. Arteriole at the hilar pole can also show similar deposits. Sometimes crescents can be seen. Peritubular, interstitial, and vascular deposits can accompany glomerular deposits and can also be seen in isolation. In the vasculature, arterioles, arteries, and even peritubular capillaries can show deposition of amyloid. Amyloid deposits stain with congo red and appear salmon pink with apple green birefringence under polarized light. Thioflavin T stain also gives green fluorescence to the amyloid deposits when viewed on immunofluorescence microscopy and may be more sensitive in picking up small amyloid deposits.

Amyloid protein can be further subtyped by using Immunofluorescence, immunohistochemistry, or mass spectrometry to identify specific types of amyloid proteins which aids in the management. AL and AA amyloid proteins are the two most common amyloid proteins identified in patients with amyloidosis other important ones being ALect2, Aβ2M, and ATTR.

On electron microscopy, amyloid deposits appear as extracellular nonbranching fibrils of 7–10 nm in diameter with random orientation. In Aβ2M short curvilinear fibrils may be seen. A case of AA amyloidosis (Fig. 17.1) and AL amyloidosis (Fig. 17.2) is illustrated.

P. Gupta, R. K. Gupta, *Pathology of Glomerular Diseases*, https://doi.org/10.1007/978-981-19-1430-0_17

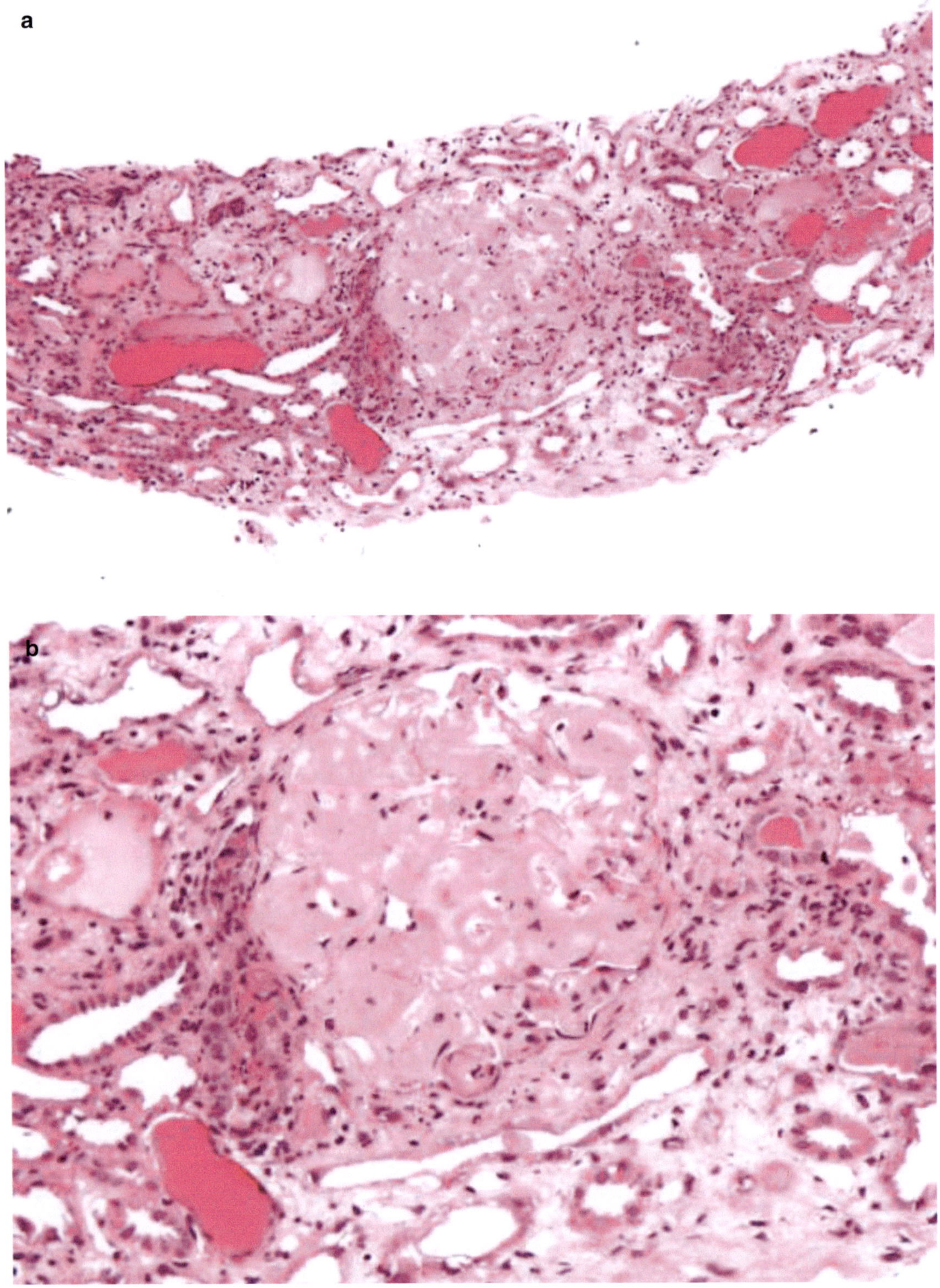

Fig. 17.1 **AA Amyloidosis.** A 58-years male patient, known to have ankylosing spondylitis since the last 10 years, presented with pedal edema. He was not hypertensive. Laboratory workup revealed massive proteinuria (urinary protein 4+) with bland urinary sediment and P/C ratio of 3.1. Serum creatinine was 2.5 mg/dl. Renal biopsy had 9 glomeruli, all of them showed mesangial expansion due to deposition of amorphous acellular eosinophilic material, at places such deposits were also evident in glomerular capillary basement membrane; the wall of the blood vessels also showed similar deposits. Renal tubules showed acute tubular injury with hyaline casts, interstitum had mild lymphocytic infiltration. IHC for serum amyloid-associated protein (AA amyloid) was strongly positive (4+). IF showed mesangial entrapment of IgM and C3 with equivocal kappa and lambda light chains; IgG, IgA, and C1q were negative. EM showed thickened and expanded glomerular capillary basement membrane with mesangial and subendothelial aggregates of randomly oriented fibrillary structures measuring about 9–12 nm in diameter. Focal effacement of visceral epithelial cell foot processes was also seen. (**a**) HE × 200, (**b**) HE × 400, (**c**) PAS × 400, (**d**) PSM × 400, (**e**) Congored × 400, (**f**) IHC for SAA × 400, and (**g, h**) EM (identity of the patient has been concealed)

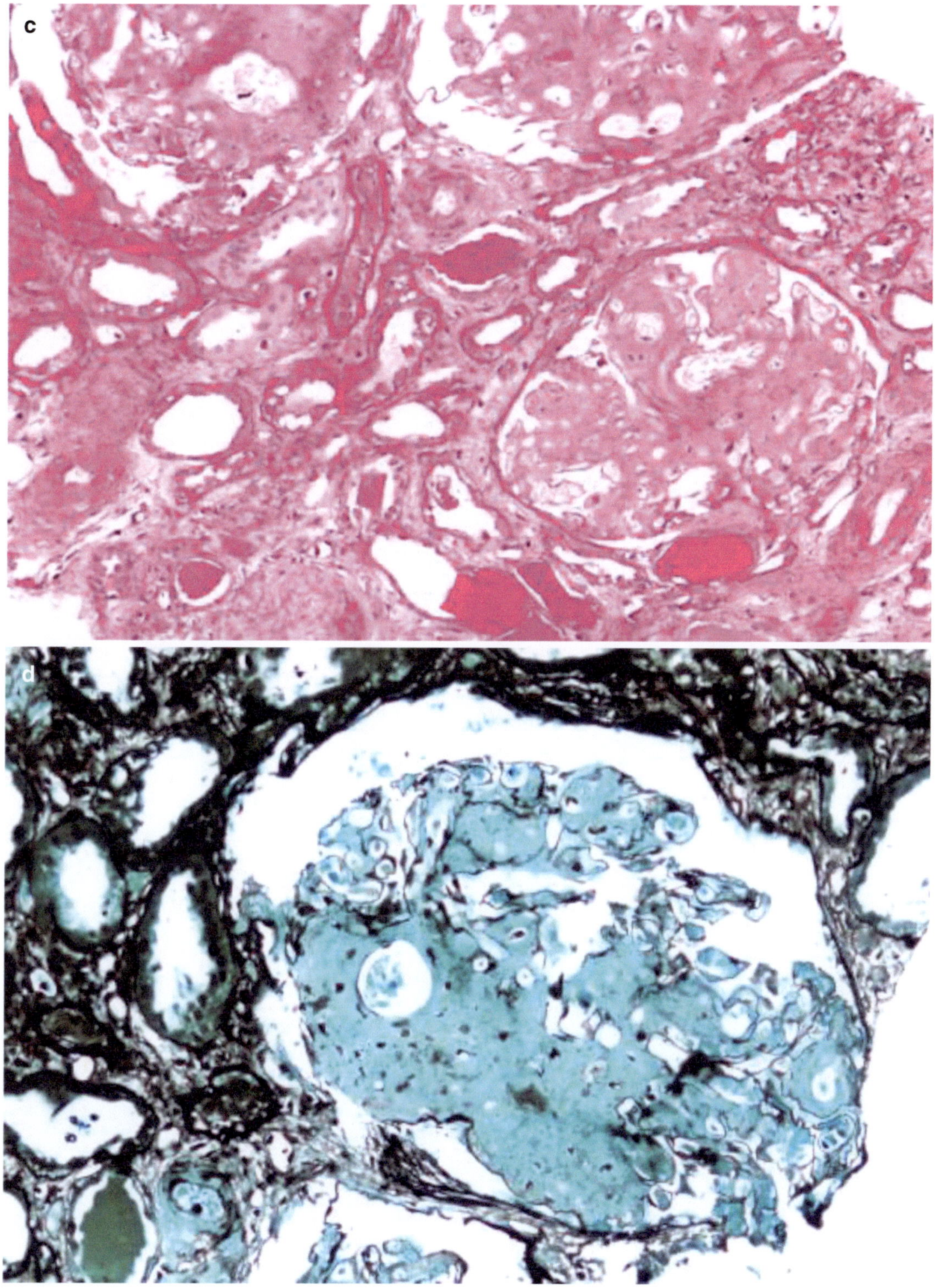

Fig. 17.1 (continued)

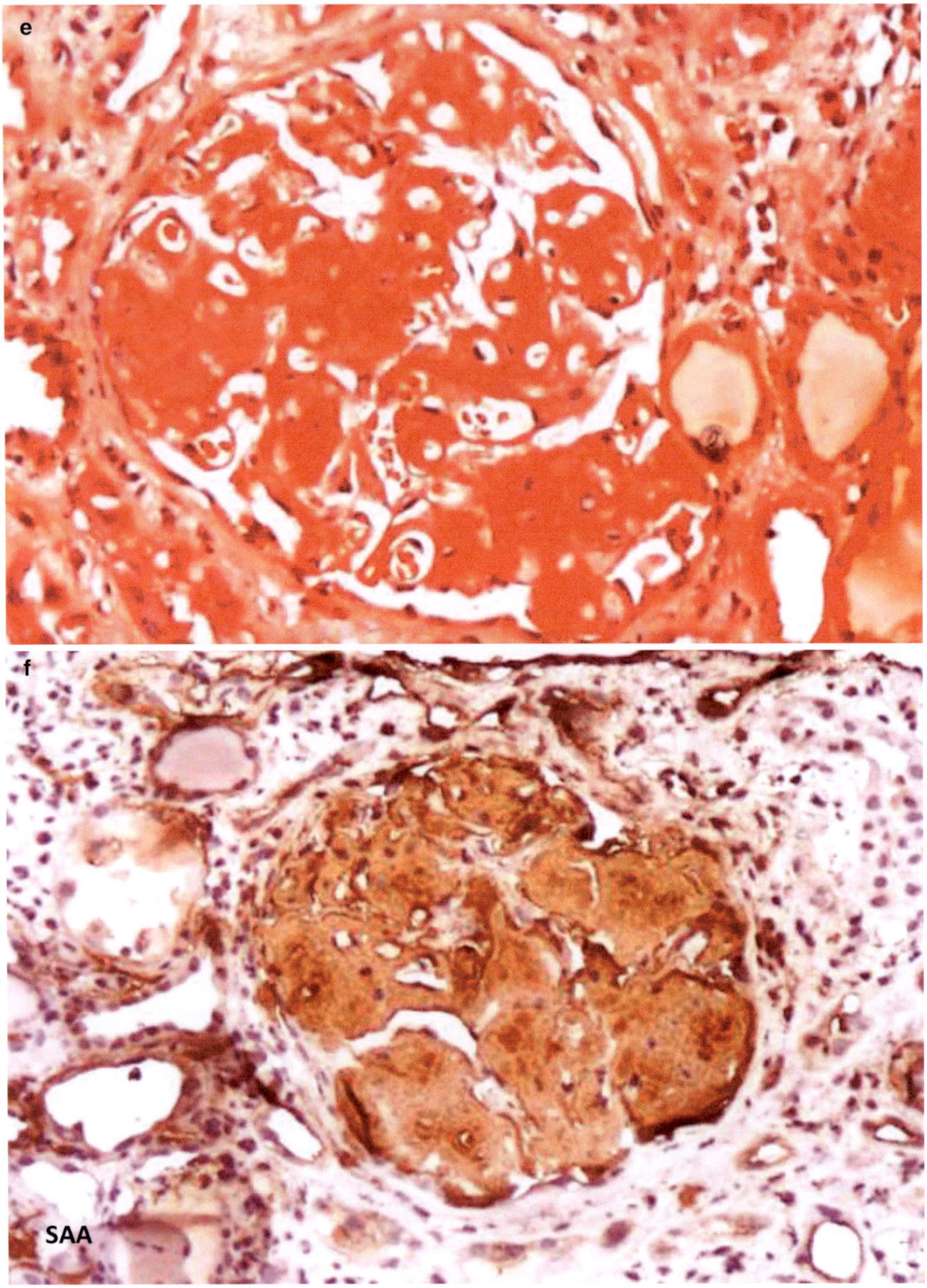

Fig. 17.1 (continued)

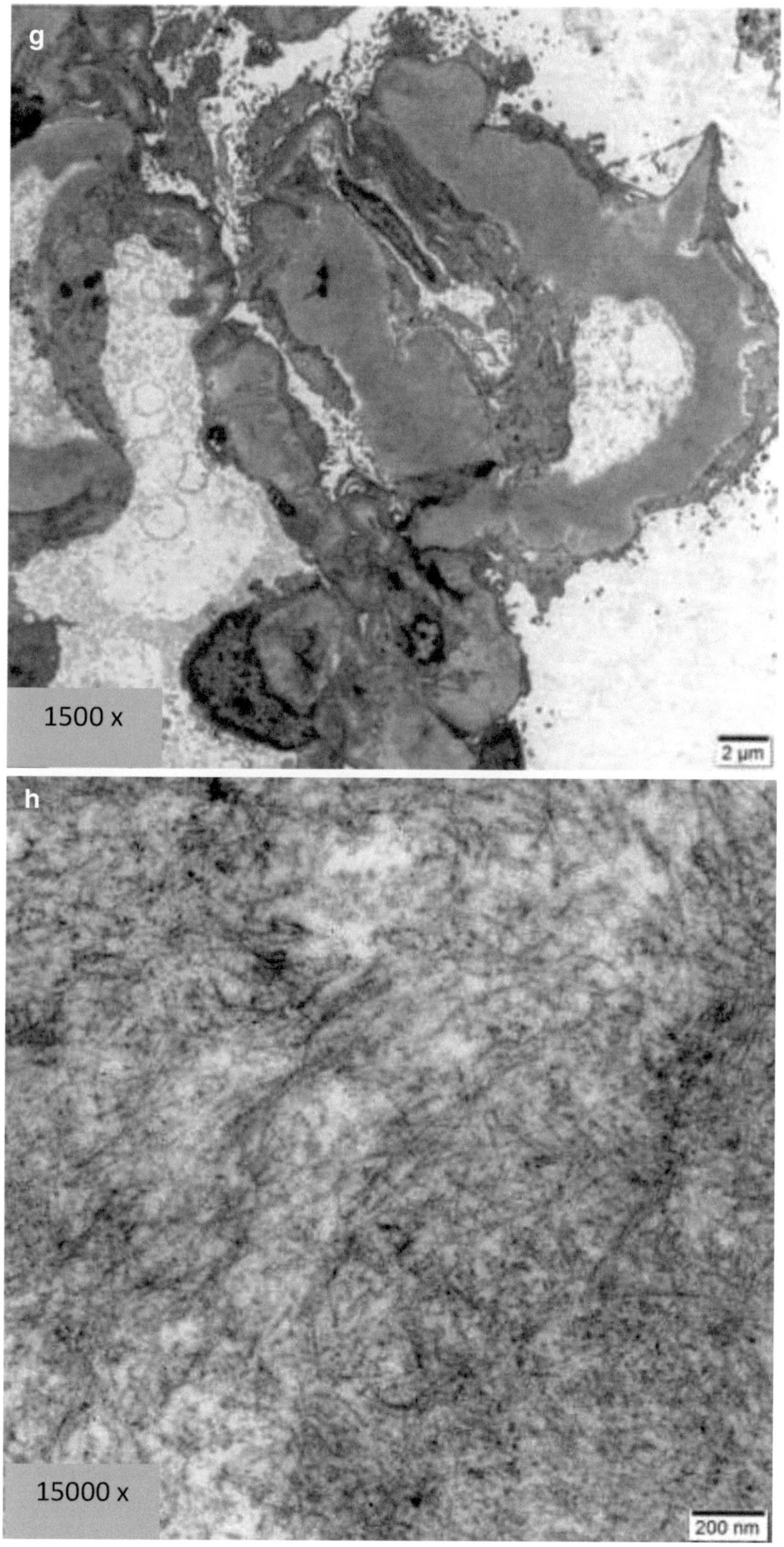

Fig. 17.1 (continued)

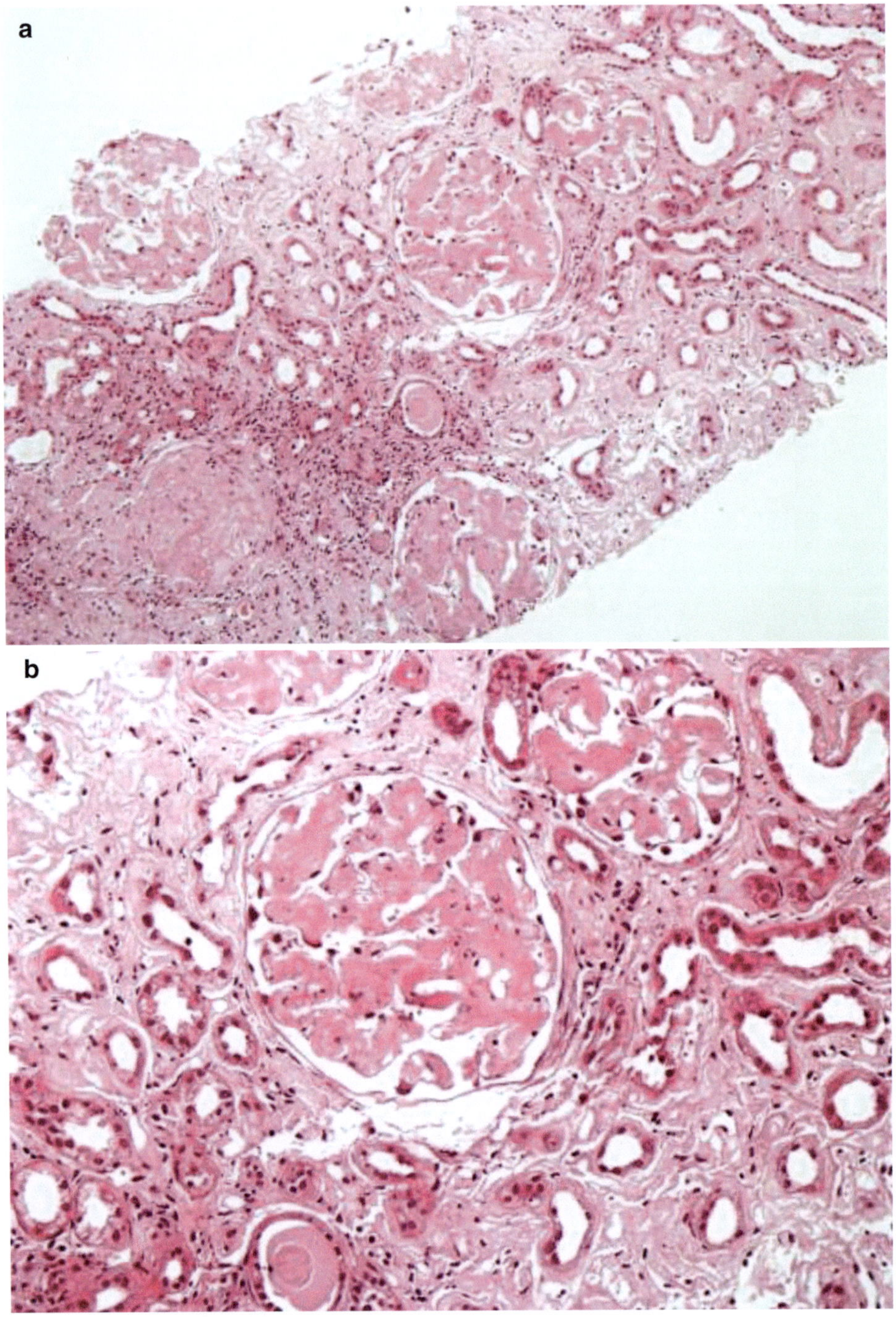

Fig. 17.2 **AL (primary) Amyloidosis.** A 63-years female patient presented with pedal edema and exertional dyspnea for 1 month. About 3 years back she was investigated for back pain and was found to have multiple myeloma. She was nondiabetic and on regular treatment for hypertension and hypothyroidism for 7 years. X-ray skull showed multiple punched-out lytic lesions, one lytic lesion was also present on left ilic bone and femur; she also had collapse of T1 vertebra. Urine analysis revealed 3+ proteinuria with 24 h urinary protein excretion being 8 g/day. She was moderately anemic with a hemoglobin content of 9.3 g/dl, total WBC count was 8.7×10^3 /cu mm, platelets were 253×10^3 /cu mm and ESR was 90 mm for the first hour (Westergren); peripheral smear showed increased rouleaux formation. Bone marrow aspiration revealed cellular marrow with 42% atypical plasma cells. Serum creatinine was 0.9 mg/dl and serum calcium was 9.1 mg/dl, serum albumin was 1.8 g/dl with A:G ratio of 0.3. Serum electrophoresis showed "M" spike 4.55 g/dl; IFE-IgG λ subtype. HbsAg and anti HCV were negative. ANA and ANCAs were negative. Serum-free light chain assay revealed kappa light chain 107.23 mg/L, lambda light chain 1853.0 mg/L with k/l ratio of 0.06. Renal biopsy had 20 glomeruli, all of them showed amorphous acellular eosinophilic congored positive deposits within mesangium and along the GBM. Similar deposits were also seen along the tubular basement membranes, interstitium, vessel wall and on congo red stain showed apple green birefringence under polarized light. Thioflavin–T stain was also positive in the deposits. Occasional foci of tubular atrophy were present. IF showed intense lambda light chain deposits (4+) in glomeruli, tubular basement membrane, interstitium and wall of blood vessels, kappa light chain showed weak positivity (+), while IgG, IgM, IgA, C3, and C1q were negative. EM showed focal effacement of visceral epithelial cell foot processes along with mesangial and subendothelial aggregates of randomly oriented fibrillary structures measuring about 9–12 nm in diameter (mean fibril diameter 10.2 nm). (**a**) HE × 100, (**b**) HE × 200, (**c**) PAS × 400, (**d**) PSM × 200, (**e**) Congo red × 400, (**f**) Polarization × 400, (**g**) Thioflavin T, (**h**) IF, (**i**, **j**) EM (identity of the patient has been concealed)

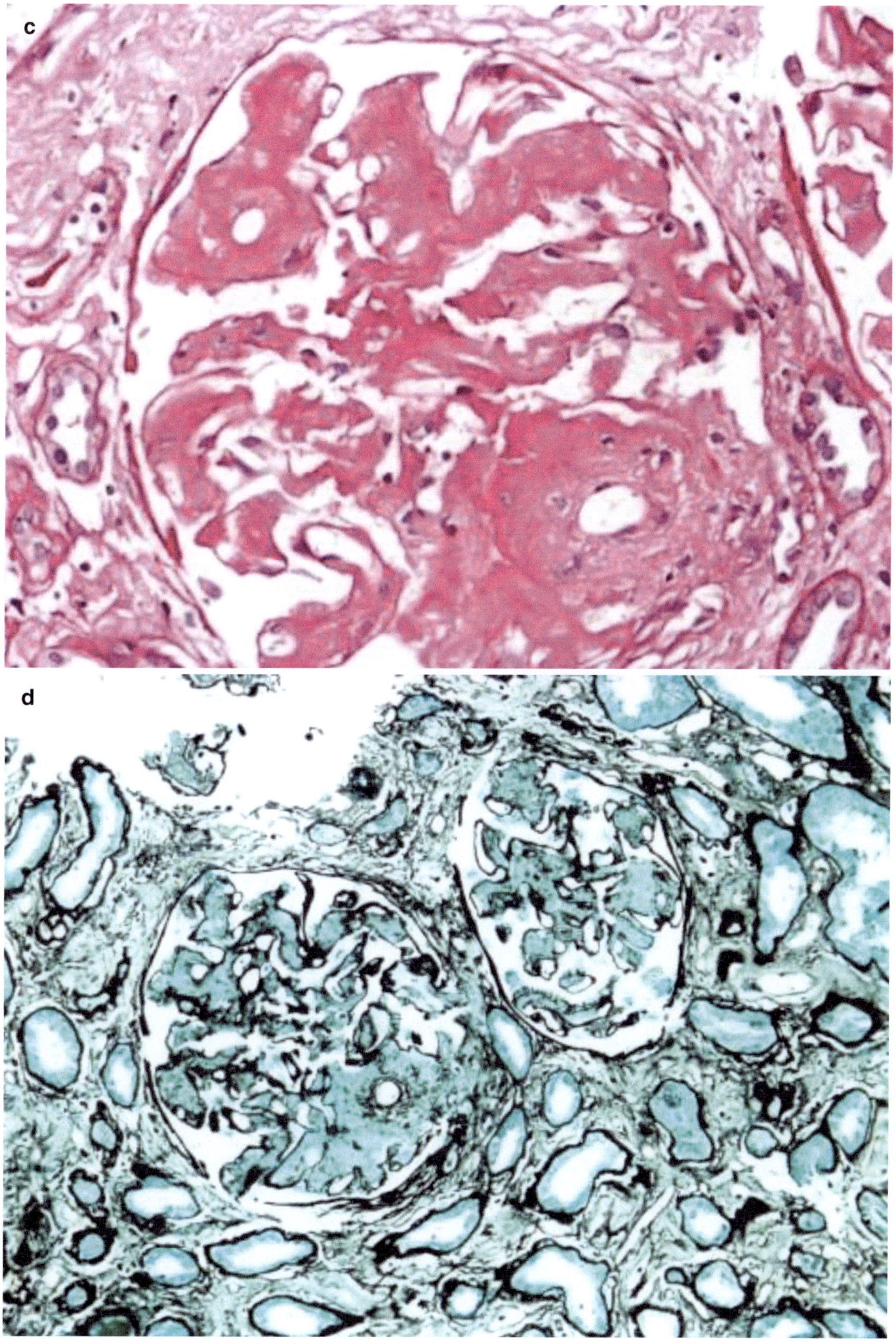

Fig. 17.2 (continued)

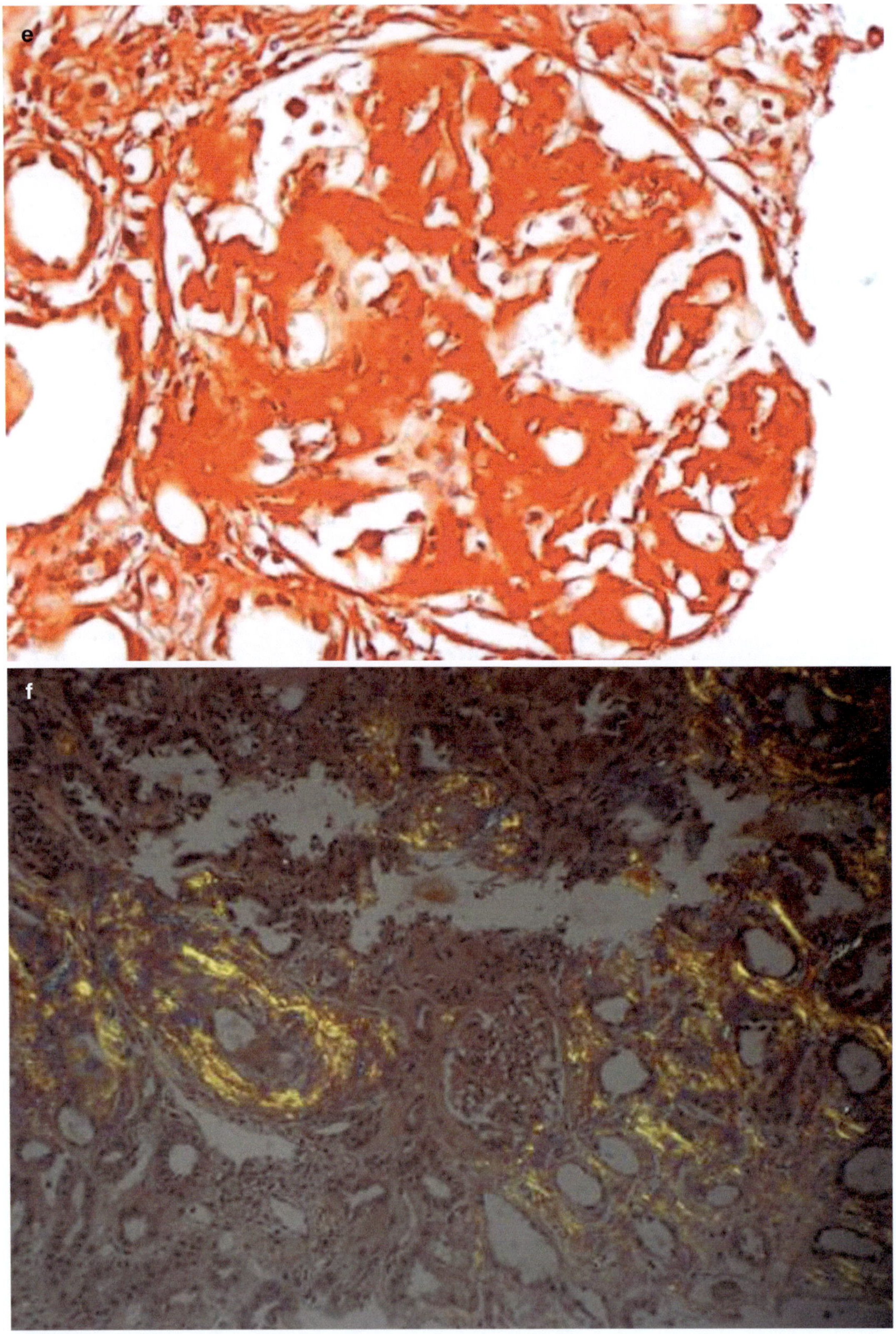

Fig. 17.2 (continued)

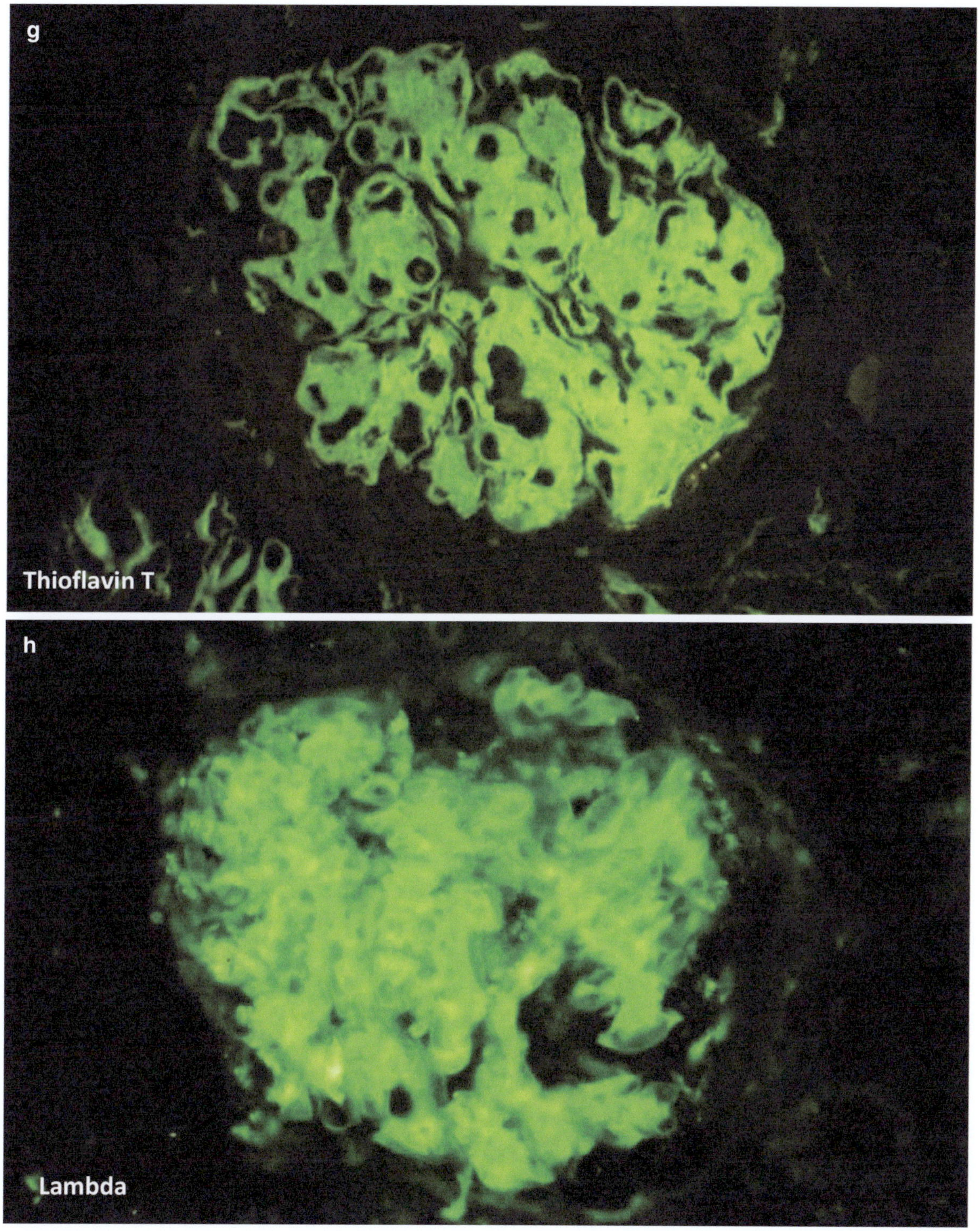

Fig. 17.2 (continued)

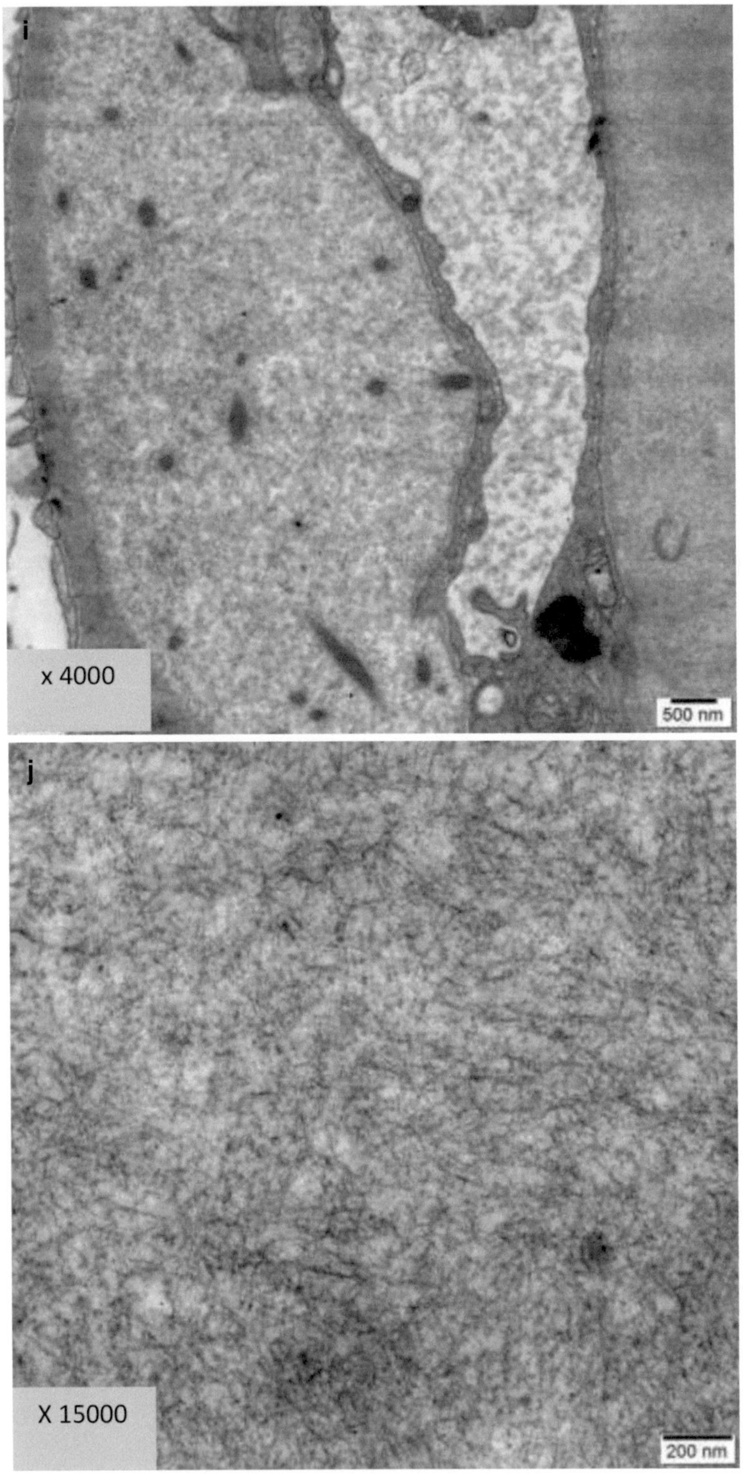

Fig. 17.2 (continued)

Further Reading

Fuah KW, Lim CTS. Renal-limited AL amyloidosis - a diagnostic and management dilemma. BMC Nephrol. 2018;19:307.

Papa R, Lachmann HJ. Secondary, AA, amyloidosis. Rheum Dis Clin N Am. 2018;44:585–603.

Ryšavá R. AL amyloidosis: advances in diagnostics and treatment. Nephrol Dial Transplant. 2019;34:1460–6.

Wechalekar AD, Gillmore JD, Hawkins PN. Systemic amyloidosis. Lancet. 2016;387(10038):2641–54.

18 Renal Involvement in Plasma Cell Dyscrasia

18.1 Myeloma Cast Nephropathy

Light chain cast nephropathy accounts for around 33% of cases of all the renal pathologies encountered in patients with multiple myeloma. The excess free light chains produced in myeloma patients exceed the endocytosis capacity of proximal tubules and can cause proximal tubulopathy or can pass into loop of Henley and distal convoluted tubules where they interact with Tamm Horsfall protein and form casts within the lumen of tubules. These abnormal light chains are tubulotoxic and can cause damage to the lining epithelium of tubules.

On Light microscopy, light chain cast nephropathy is seen as pale casts within the renal tubules particularly distal tubules which have lamellated or fractured appearance. They appear pale and weakly PAS-positive as compared to hyaline casts but sometimes PAS-positive casts can also be seen. These casts can lead to damage to tubular lining epithelium leading to acute tubular injury and also incite inflammatory cell reaction and giant cell reaction around them.

On Immunofluorescence, these casts show light chain restriction which is more commonly kappa light chain. Other immunoglobulins are absent. Monoclonality in casts can be demonstrable when they have formed acutely. Sometimes trapping of both light chains is seen and so monoclonal light chain restriction may not be identified on immunofluorescence.

On electron microscopy casts show either fibrillar material, cellular debris, or granular electron-dense material. Some cases can show crystalline structures.

Some cases of cast nephropathy can be associated with amyloidosis. Amyloid deposits can both be seen within tubular casts and glomeruli. A case of light chain cast nephropathy is illustrated (Fig. 18.1).

P. Gupta, R. K. Gupta, *Pathology of Glomerular Diseases*, https://doi.org/10.1007/978-981-19-1430-0_18

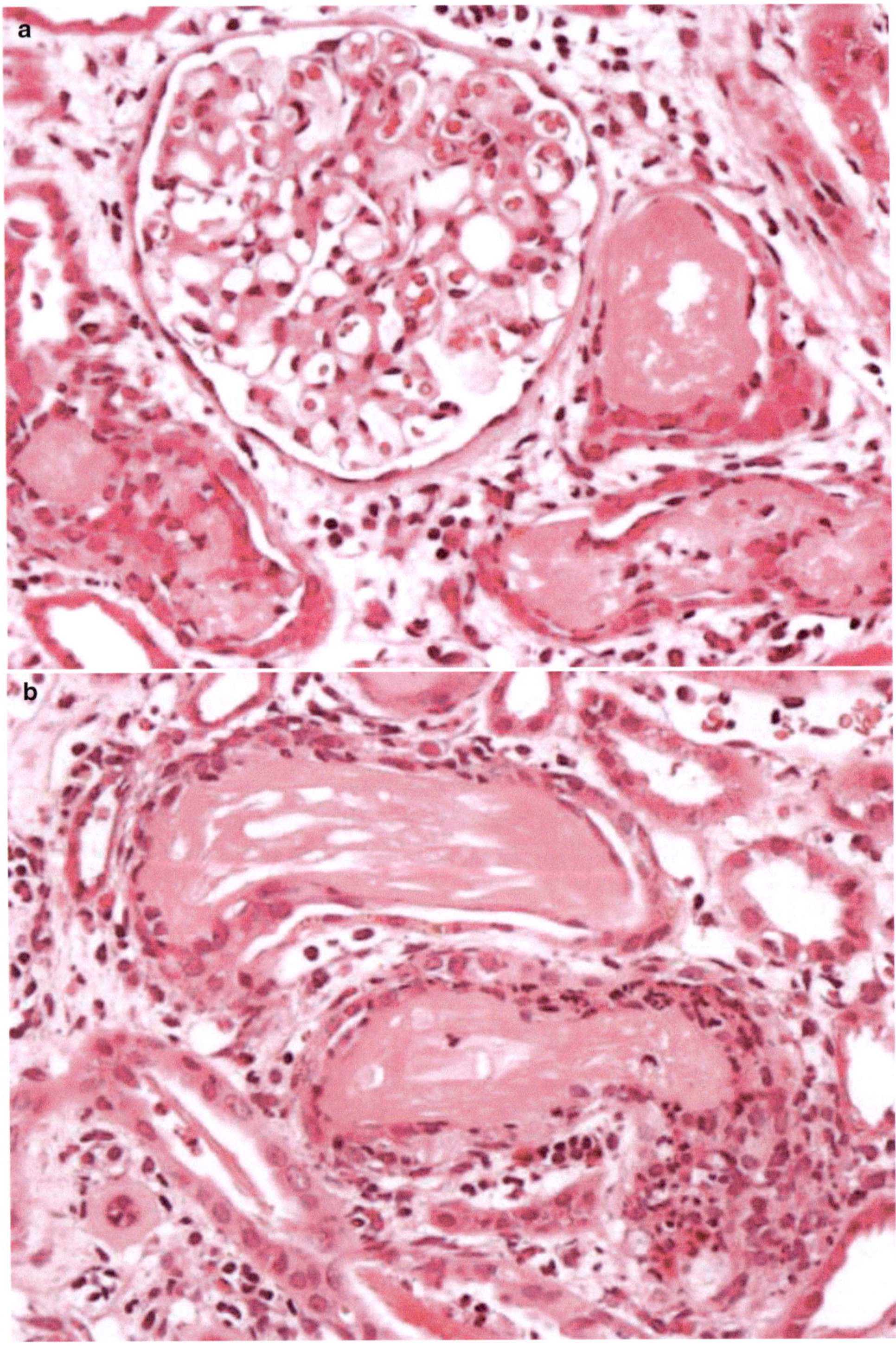

Fig. 18.1 Light Chain Cast Nephropathy. A 63-years male patient, treated case of pulmonary tuberculosis and known to have a positive history of coronary heart disease with type II DM and HTN since last 10 years, presented with rapidly progressive renal failure. Serum creatinine rose from 0.8 to 10 mg/dL in 3 months. Patient had a history of NSAID intake for 4 days prior to admission. Laboratory workup revealed Hb level of 10.5 g/dL and ESR was 56 mm for first hour (Westergren). Urine examination showed albumin +, WBC 3–5/hpf, and no RBC. Urine P:C ratio was 1.4. Total serum protein was 6.40 g/dL with serum albumin 3.72 g/dl and serum globulin 2.68 g/dl; A/G ratio was 2:1. Serum beta 2 microglobulin was 24.11 mg/L. Serum C3 was 1291 mg/L and serum C4 was 440 mg/L. c-ANCA, p-ANCA and ANA were negative by IIF. Serum kappa light chain was 18.85 mg/L and lambda light chain was 11722 mg/L with kappa-lambda ratio of 0.002. Renal biopsy had 10 glomeruli. Renal tubules had multiple intratubular fractured and lamellated casts with denudation of lining epithelium associated with inflammatory reaction around the casts and occasional giant cells; casts were PAS and congored negative. Tubulointerstitial changes were also present. Glomeruli did not show any amyloid deposits. IF showed lambda light chain restriction within the casts. (**a** and **b**) HE × 400, (**c**) PAS × 200, and (**d**) IF × 400

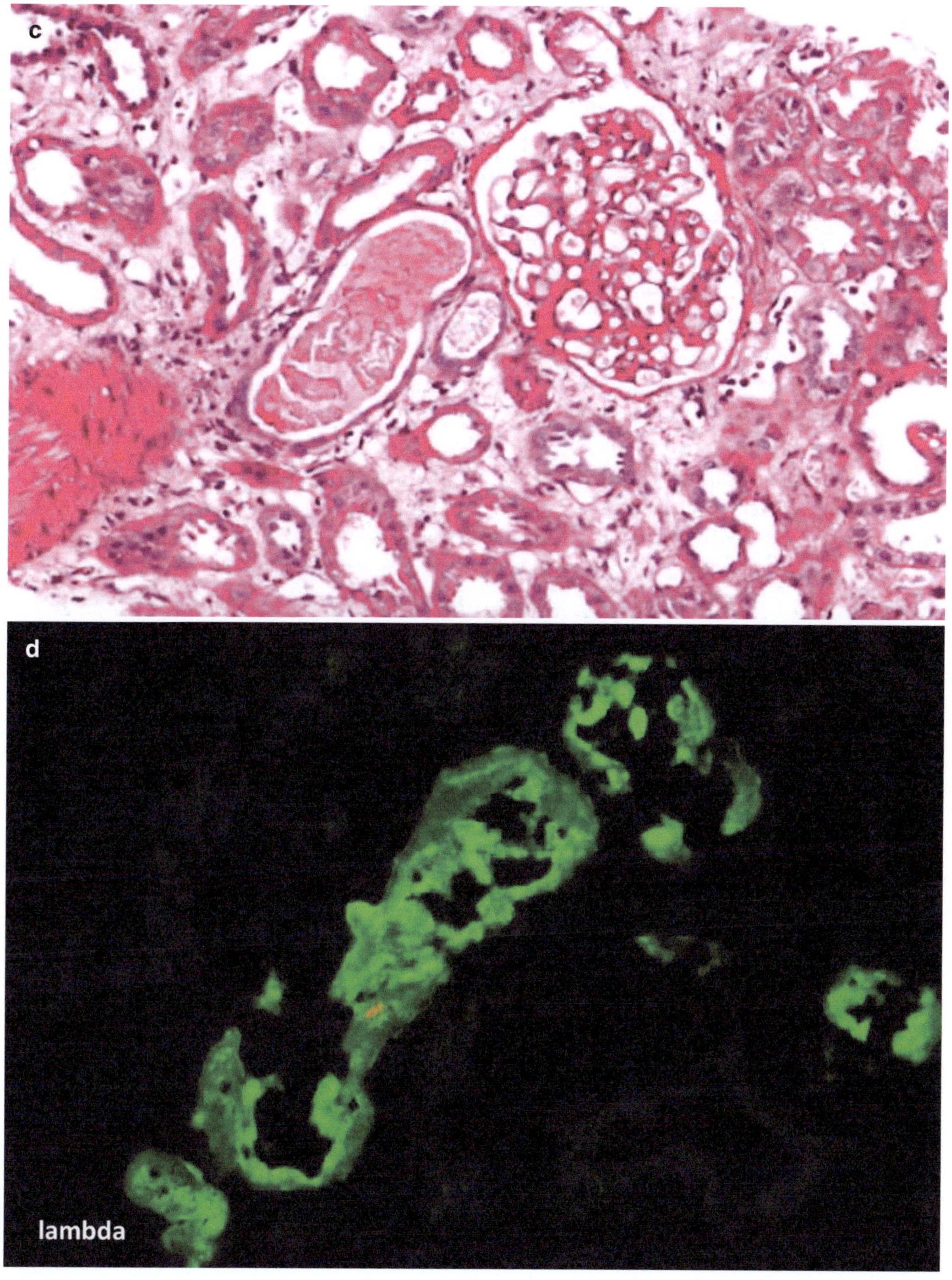

Fig. 18.1 (continued)

18.2 Monoclonal Immunoglobulin Deposition Disease (MIDD)

Monoclonal immunoglobulin deposition disease (MIDD) comprises light chain deposition disease (LCDD), heavy chain deposition disease (HCDD), and combined light and heavy chain deposition disease.

18.2.1 Light Chain Deposition Disease (LCDD)

It can be seen in the setting of myeloma and also in cases of monoclonal gammopathy of renal significance (MGRS). It is usually seen in patients >50 years of age. Patients present with proteinuria usually in the nephrotic range and may be accompanied by hypertension, hematuria, and renal insufficiency. There can be associated cast nephropathy.

Renal biopsy shows nodular glomerulopathy with even distribution of PAS-positive and argyrophilic nodules. Mesangial proliferation and MPGN pattern may be seen. Thickened and tortuous tubular basement membrane can be appreciated. On Immunofluorescence light chain deposits can be seen in glomerular capillary basement membrane, tubular basement membrane, and vessel wall. Electron microscopy shows powdery to punctate electron-dense deposits at the site of light chain deposition in glomeruli (lamina rara interna or subendothelial), tubular basement membranes, or vessel walls.

Recurrence of disease can be seen in the transplanted kidney.

18.2.2 Heavy Chain Deposition Disease (HCDD)

Heavy chain deposition disease (HCDD) is a type of monoclonal immunoglobulin deposition disease in which patients have glomerular deposition of truncated heavy chains. It is a rare complication of plasma cell neoplasm and patients present with proteinuria which may be in the nephrotic range or nephrotic syndrome along with hematuria, hypertension, and progressive loss of renal function. Reduced complement levels can be seen. At the time of diagnosis, monoclonal gammopathy by serum or urine electrophoresis may be present in 50–60% of cases. On light microscopy similar to LCDD nodular glomerular morphology is appreciated. Nodules are PAS and silver positive. On Immunofluorescence monoclonal IgG deposits (IgG1 most common, IG2, IgG3, or IgG4 subclasses) are seen within the nodules without any light chain deposits. Less commonly monoclonal IgA and IgM deposits may be seen. On electron microscopy linear to granular electron-dense deposits without any substructure can be observed along the glomerular capillary basement membrane and tubular basement membranes. Mesangial powdery electron-dense deposits can also be seen. In patients treated with chemotherapy, complete hematologic response and improvement in renal function are observed. Untreated patients progress to end-stage renal disease and have a poor prognosis. A case of combined light and heavy chain deposition disease (LCHDD) is illustrated (Fig. 18.2).

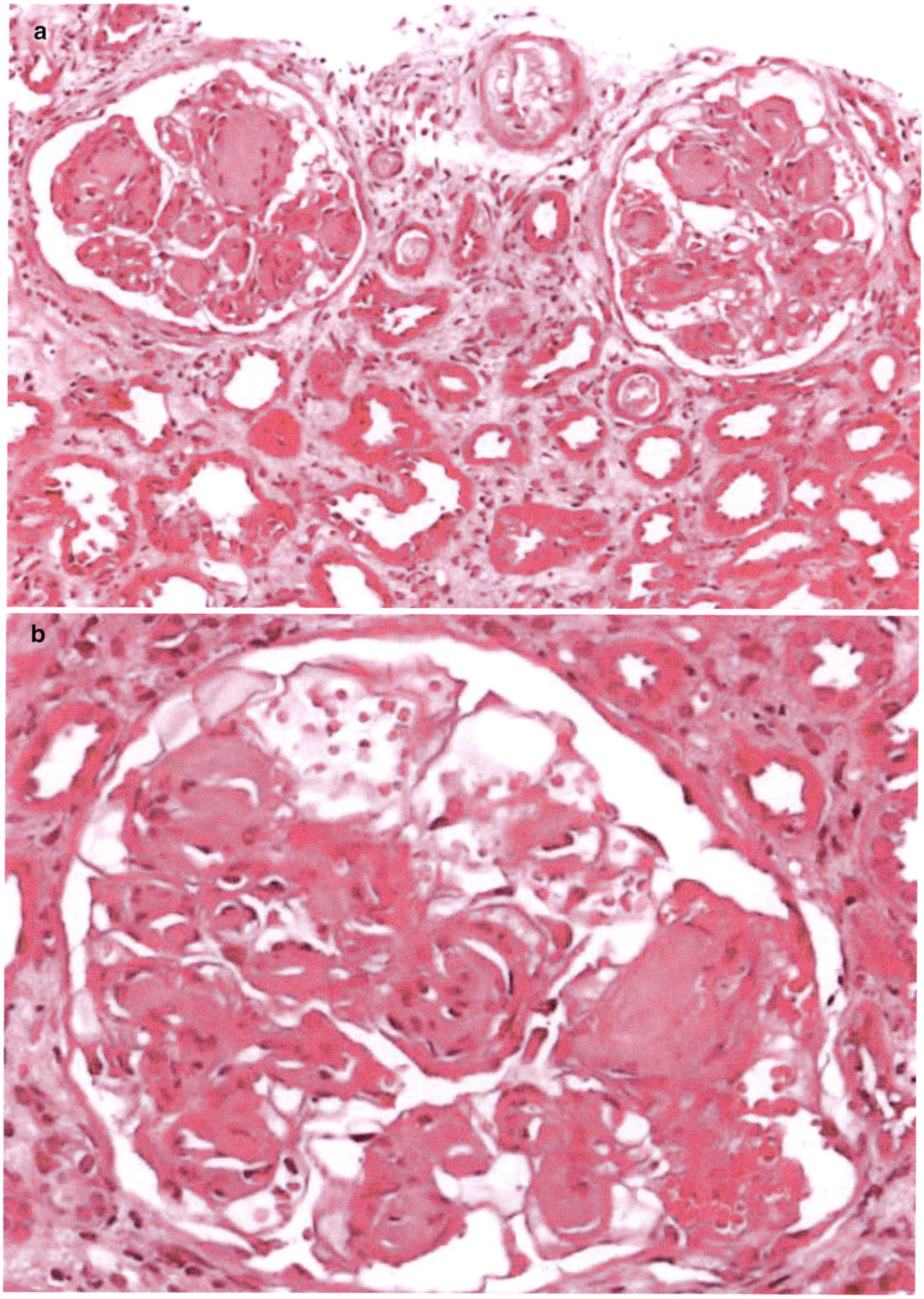

Fig. 18.2 Combined Light Chain and Heavy Chain Deposition Disease (LCHDD). A 72-years male patient, recently diagnosed as HTN associated with renal dysfunction. USG showed B/L kidneys normal in size and shape. Right kidney was 10 × 5.3 cm and the left kidney was 9.4 × 4.7 cm in size; besides the right kidney had a 6 mm mid-pole calculus. Urine examination revealed albumin 3+, pus cells 10–12/hpf, RBC 30–35/hpf, granular cast +, leucocyte esterase +. Urine P:C ratio: 8.54. Serum creatinine 6.2 mg/dl which increased to 8.6 mg/dl in 2 weeks. Lipid profile showed serum cholesterol 348 mg/dl, TG 268 mg/dl, LDL 248 mg/dl, VLDL 54 mg/dl. c-ANCA and p-ANCA were negative. Following biopsy, urine electrophoresis showed M band. Serum immunofixation electrophoresis showed that the monoclonal band corresponds to IgG-kappa. Free kappa light chain was 687.08 mg/L, free lambda light chain was 60.52 mg/L; kappa: lambda free light chain ratio: 11.35:1. Serum Beta 2 microglobulin was 19,926 ng/ml and serum calcium was 8.26 mg/dl. Renal biopsy showed glomerular enlargement and nodular glomerulosclerosis along with tubulointerstitial and vascular changes. The nodules were PAS-positive and silver positive; the GBM also showed splitting (arrows). On IF the nodules, mesangium, tubular basement membrane and the blood vessel wall were positive for IgG and the deposits showed kappa light chain restriction. IF for IgM, IgA, C3 and lambda light chain was negative. EM showed powdery to granular electron-dense deposits in mesangial area and along GBM. (**a**) HE × 100 and (**b**) HE × 400. (**c**) PAS × 400. (**d**) PSM × 400. (**e**–**g**) IF × 400. (**h**) EM × 2500 (identity of the patient has been concealed)

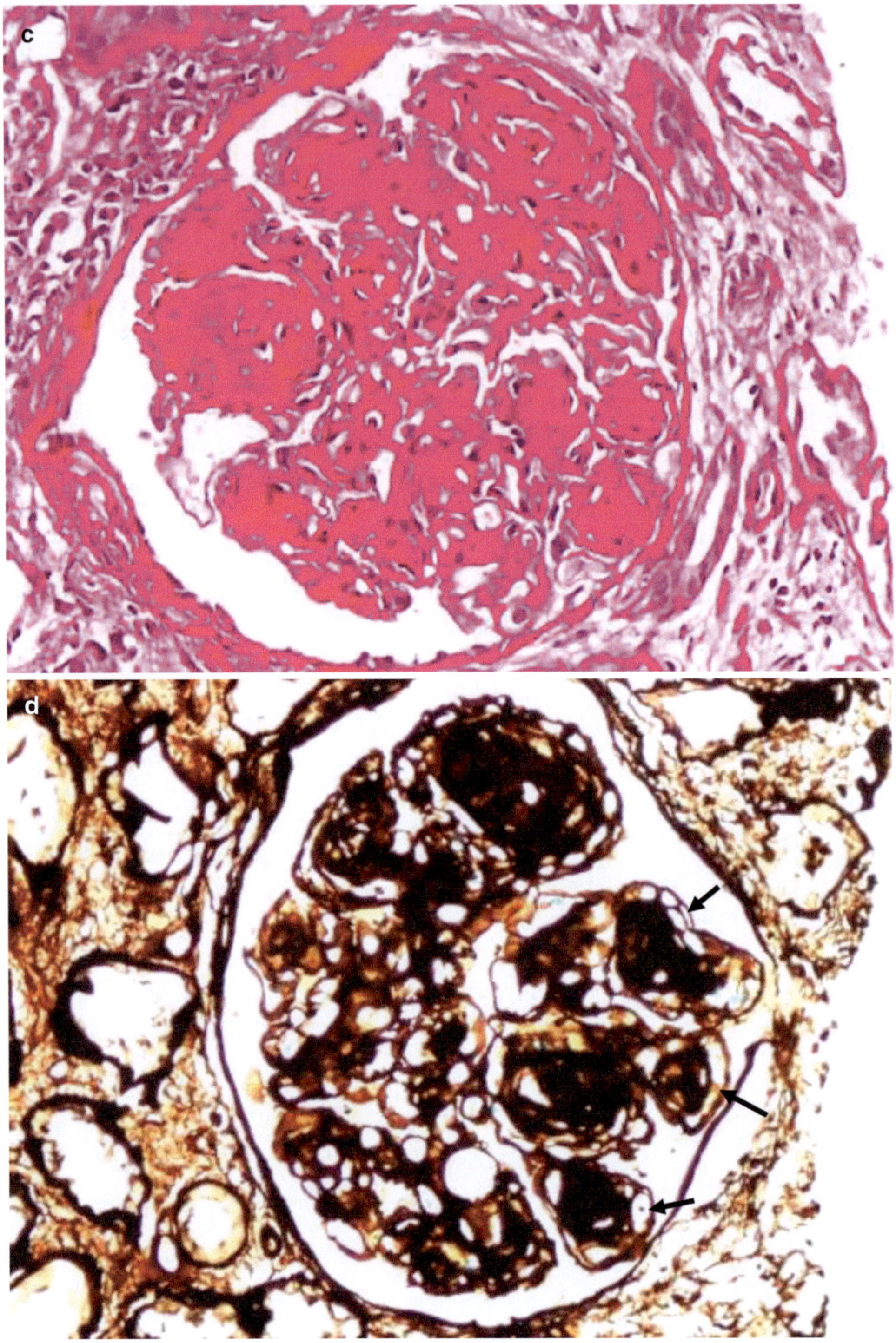

Fig. 18.2 (continued)

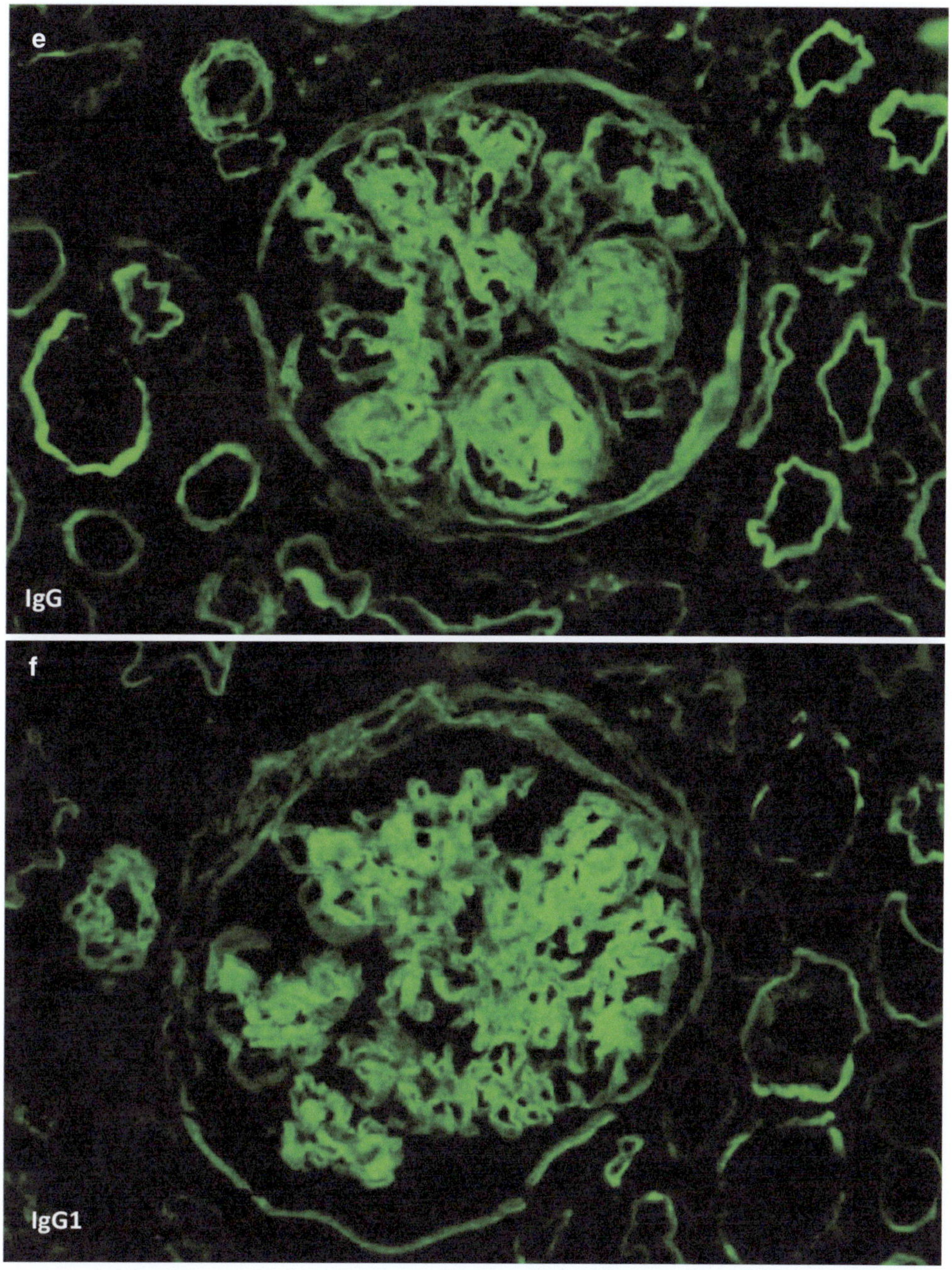

Fig. 18.2 (continued)

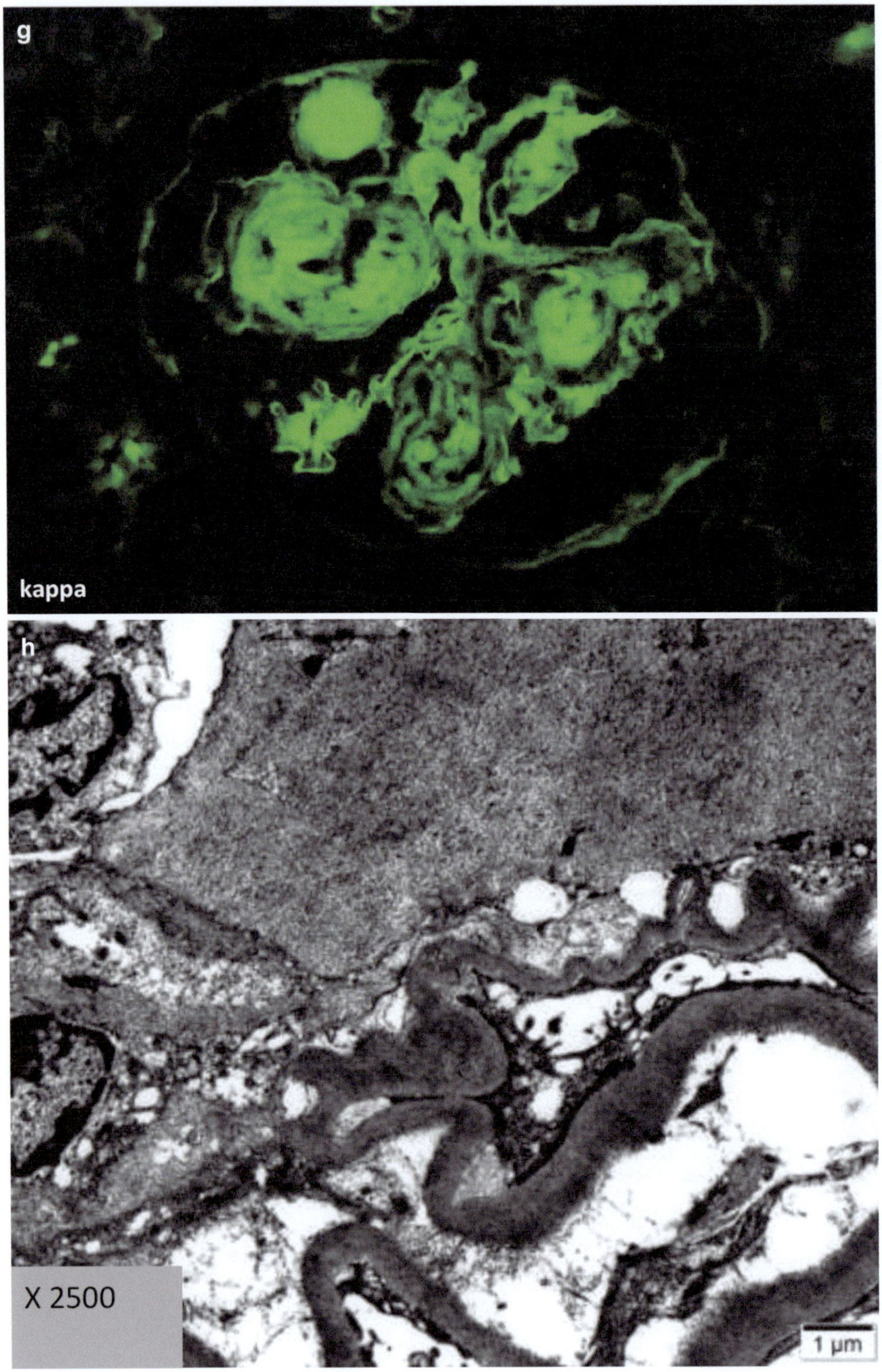

Fig. 18.2 (continued)

18.3 Proliferative Glomerulonephritis with Monoclonal Immunoglobulin Deposits (PGNMID)

It is characterized by proliferative glomerular morphology most commonly membrano-proliferative or endocapillary proliferative pattern of injury with monoclonal light chain and heavy chain deposits in the glomeruli in a pattern similar to immune complex-mediated glomerulonephritis. Patients affected with this disease are usually <50 years of age although cases have also been described in children and young adults. Patients present with nephrotic range proteinuria, variable hematuria, and can have renal dysfunction. One-third of patients can have low serum complements C3 and C4. Exact pathogenesis of this condition is unknown and only 30% patients will have evidence of dysproteinemia at presentation. Multiple myeloma is not seen in these patients at presentation or follow up and they form part of spectrum of lesions seen in monoclonal gammopathy of renal significance (MGRS). Many patients do not have detectable M protein in serum or urine. On light microscopy membranoproliferative, endocapillary proliferative, mesangioproliferative or rarely membranous pattern may be seen. On immunofluorescence, mesangial and capillary wall (usually subendothelial but occasionally subepithelial) deposits of immunoglobulin light chain and monoclonal heavy chain usually IgG of one particular subclass (IgG3 most commonly) are seen. The deposits are confined to glomeruli. Rarely IgA and even rarer IgM monoclonal deposits may be seen. On electron microscopy electron-dense deposits similar to immune-complex mediated glomerulonephritis are seen in subendothelial and mesangial region and rarely in subepithelial region. Glomerular capillary double contours may be appreciated. Two cases of PGNMID have been illustrated (Figs. 18.3 and 18.4). Some authors have described early recurrence of this condition in renal allograft.

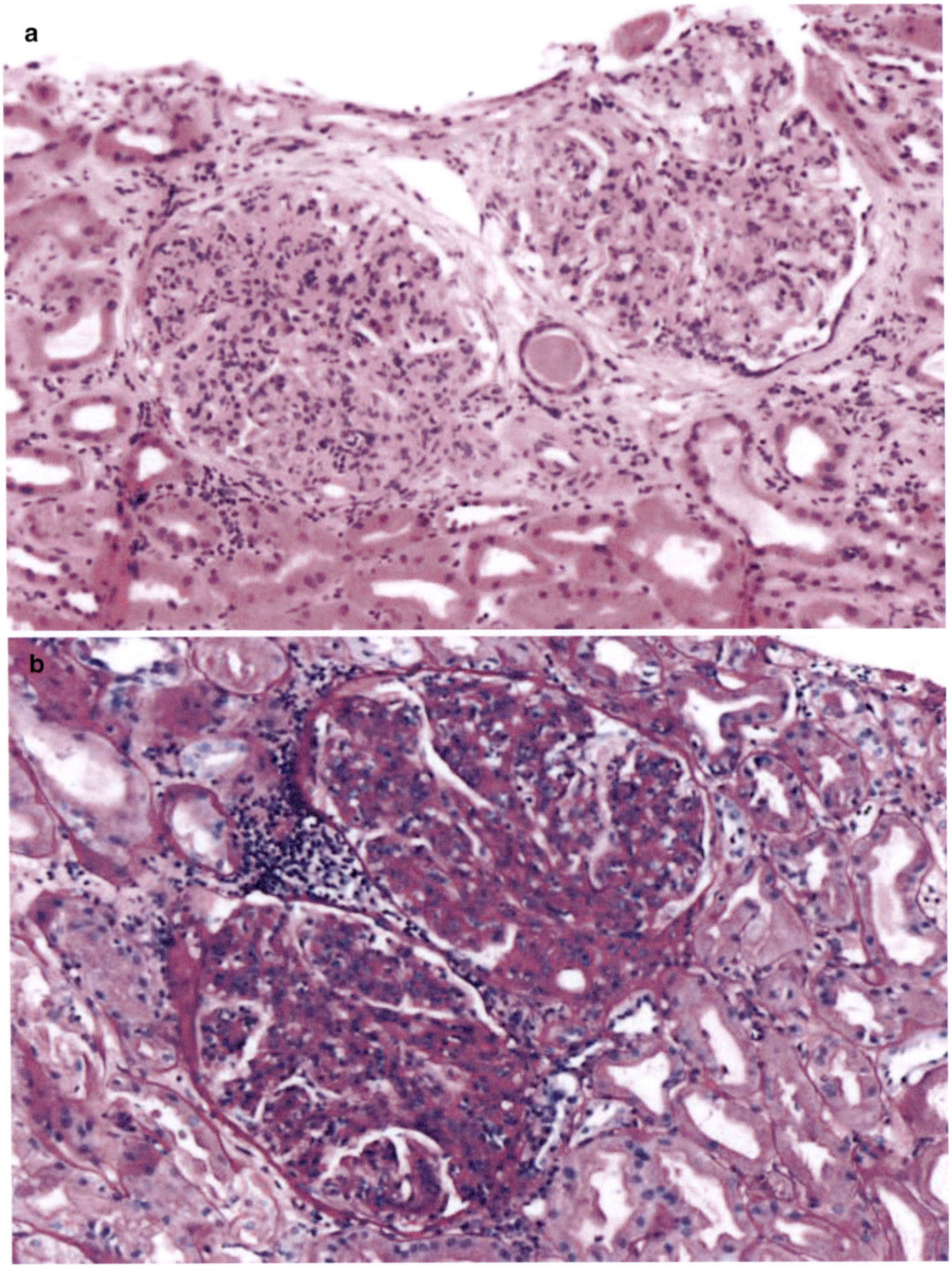

Fig. 18.3 Proliferative Glomerulonephritis with Monoclonal Immunoglobulin Deposits (PGNMID). A 65-years female patient, 2 years post-renal transplant (HLA identical donor) presented with proteinuria 3 g/24 h; urinary sediment had 300 dysmorphic RBC/μl. Post-transplant serum immunofixation revealed M-protein + IgG lambda. Renal allograft biopsy revealed MPGN pattern with mesengial hypercellularity, endocapillary proliferation as well as double contour formation of GBM. There was moderate tubular atrophy with interstitial inflammatory infiltrate and interstitial fibrosis. There was no evidence of rejection. IF showed mesangial and subendothelial deposits of IgG, lambda and complement C3; IgA, IgM, kappa, C1q and C4d were negative. EM performed on FFPE material showed mesangial and subendothelial electron-dense deposits without fibrillary substructures and duplication of GBM. (**a**) HE × 400, (**b**) PAS × 400, (**c**) Jones × 400, (**d–f**) IF × 400, and (**g**) EM × 11000. (Contributor–Dr. Joris J. Roelofs, Department of Pathology, Amsterdam University Medical Centers, Amsterdam, The Netherlands)

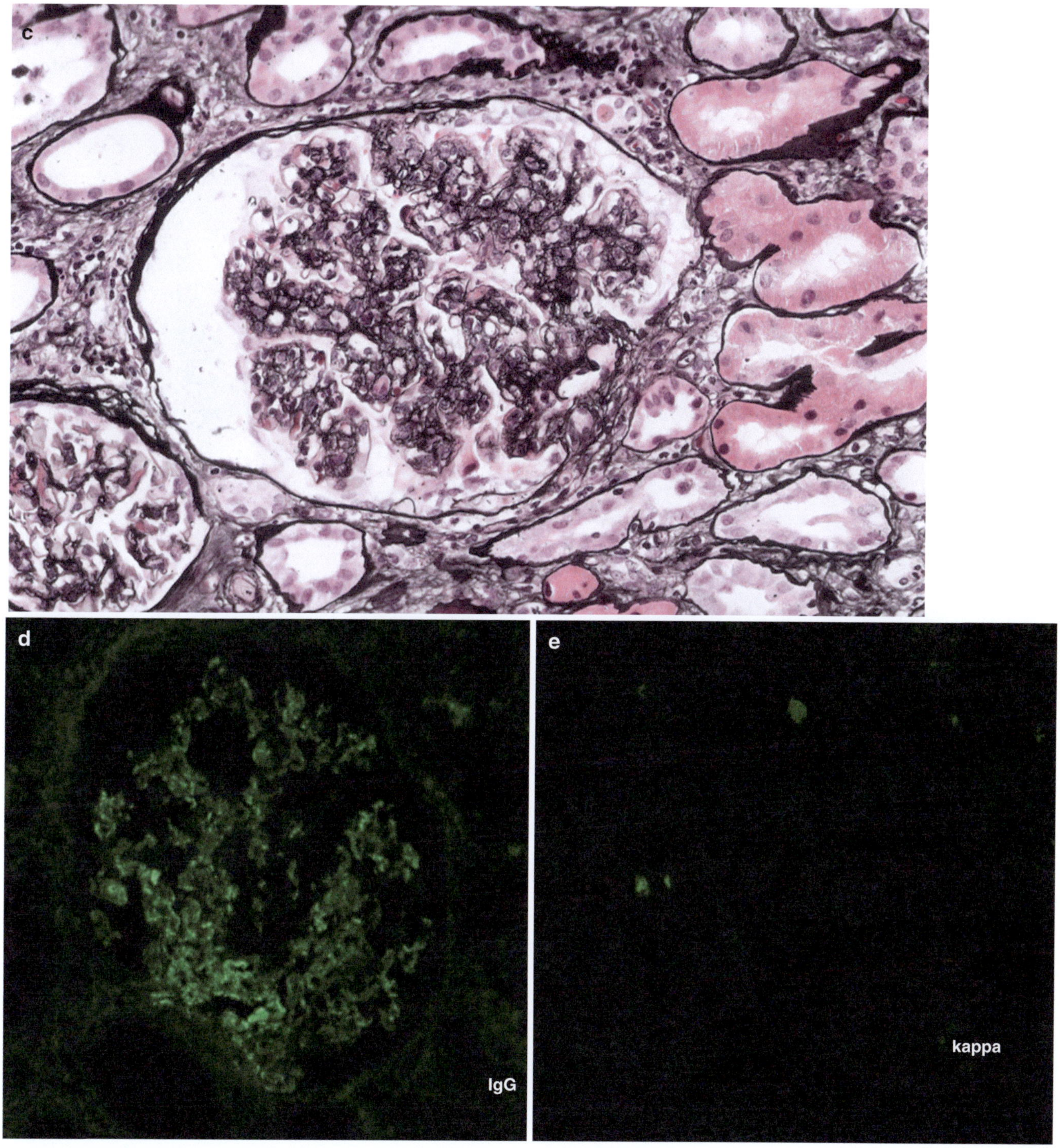

Fig. 18.3 (continued)

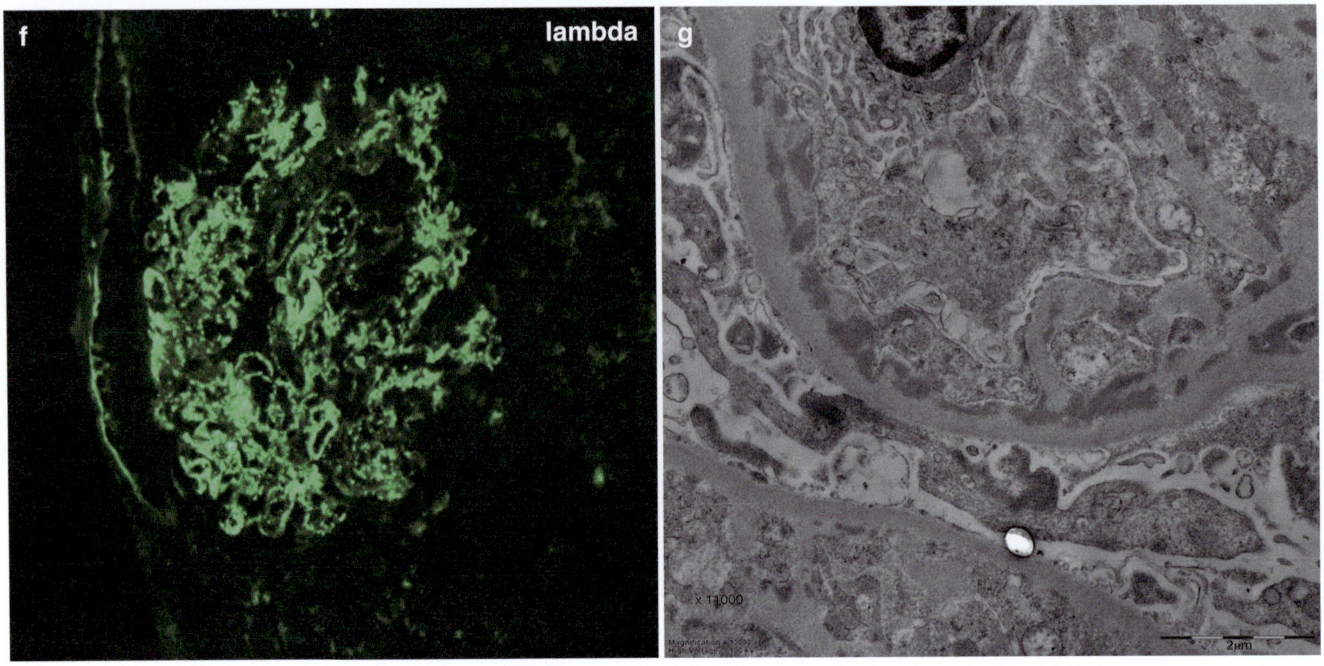

Fig. 18.3 (continued)

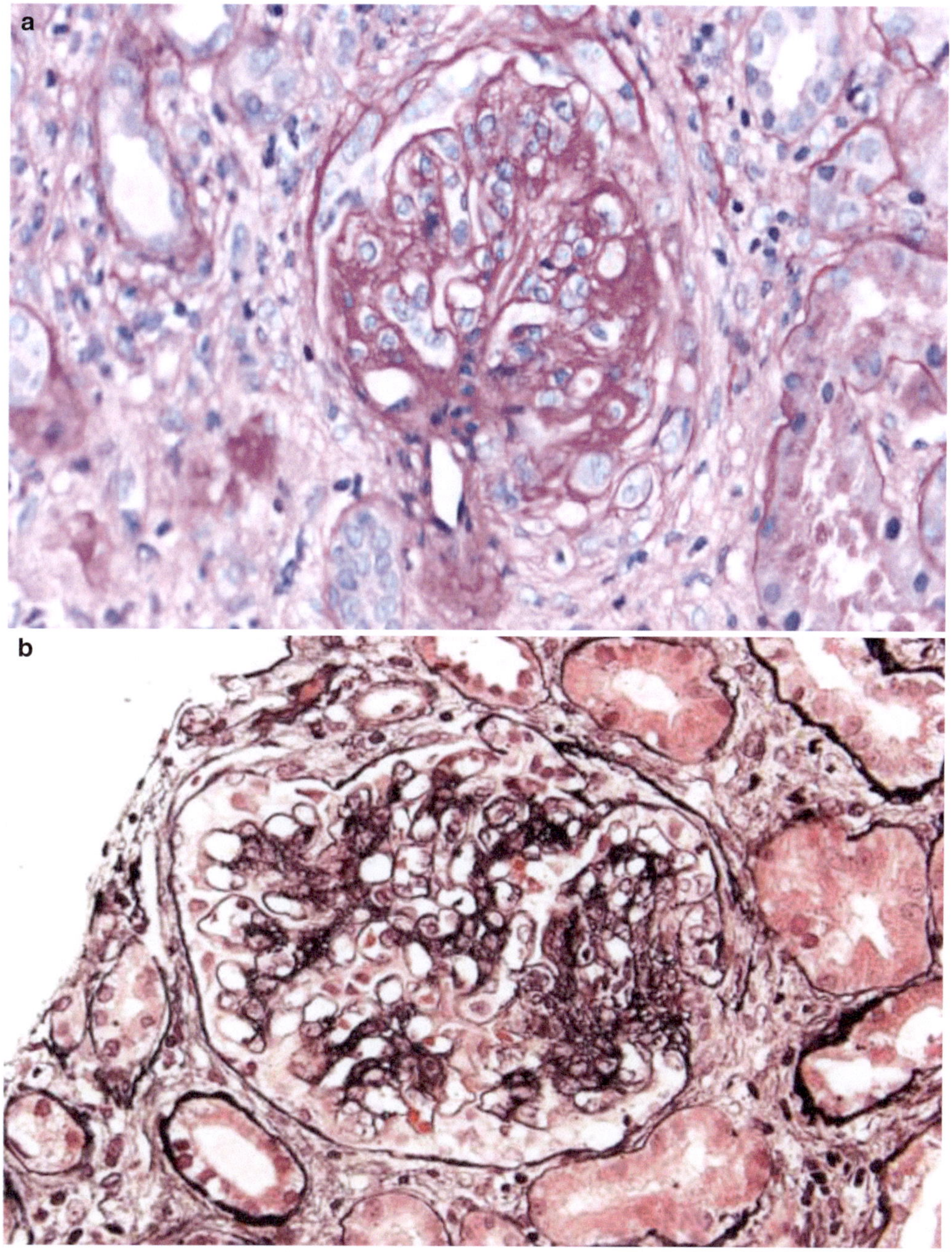

Fig. 18.4 Proliferative Glomerulonephriis with Monoclonal Immunoglobulin Deposits (PGNMID). A 26-years asthmatic male patient presented with h/o weight gain of 7 kg in 1 year and ankle edema. Urine examination revealed proteinuria of 8.5 g/24 h with 5–10 RBC/hpf. Serum albumin was 3.2 g/dl and serum creatinine was 500 µmol/l. No M band on electrophoresis and ANA, ANCA, Hep B, Hep C, HIV, and cryoglobulins were negative. Renal biopsy had 11 glomeruli, 2 were globally sclerosed and 7 showed segmental sclerosis associated with tubular atrophy and interstitial fibrosis accompanied by a dense interstitial inflammatory infiltrate. Other two glomeruli showed mesangial expansion, endocapillary hypercellularity, double countours, and immune deposits along the capillary walls. IF showed mesangial and subendothelial deposits of IgA, C3, and kappa. EM showed mesangial, subendothelial, subepithelial, and intramembranous electron-dense deposits with duplication of GBM. There was widespread effacement and microvillous transformation of podocytes. (**a**) PAS × 200, (**b** and **c**) Jones × 400, (**d–i**) IF × 400 and (**j–l**) EM (Contributor—Dr. Joris J. Roelofs, Department of Pathology, Amsterdam University Medical Centers, Amsterdam, The Netherlands)

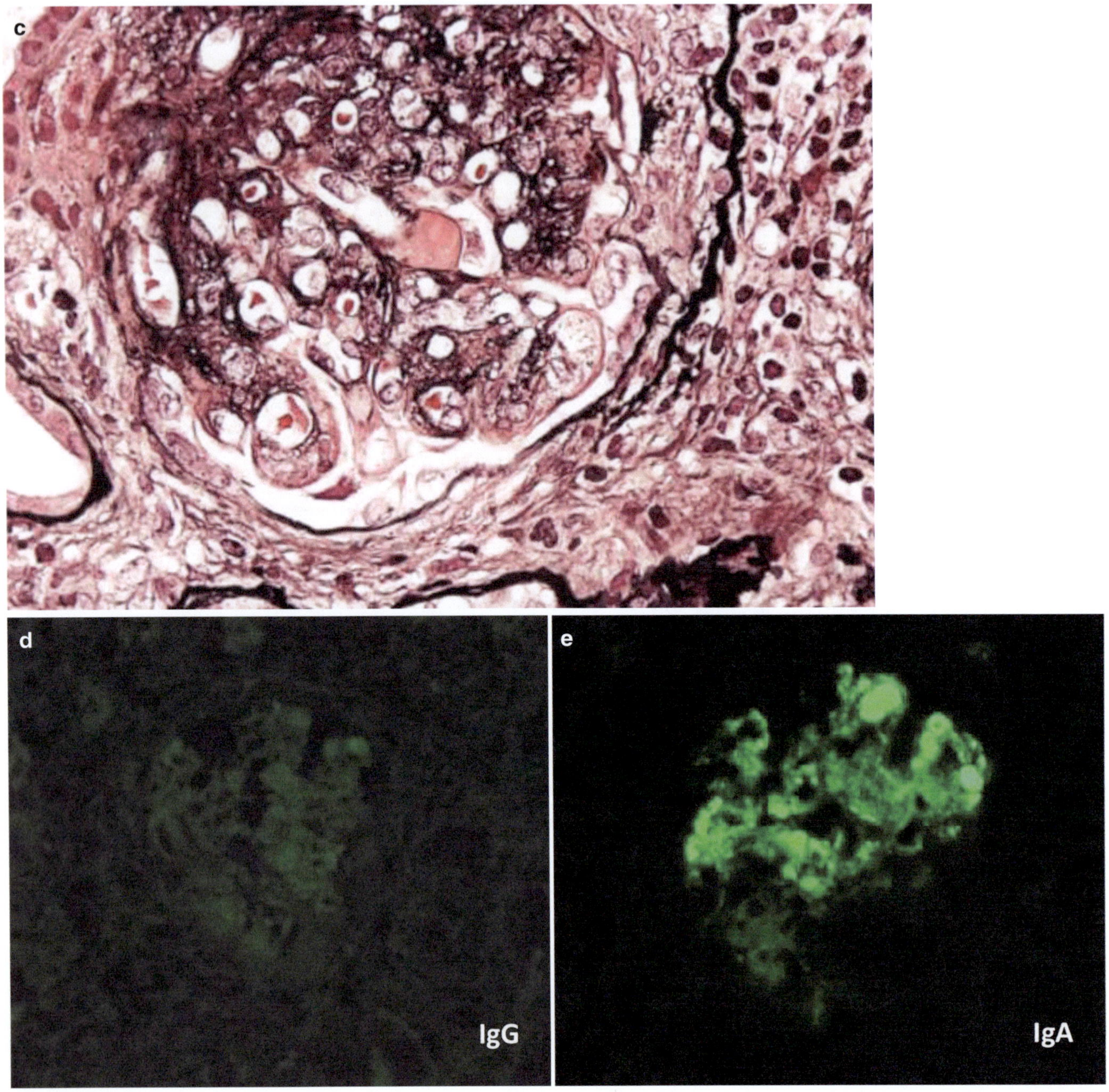

Fig. 18.4 (continued)

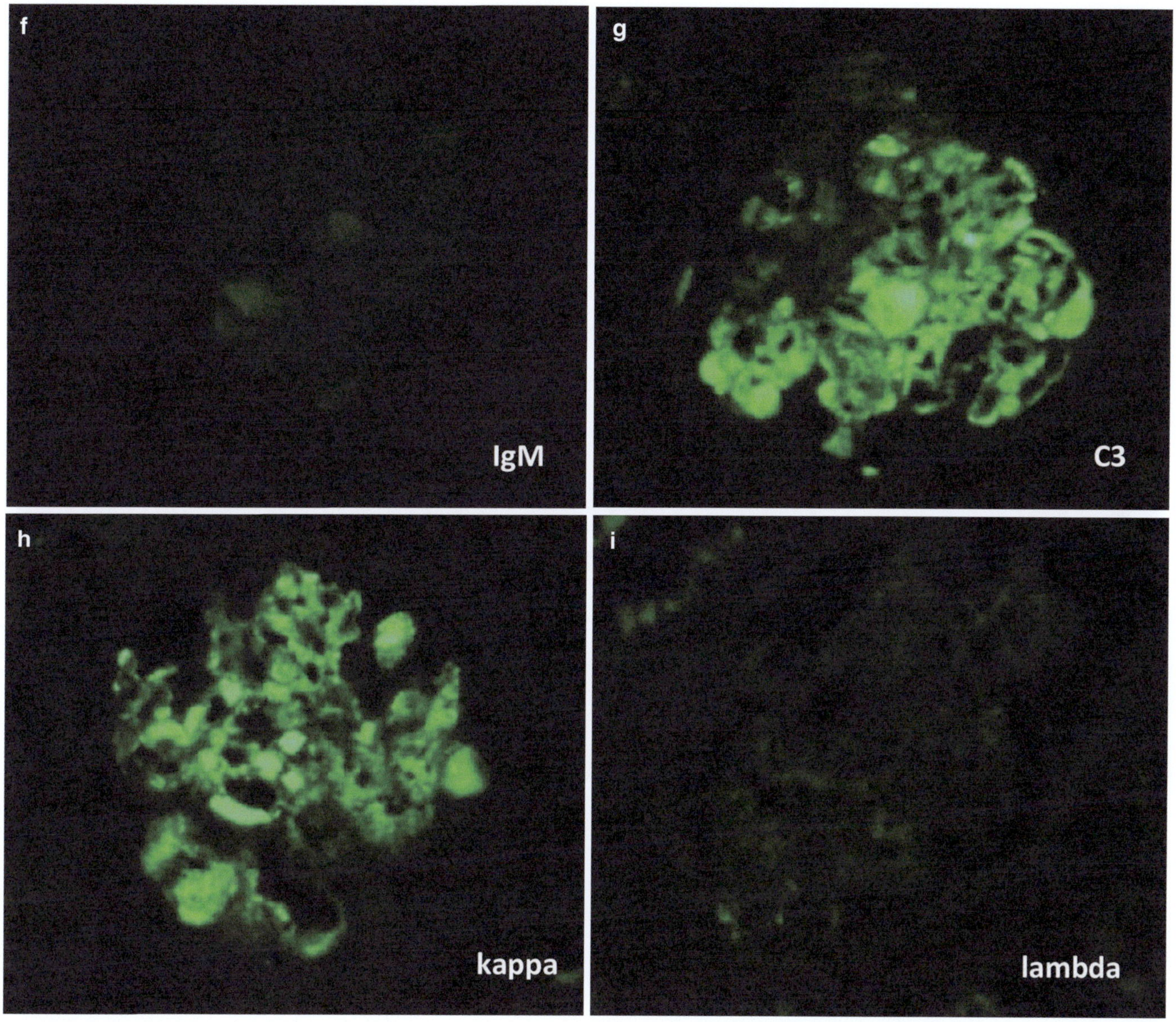

Fig. 18.4 (continued)

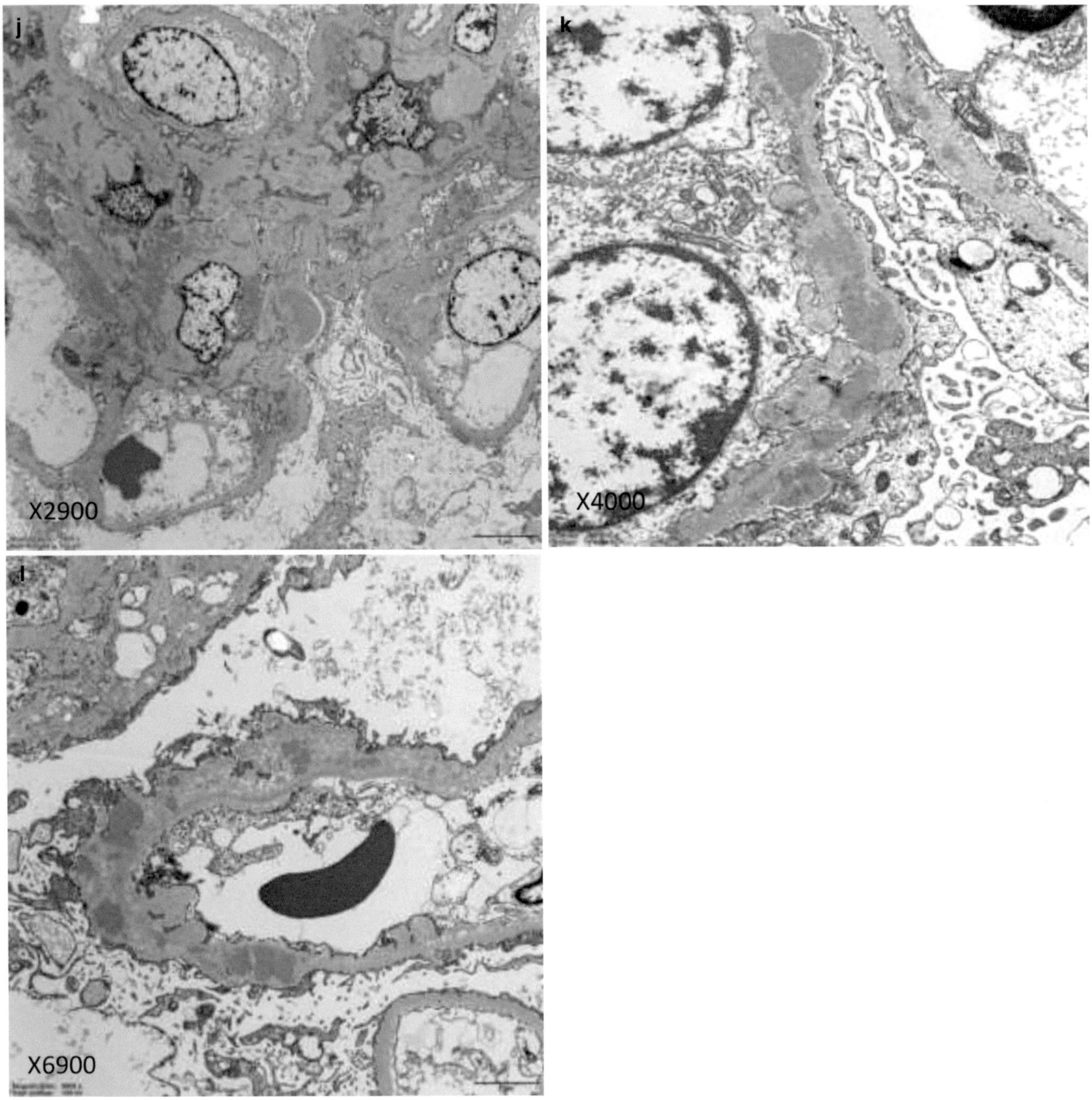

Fig. 18.4 (continued)

18.4 Monoclonal Gammopathy of Renal Significance (MGRS)

Monoclonal gammopathy of renal significance (MGRS) is characterized by the production of nephrotoxic monoclonal light chains or heavy chains by small neoplastic clonal proliferation of plasma cells or other hematolymphoid neoplasms which would otherwise not require treatment according to current disease-specific hematological criteria. Hematological assessment of these patients often shows <10% clonal plasma cells in the bone marrow with <30 g/L of serum monoclonal immunoglobulin. Renal manifestations of MGRS can be diverse in the form of monoclonal immunoglobulin deposition disease (MIDD), Proliferative glomerulonephritis with monoclonal immunoglobulin deposits (PGNMID), amyloidosis, fibrillary glomerulonephritis, immunotactoid glomerulonephritis, cryoglobulinemia, C3 glomerulopathy, thrombotic microangiopathy, light chain proximal tubulopathy or crystaglobulin induced nephropathy. Clinical manifestations would be according to the specific form of renal disease involving the kidney. These patients of MGUS/smoldering myeloma/smoldering Waldenstrom's macroglobulinemia with renal involvement (MGRS) would require treatment so as to halt the progression of renal disease and prevent the development of end-stage renal disease as they do not undergo spontaneous remission. These disorders also have very high chances of recurrence after transplantation if left untreated. Renal biopsy along with immunofluorescence microscopy and electron microscopy plays a crucial role in the diagnosis of monoclonal gammopathy of renal significance. A case of light chain deposition disease, LCDD (Fig. 18.5), and heavy chain deposition disease, HCDD (Fig. 18.6) in the setting of MGRS have been illustrated.

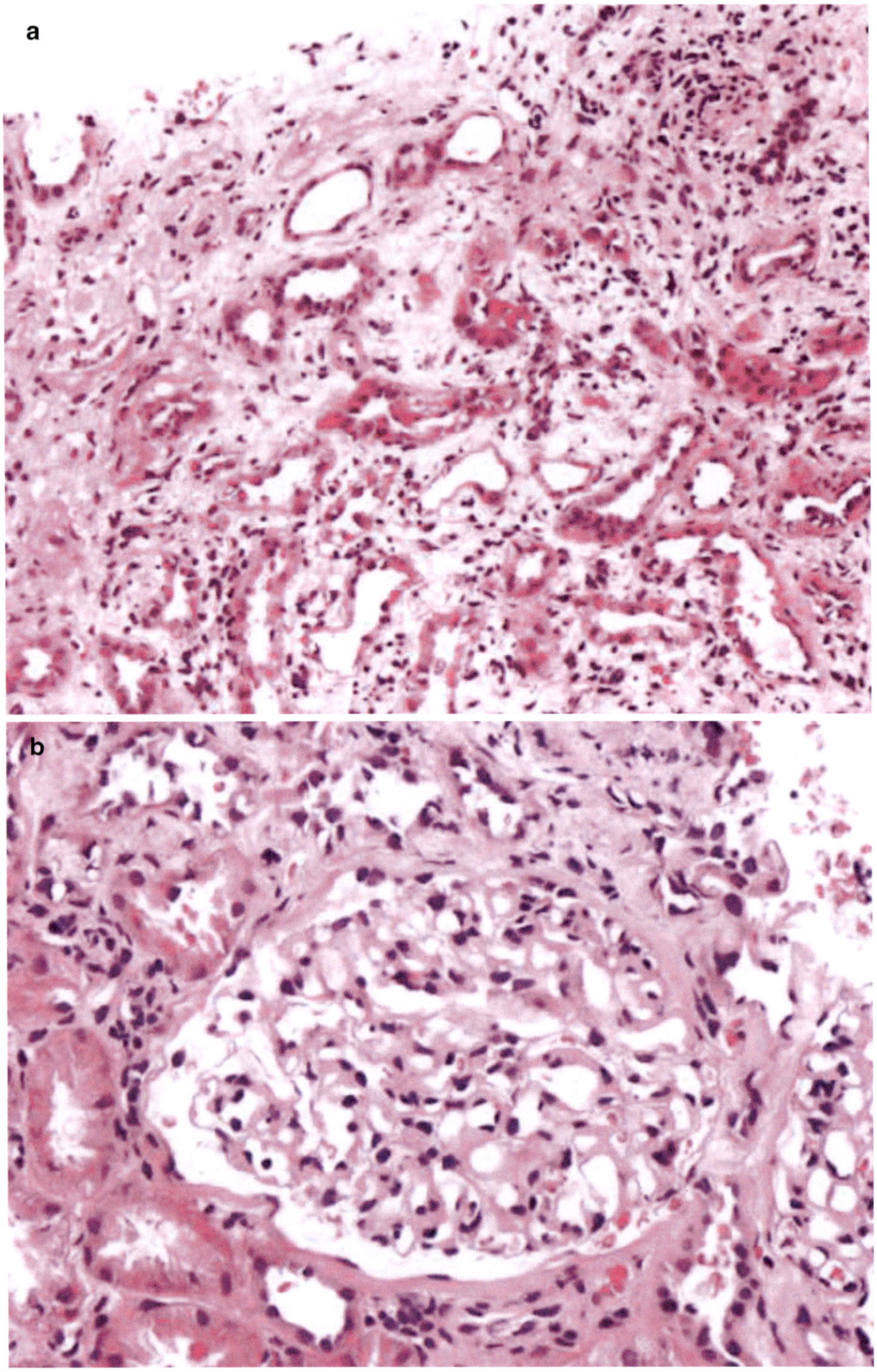

Fig. 18.5 LCDD in MGRS A 61-years male patient presented with generalized weakness and reduced appetite for 1 month. He was nondiabetic and nonhypertensive. There was no history of backache, arthralgia, or NSAID intake. On examination, there was no pedal edema or facial swelling. His hemoglobin was 11 g/dl, serum calcium was 9 mg/dl and serum creatinine was 4.5 mg/dl. Urine analysis showed absence of protein or sugar and microscopy showed 2–4 RBC/hpf. ANA, c-ANCA and p-ANCA were all negative. Serum protein electrophoresis was negative. Serum immunofixation electrophoresis revealed a monoclonal band corresponding to IgA-kappa. Serum-free light chain assay showed kappa/lambda ratio of 11.17 with markedly elevated kappa light chains (333 mg/L). Bone marrow aspiration showed just 7% plasma cells. Renal biopsy revealed 10 glomeruli; mild mesangial expansion was seen in few glomeruli. Nodular configuration, endocapillary hyperplasia, increased mesangial cellularity or MPGN pattern was not seen. Few glomeruli showed thickening of Bowman's capsule and periglomerular fibrosis. Few of tubules showed thickening of basement membranes by PAS and silver positive deposits. Lining epithelium of few tubules was infiltrated by lymphocytes. Interstitium showed lymphoplasmacytic infiltrate and occasional eosinophils and edema. Focal tubular atrophy and interstitial fibrosis were seen. Blood vessels were unremarkable. IF showed glomerular mesangial and capillary wall deposits of kappa light chain. Similar deposits were seen along tubular basement membrane and in interstitium. IgG, IgA, IgM, C3, C1q, and lambda were negative. EM showed powdery electron-dense deposits in subendothelial and mesangial areas of glomeruli. Similar deposits were also seen along Bowman's capsule of glomeruli and tubular basement membranes. (**a–c**) HE × 400, (**d–e**) PAS × 400, (**f**) PSM × 200, (**g**) IF × 200, (**h–j**) EM

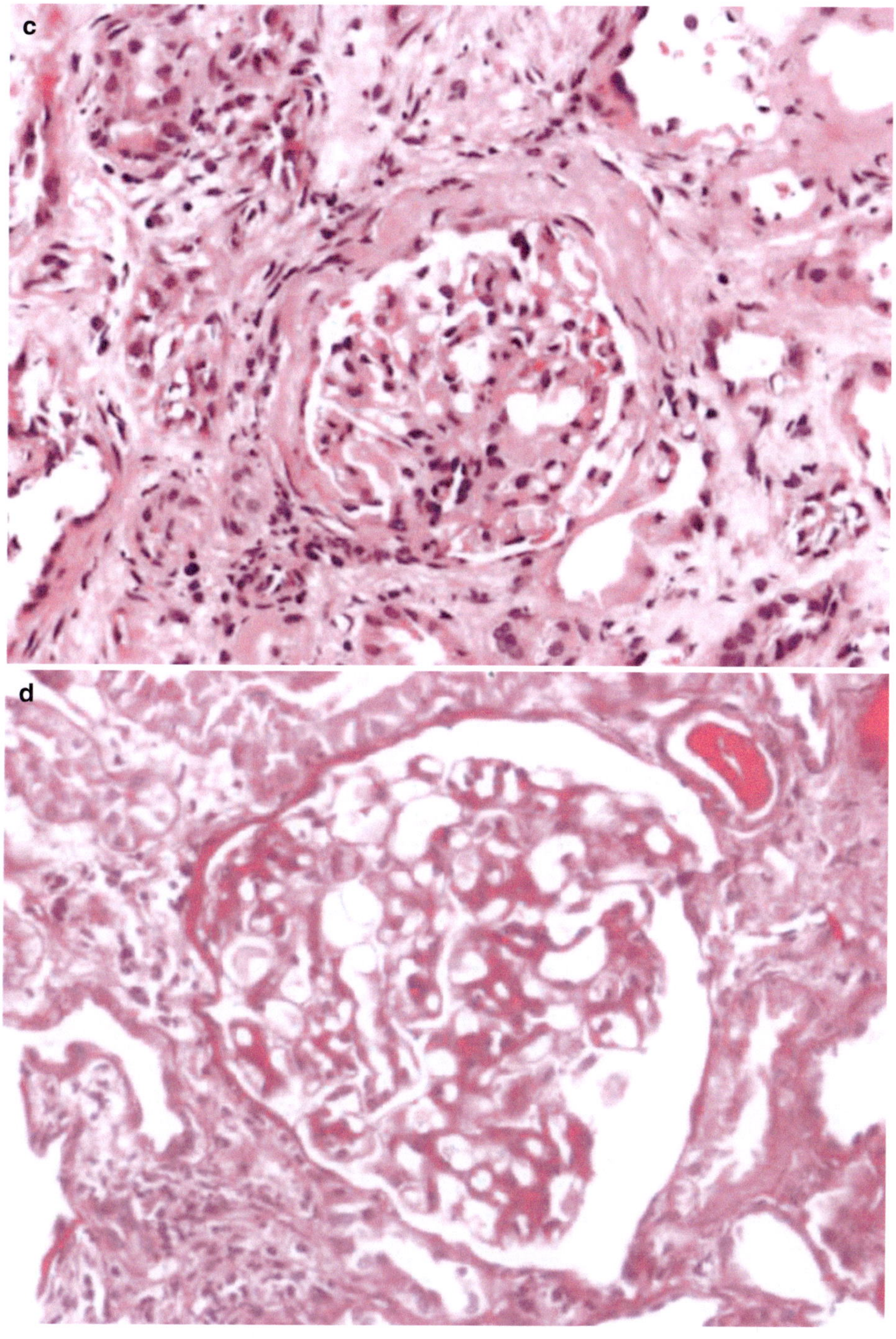

Fig. 18.5 (continued)

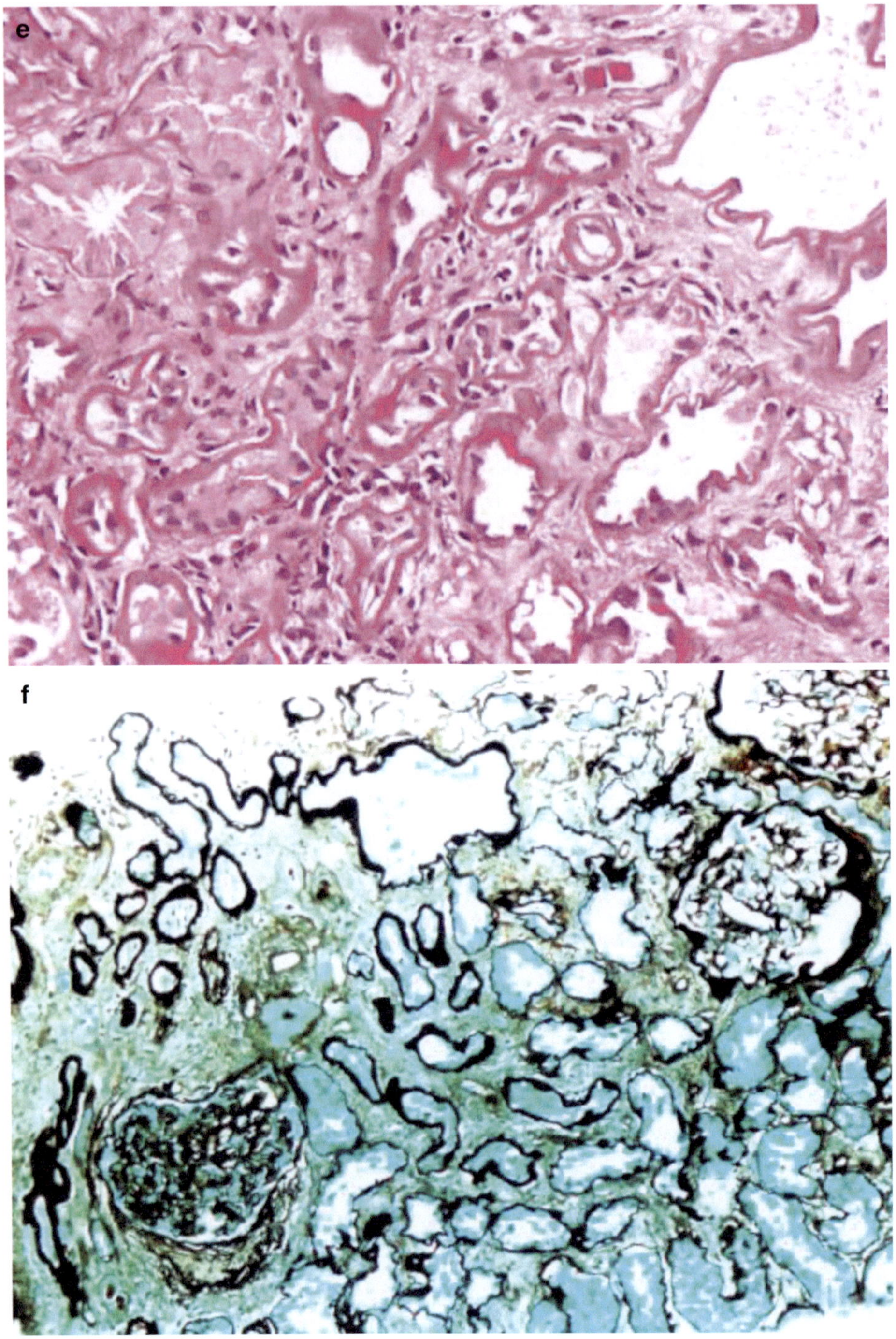

Fig. 18.5 (continued)

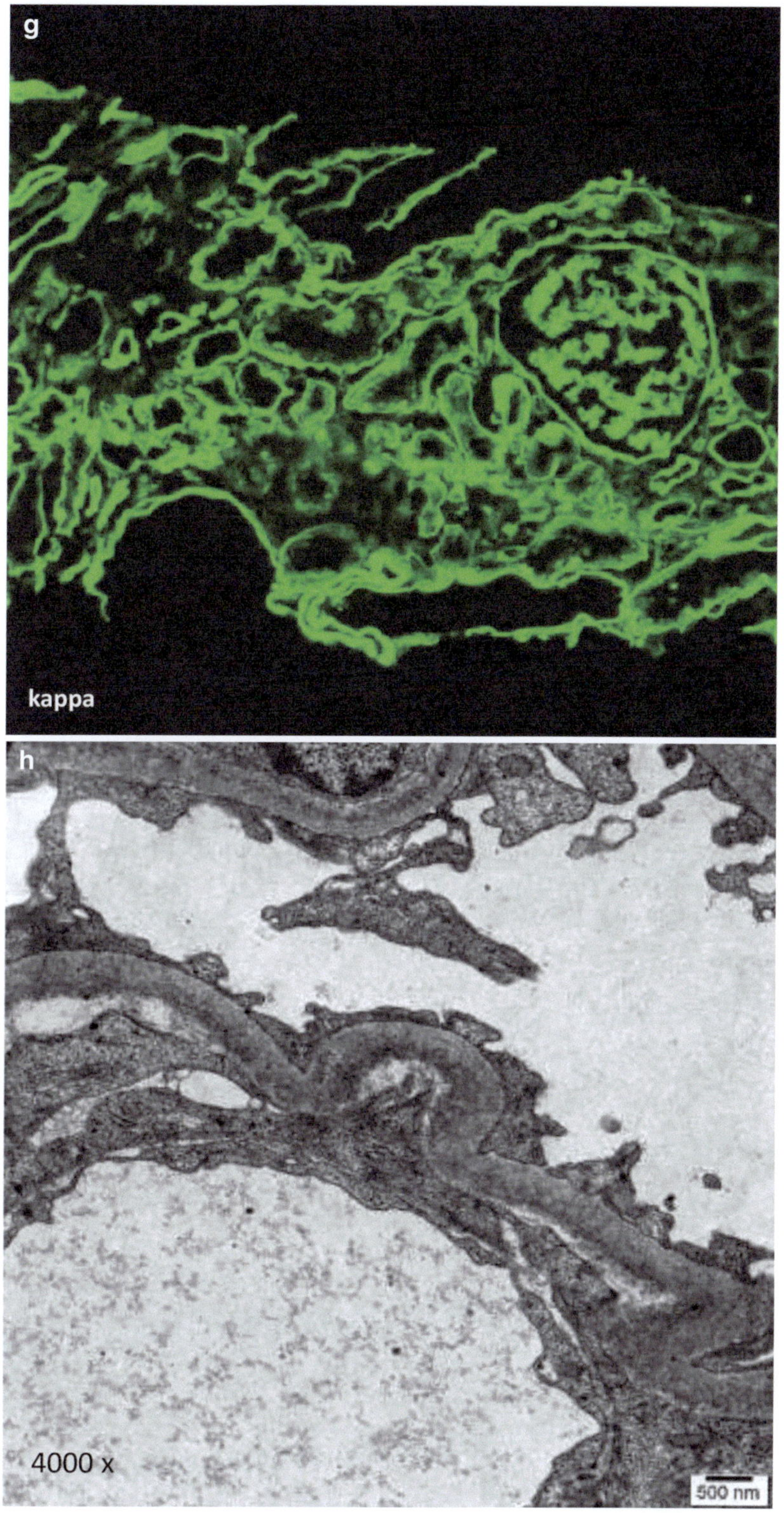

Fig. 18.5 (continued)

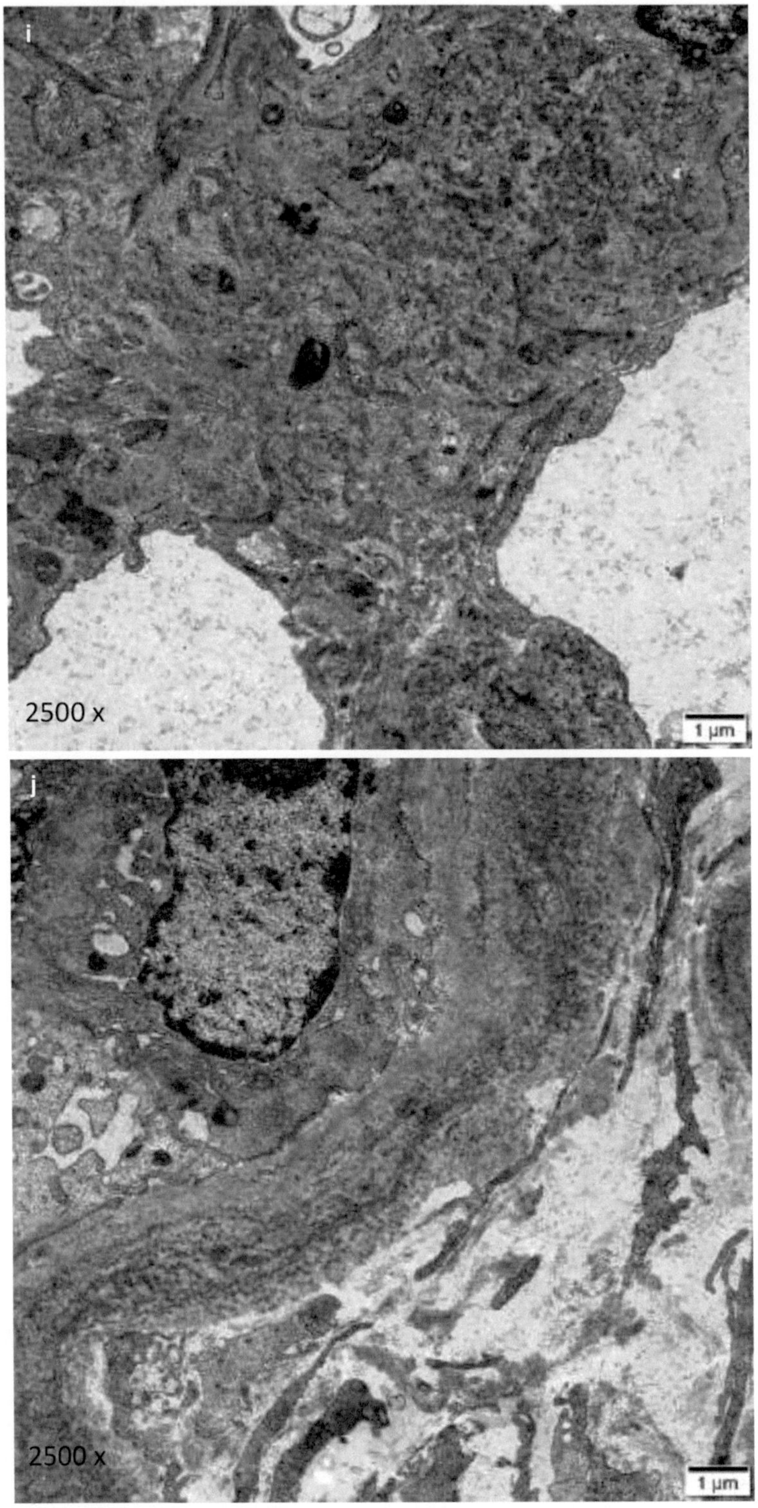

Fig. 18.5 (continued)

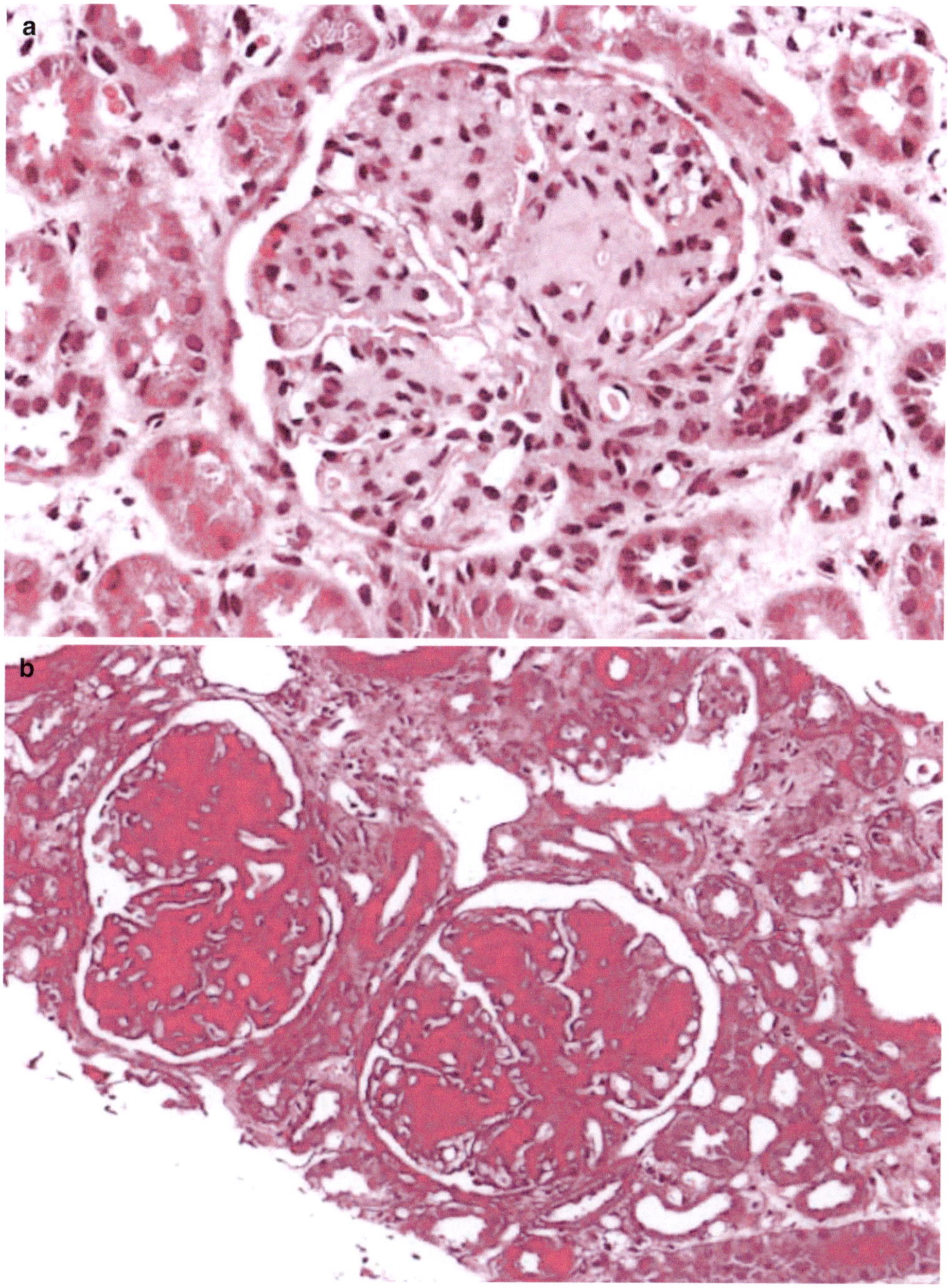

Fig. 18.6 **HCDD in MGRS** A 35-years non-diabetic male patient presented with bilateral pedal edema and hypertension for past 2 months. His urine analysis revealed albumin ++, RBC 3-5 and WBC 10–15/hpf. Urinary P/C ratio was 2.1. His glycosylated hemoglobin was 4.7%. Serum complements were wnl and ASO titer was negative. Immunofixation electrophoresis did not show any monoclonal band. Serum IgG was 5.35 g/L, serum IgA was 2.69 g/L and serum IgM was 0.34 g/L. Renal biopsy had 13 glomeruli, none of them had segmental or global glomerulosclerosis. All the glomeruli showed mesangial expansion with the formation of mesangial nodules and patent capillary loops. The nodules were PAS and PSM positive and congo red negative. Any reduplication of the capillary basement membrane was not evident. Some of the renal tubules had thickened PAS-positive basement membrane and the interstitium had mild lymphocytic infiltration. Blood vessels showed mild arteriosclerosis. IF showed positivity for IgG (4+) which was a monoclonal IgG1 subtype along the glomerular mesangium and capillary basement membrane and the tubular basement membrane; all other IgG subclasses including IgG2, IgG3, and IgG4, IgM, IgA, C3, C1q and kappa and lambda light chains were negative in glomeruli. EM revealed subendothelial electron-dense deposits in GBM along with focal loss of foot processes, mesangial areas were also expanded and showed electron-dense deposits. Tubules also showed electron-dense deposits along the basement membrane. (**a**) HE × 400, (**b**) PAS × 400, (**c**) PSM × 400, (**d**, **e**) IF × 400 and (**f**, **g**) EM (identity of the patient has been concealed)

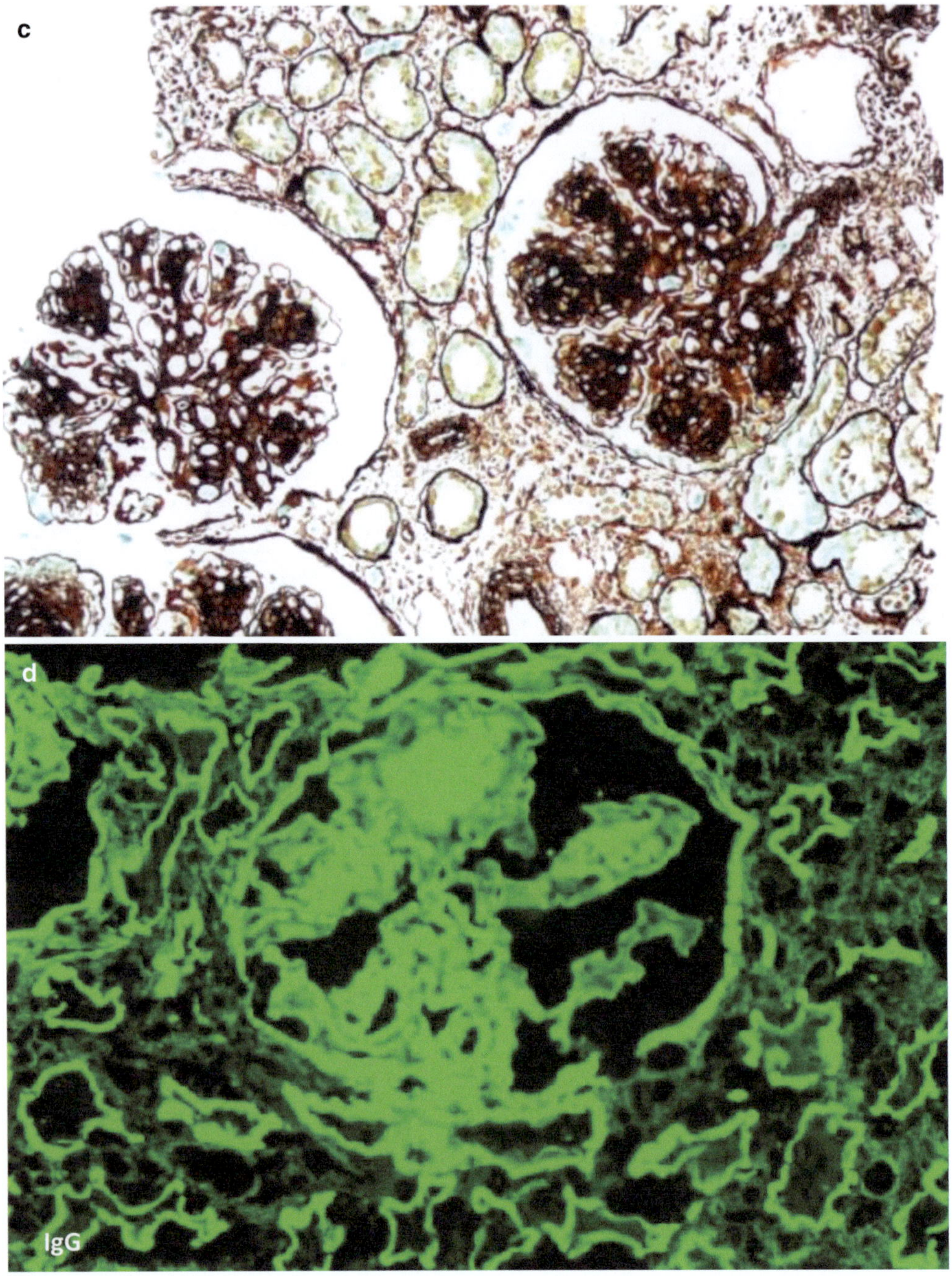

Fig. 18.6 (continued)

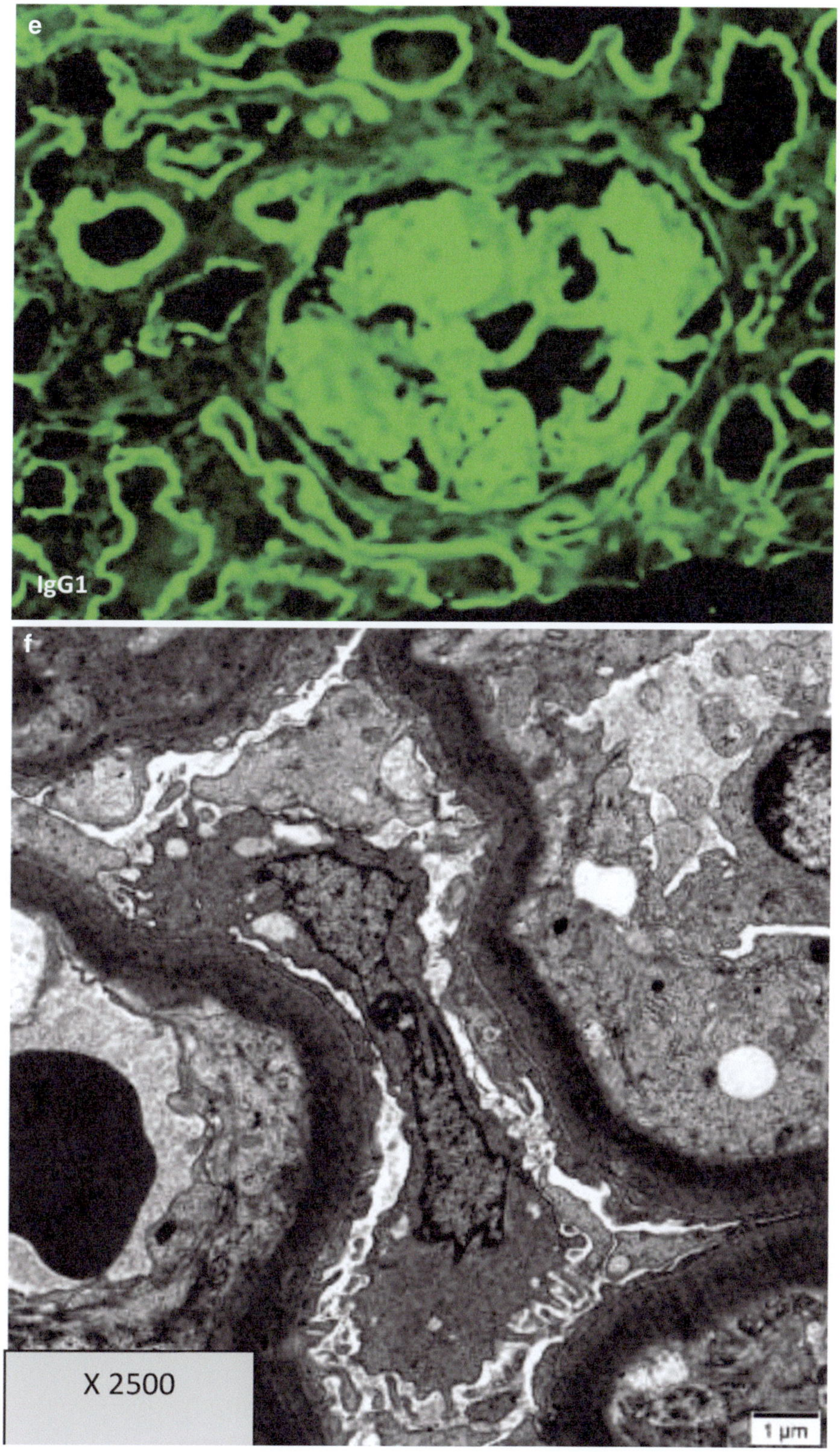

Fig. 18.6 (continued)

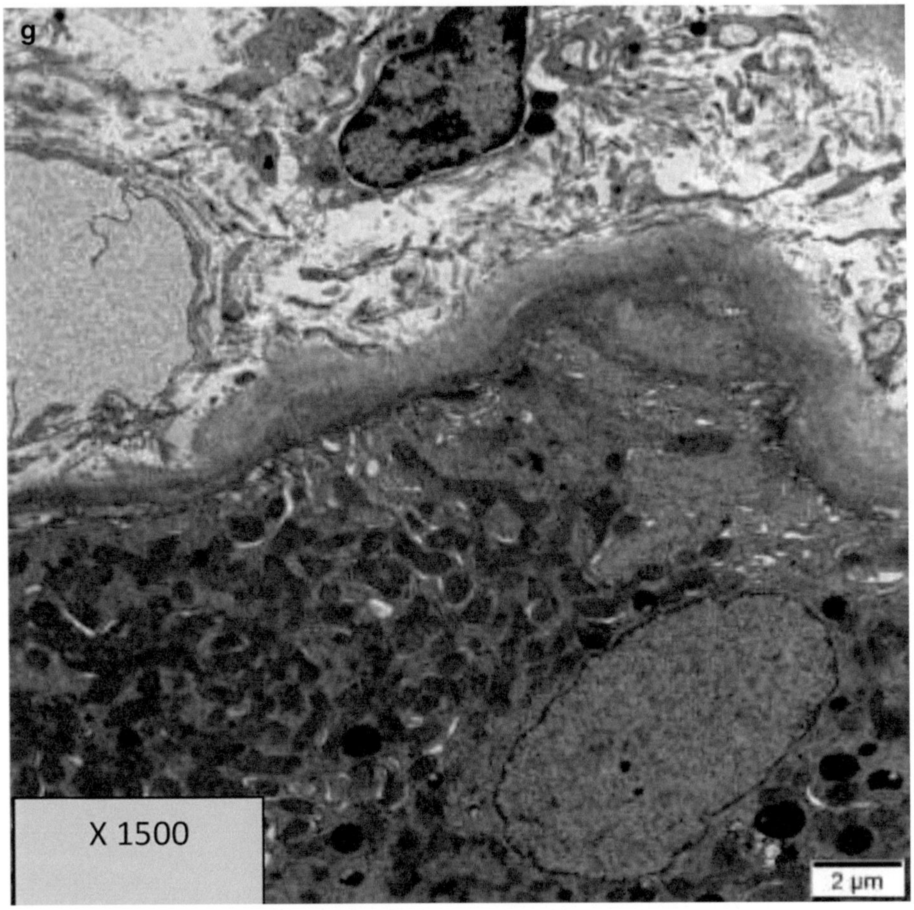

Fig. 18.6 (continued)

Further Reading

Myeloma Cast Nephropathy

Manohar S, Nasr SH, Leung N. Light chain cast nephropathy: practical considerations in the management of myeloma kidney-what we know and what the future may hold. Curr Hematol Malig Rep. 2018;13:220–6.

Nasr SH, Valeri AM, Sethi S, Fidler ME, Cornell LD, Gertz MA, Lacy M, Dispenzieri A, Rajkumar SV, Kyle RA, Leung N. Clinicopathologic correlations in multiple myeloma: a case series of 190 patients with kidney biopsies. Am J Kidney Dis. 2012;59:786–94.

Santos A, Soto K, Sis B, Touchard G, Venner CP, Bridoux F. Clinicopathologic predictors of renal outcomes in light chain cast nephropathy: a multicenter retrospective study. Blood. 2020;21(135):1833–46.

Sathick IJ, Drosou ME, Leung N. Myeloma light chain cast nephropathy, a review. J Nephrol. 2019;32:189–98.

Light Chain Deposition Disease (LCDD)

Kanzaki G, Okabayashi Y, Nagahama K, Ohashi R, Tsuboi N, Yokoo T, Shimizu A. Monoclonal immunoglobulin deposition disease and related diseases. J Nippon Med Scheme. 2019;86:2–9.

Sayed RH, Wechalekar AD, Gilbertson JA, Bass P, Mahmood S, Sachchithanantham S, Fontana M, Patel K, Whelan CJ, Lachmann HJ, Hawkins PN, Gillmore JD. Natural history and outcome of light chain deposition disease. Blood. 2015;126:2805–10.

Sethi S, Rajkumar SV, D'Agati VD. The complexity and heterogeneity of monoclonal immunoglobulin-associated renal diseases. J Am Soc Nephrol. 2018;29:1810–23.

Wang Q, Jiang F, Xu G. The pathogenesis of renal injury and treatment in light chain deposition disease. J Transl Med. 2019;17:387.

Heavy Chain Deposition Disease (HCDD)

Bridoux F, Javaugue V, Bender S, Leroy F, Aucouturier P, Debiais-Delpech C, Goujon JM, Quellard N, Bonaud A, Clavel M, Trouillas P, Di Meo F, Gombert JM, Fermand JP, Jaccard A, Cogné M, Touchard G, Sirac C. Unravelling the immunopathological mechanisms of heavy chain deposition disease with implications for clinical management. Kidney Int. 2017;91:423–34.

Cohen C, El-Karoui K, Alyanakian MA, Noel LH, Bridoux F, Knebelmann B. Light and heavy chain deposition disease associated with CH1 deletion. Clin Kidney J. 2015;8:237–9.

Oe Y, Soma J, Sato H, Ito S. Heavy chain deposition disease: an overview. Clin Exp Nephrol. 2013;17:771–8.

Zhang Y, Li X, Liang D, Xu F, Liang S, Zhu X, Zheng N, Huang X, Liu Z, Zeng C. Heavy chain deposition disease: clinicopathologic characteristics of a Chinese cases series. Am J Kidney Dis. 2020;75:736–43.

Proliferative Glomerulonephritis with Monoclonal Immunoglobulin Deposits (PGNMID)

Leung N, Bridoux F, Batuman V, et al. The evaluation of monoclonal gammopathy of renal significance: a consensus report of the International Kidney and Monoclonal Gammopathy Research Group. Nat Rev Nephrol. 2009;15:45–59.

Nasr SH, Satoskar A, Markowitz GS, et al. Proliferative glomerulonephritis with monoclonal IgG deposits. J Am Soc Nephrol. 2009;20:2055–64.

Said SM, Cosio FG, Valeri AM, Leung N, Sethi S, Salameh H, Cornell LD, Fidler ME, Alexander MP, Fervenza FC, Drosou ME, Zhang D, D'Agati VD, Nasr SH. Proliferative glomerulonephritis with monoclonal immunoglobulin G deposits is associated with high rate of early recurrence in the allograft. Kidney Int. 2018;94:159–69.

Sethi S, Vincet S, Rajkumar VD, D'Agati VD. The complexity and heterogeneity of monoclonal immunoglobulin-associated renal diseases. JASN. 2018;29:1810–23.

Xing G, Gillespie R, Bedri B, Quan A, Zhang P, Zhou XJ. Proliferative glomerulonephritis with monoclonal IgG deposits in children and young adults. Pediatr Nephrol. 2018;33:1531–8.

Monoclonal Gammopathy of Renal Significance (MGRS)

Amaador K, Peeters H, Minnema MC, Nguyen TQ, Dendooven A, Vos JMI, Croockewit AJ, van de Donk NWCJ, Jacobs JFM, Wetzels JFM, Sprangers B, Abrahams AC. Monoclonal gammopathy of renal significance (MGRS) histopathologic classification, diagnostic workup, and therapeutic options. Neth J Med. 2019;77:243–54.

Jain A, Haynes R, Kothari J, Khera A, Soares M, Ramasamy K. Pathophysiology and management of monoclonal gammopathy of renal significance. Blood Adv. 2019;3:2409–23.

Leung N, Bridoux F, Batuman V, Chaidos A, Cockwell P, D'Agati VD, Dispenzieri A, et al. The evaluation of monoclonal gammopathy of renal significance: a consensus report of the International Kidney and Monoclonal Gammopathy Research Group. Nat Rev Nephrol. 2019;15:45–59.

Leung N, Bridoux F, Nasr SH. Monoclonal gammopathy of renal significance. N Engl J Med. 2021;384:1931–41.

19 Cryoglobulinemic, Fibrillary, and Collagenofibrotic Glomerulopathy

19.1 Cryoglobulinemic Glomerulonephritis

Cryoglobulinemia is characterized by the presence of cryoglobulins in the serum. Cryoglobulinemic vasculitis can show involvement of skin, joints, kidney, peripheral nerves, etc. Cryoglobulinemic glomerulonephritis is seen in patients with type II (hepatitis C, connective tissue disorders) and type III (chronic hepatitis B and C, mixed connective tissue diseases) mixed cryoglobulinemia and in patients with type I cryoglobulinemia with monoclonal IgG3 or IgG1 (associated with MGUS, lymphoma or multiple myeloma). Cryoglobulinemic glomerulonephritis is most commonly seen in the setting of type II cryoglobulinemia. These patients can have reduced serum C3 and C4 levels.

Patients with renal involvement commonly present with hematuria, hypertension, proteinuria, and renal insufficiency. Up to 50% of patients can have nephrotic range proteinuria.

Light microscopy shows MPGN type I pattern (majority of patients) with lobular accentuation, endocapillary hyperplasia, and hyaline thrombi (PAS-positive) within the lumen of glomerular capillary loops. The endocapillary hyperplasia is because of mesangial cell interposition or monocytes/macrophages.

Other than MPGN pattern, endocapillary proliferative pattern, mesangioproliferative pattern, or crescentic glomerulonephritis can also be seen.

On immunofluorescence, granular IgG and IgM staining can be seen along glomerular capillary walls, mesangium, and within hyaline thrombi. Cases that are associated with monoclonal gammopathy will show monoclonal kappa or lambda light chain along the glomerular capillary wall and in thrombi.

On electron microscopy, amorphous deposits, short and curved microtubules, or annular profiles of microtubules can be seen. They can be seen in subendothelial location, mesangium, or within the capillary lumen. A case of cryoglobulinemic glomerulonephritis is illustrated (Fig. 19.1).

P. Gupta, R. K. Gupta, *Pathology of Glomerular Diseases*, https://doi.org/10.1007/978-981-19-1430-0_19

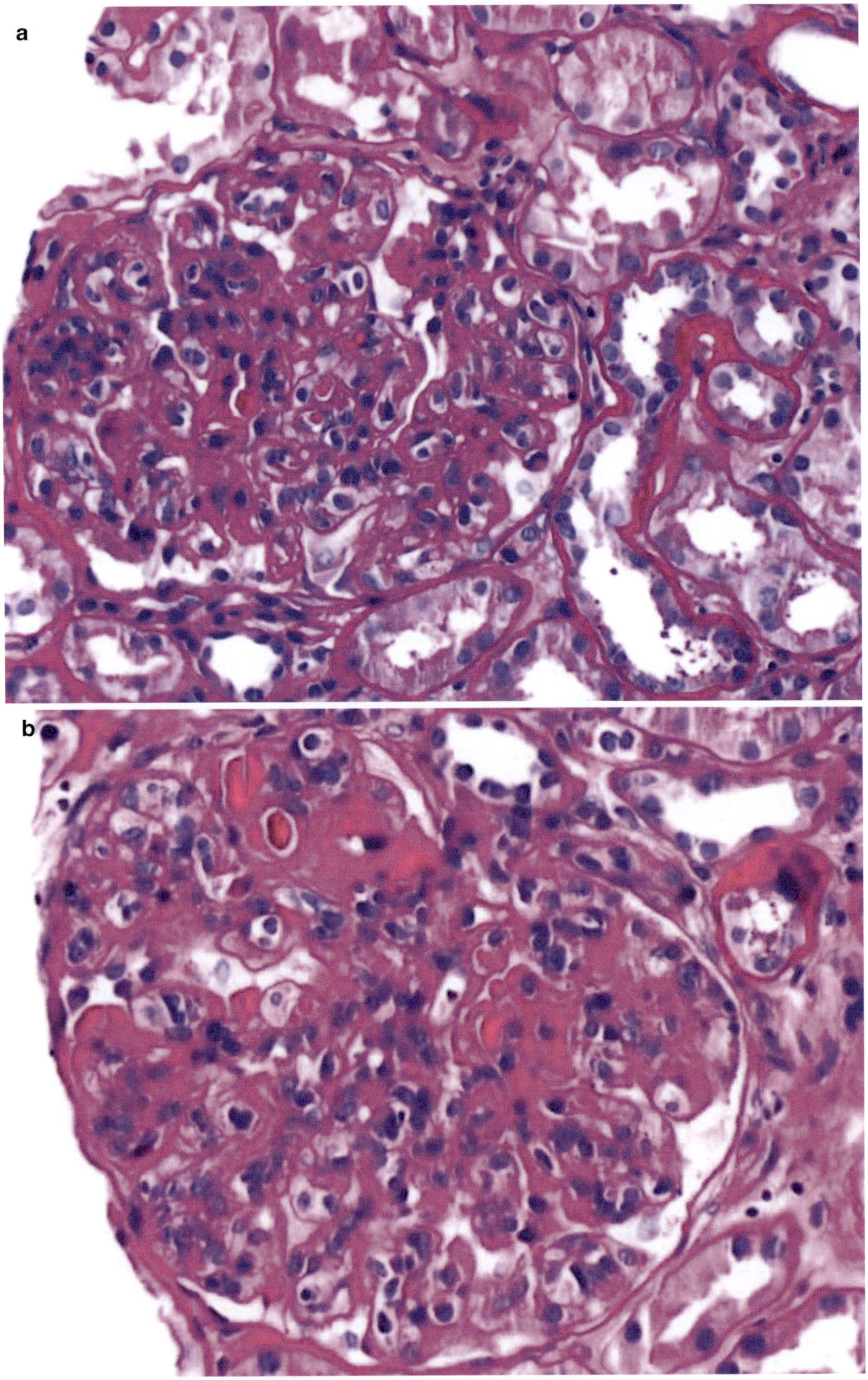

Fig. 19.1 **Cryoglobulinemic Glomerulonephritis** A 70-years African American male patient with a history of diabetes mellitus, hypertension, liver disease, congestive heart failure, chronic kidney disease, and hepatitis C infection with cryoglobulinemia, presented with gastrointestinal bleeding, anemia and acute kidney injury. Serum creatinine was 3.5 mg/dL. Renal biopsy revealed that the glomeruli were enlarged with endocapillary hyperplasia and intravascular fibrin thrombi. IF showed positivity for IgG, IgM, kappa and lambda. EM showed intramembranous electron-dense deposits. (**a**) PAS × 200, (**b**) PAS × 400, (**c**–**f**) IF × 400, (**g**–**i**) EM. (Contributor—Helen Liapis, Professor of Pathology and Immunology and Internal Medicine (Renal) retired, Washington University School of Medicine, Saint Louis, MO, USA)

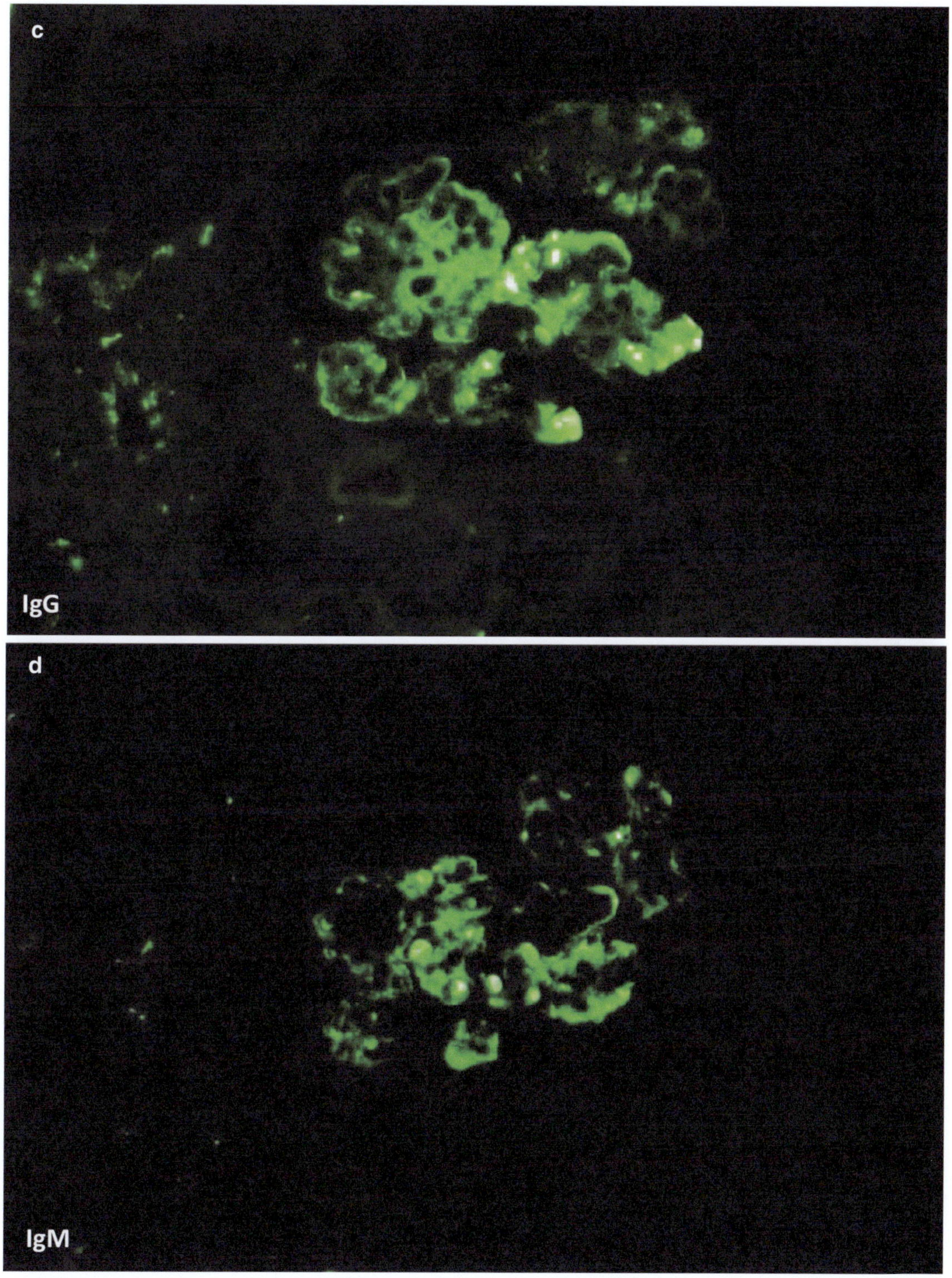

Fig. 19.1 (continued)

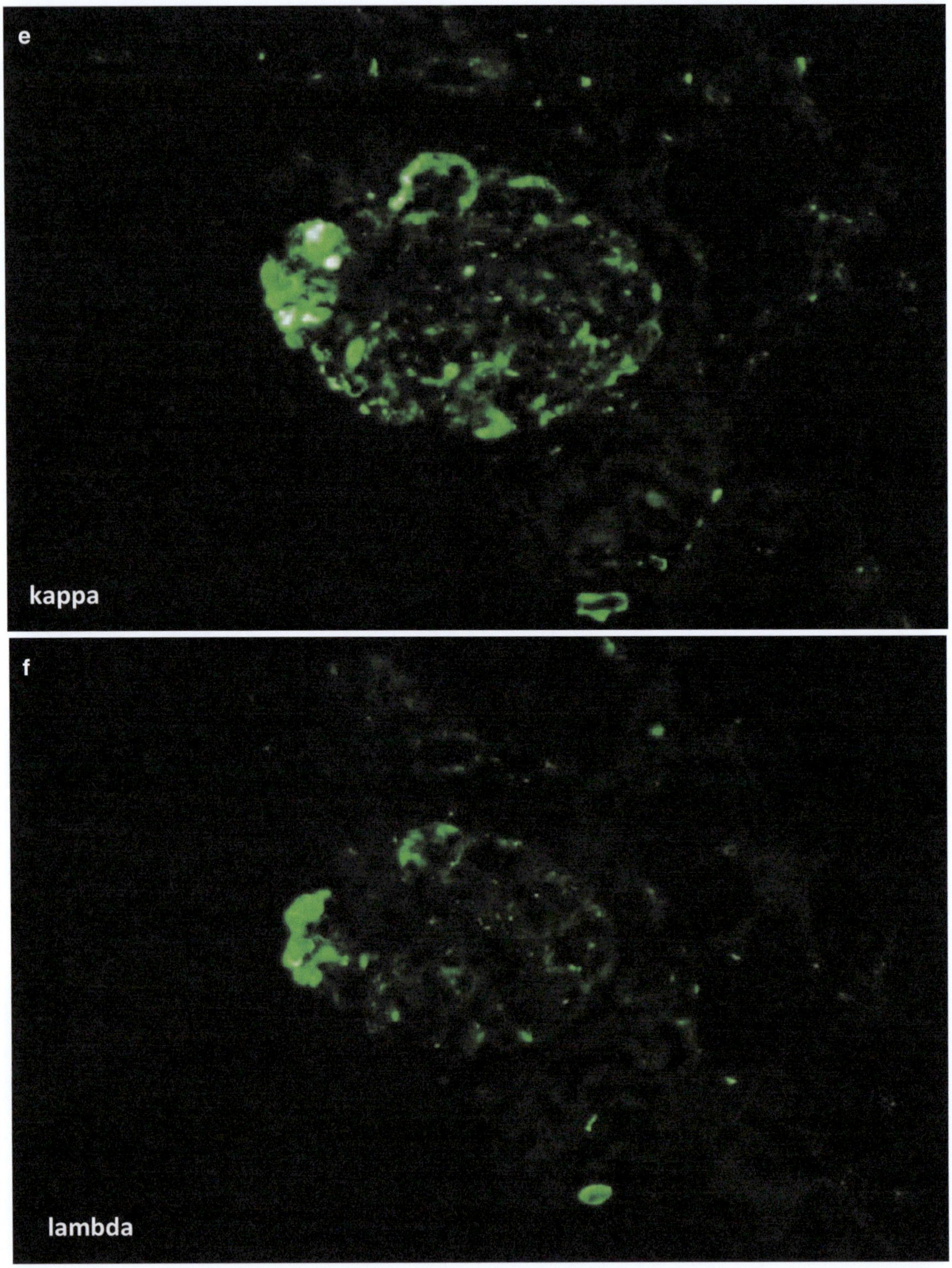

Fig. 19.1 (continued)

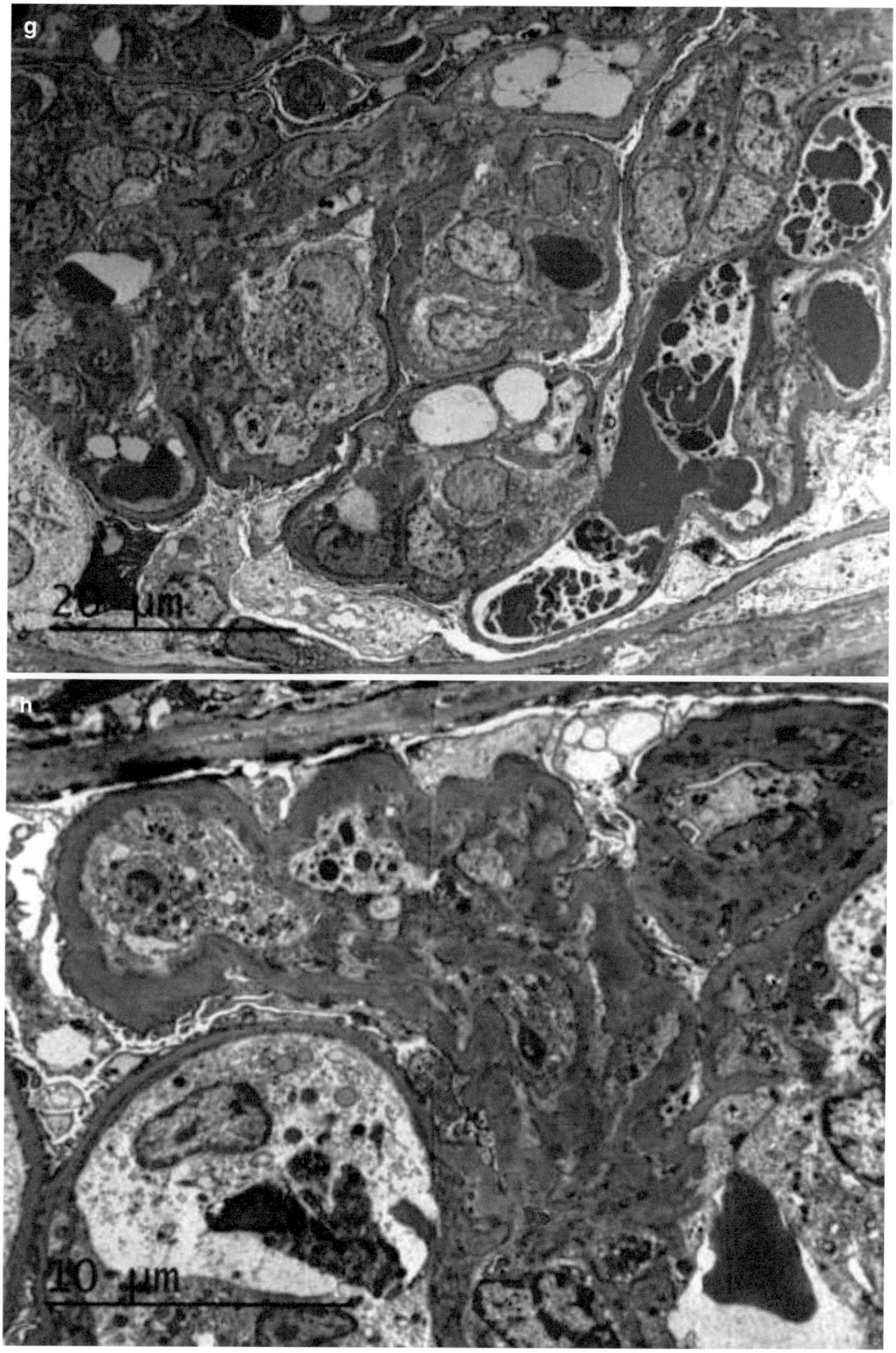

Fig. 19.1 (continued)

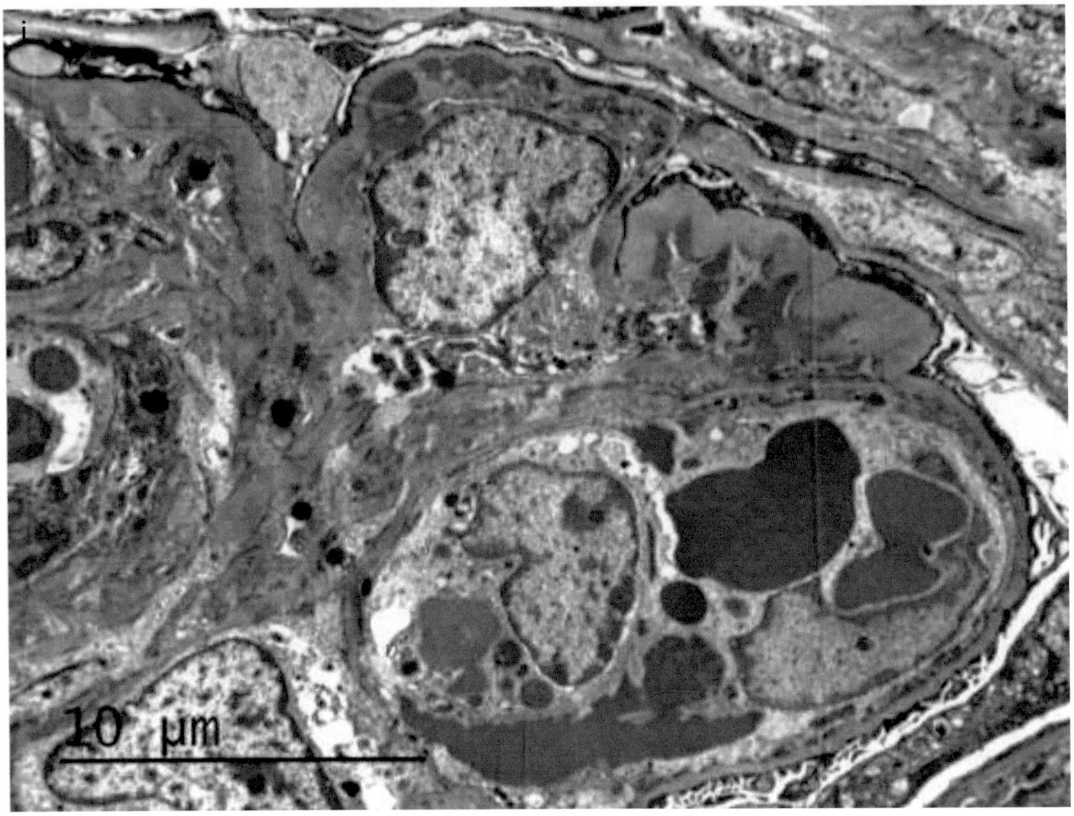

Fig. 19.1 (continued)

19.2 Fibrillary Glomerulonephritis

Patients with fibrillary glomerulonephritis present clinically with nephrotic range proteinuria accompanied by hematuria. Patient may have evidence of renal insufficiency. Majority of patients are beyond fifth decade of life and females are more commonly involved than males. On light microscopy, renal biopsy may have mesangioproliferative, membranoproliferative, or diffuse endocapillary proliferative pattern. Rarely membranous pattern or diffuse sclerosing pattern may also be seen. Pale PAS nonargyrophilic weakly eosinophilic material is seen to be deposited in mesangium which can also be seen along the glomerular capillary basement membrane. These deposits may appear smudgy on immunofluorescence. IgG, C3, kappa and lambda are positive in the glomerular deposits. In cases that are secondary to paraproteinemia, light chain restriction may be seen. Rarely tubular basement membrane deposits can also be seen. On electron microscopy, randomly oriented nonbranching fibrils are seen which are 15–25 nm in diameter and are larger in size than amyloid fibrils. These are distributed within the mesangium but can also be seen within lamina densa of glomerular capillary basement membrane with rare subepithelial and subendothelial deposits. Sometimes small conventional electron dense deposits can also be identified. Laser microdissection and mass spectrometry studies have identified DNAJB9 as chief protein in deposits of fibrillary glomerulonephritis. Immunohistochemistry for DNAJB9 is available and helps in confirming the diagnosis in these cases. Prognosis of fibrillary glomerulonephritis is poor with a significant proportion of cases progressing to ESRD. Fibrillary glomerulonephritis can reoccur in renal transplants although limited data is available. Two cases of fibrillary glomerulonephritis are illustrated (Figs. 19.2 and 19.3).

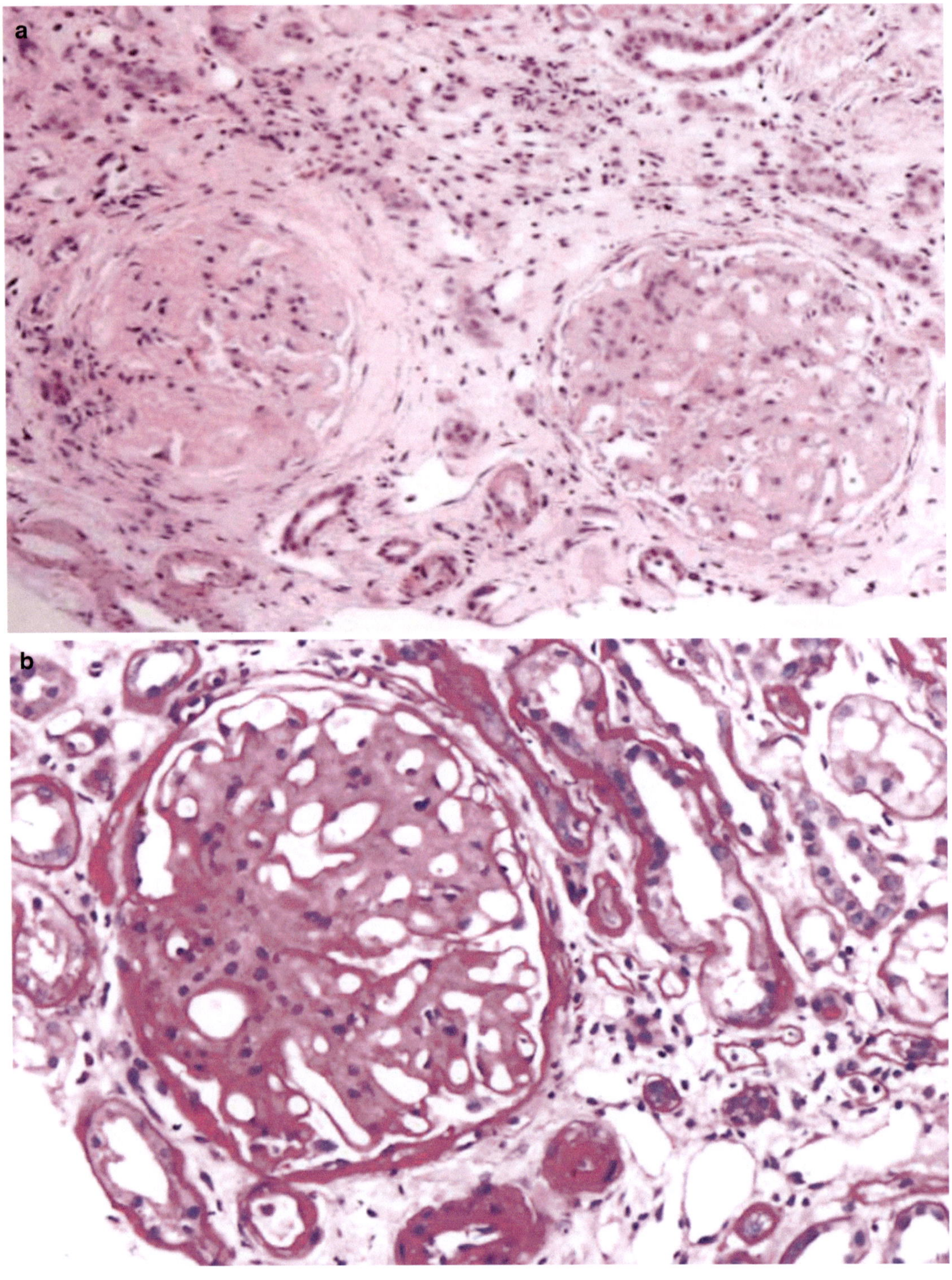

Fig. 19.2 Fibrillary Glomerulonephritis A 42-years non-diabetic male patient presented with nephritic syndrome and hypertension. His urinary albumin was 3+ with blend urinary sediment. Serum albumin was 2.2 gm/dl and serum cholesterol was 300 mg/dl. Serum complement C3 and C4 were wnl. Two core renal biopsy was obtained which contained 40 glomeruli, 16 of them were globally sclerosed. Other glomeruli showed diffuse mesangial expansion by eosinophilic, weakly PAS-positive, variably argyrophilic, non-congophilic material with segmental capillary wall deposits. Variable mesangial hypercellularity was also noted. Any endocapillary hypercellularity, neutrophil infiltration, or crescents were not seen. Blood vessels were unremarkable. About 50% of tubules showed atrophy and the interstitial fibrosis involved about 50% of the cortex. Woolly polyclonal IgG deposition was seen in mesangial and capillary wall locations. IHC was positive for DNAJB9. EM showed randomly arranged fibrils of 10–20 nm. (**a**) HE × 200, (**b**) PAS × 400, (**c**) Jones × 400, (**d**) IF for polyclonal IgG × 400, (**e**) IHC for DNAJB9 × 400 and (**f**) EM (Contributor—Dr. Geetika Singh, Additional Professor, All India Institute of Medical Sciences, New Delhi, India)

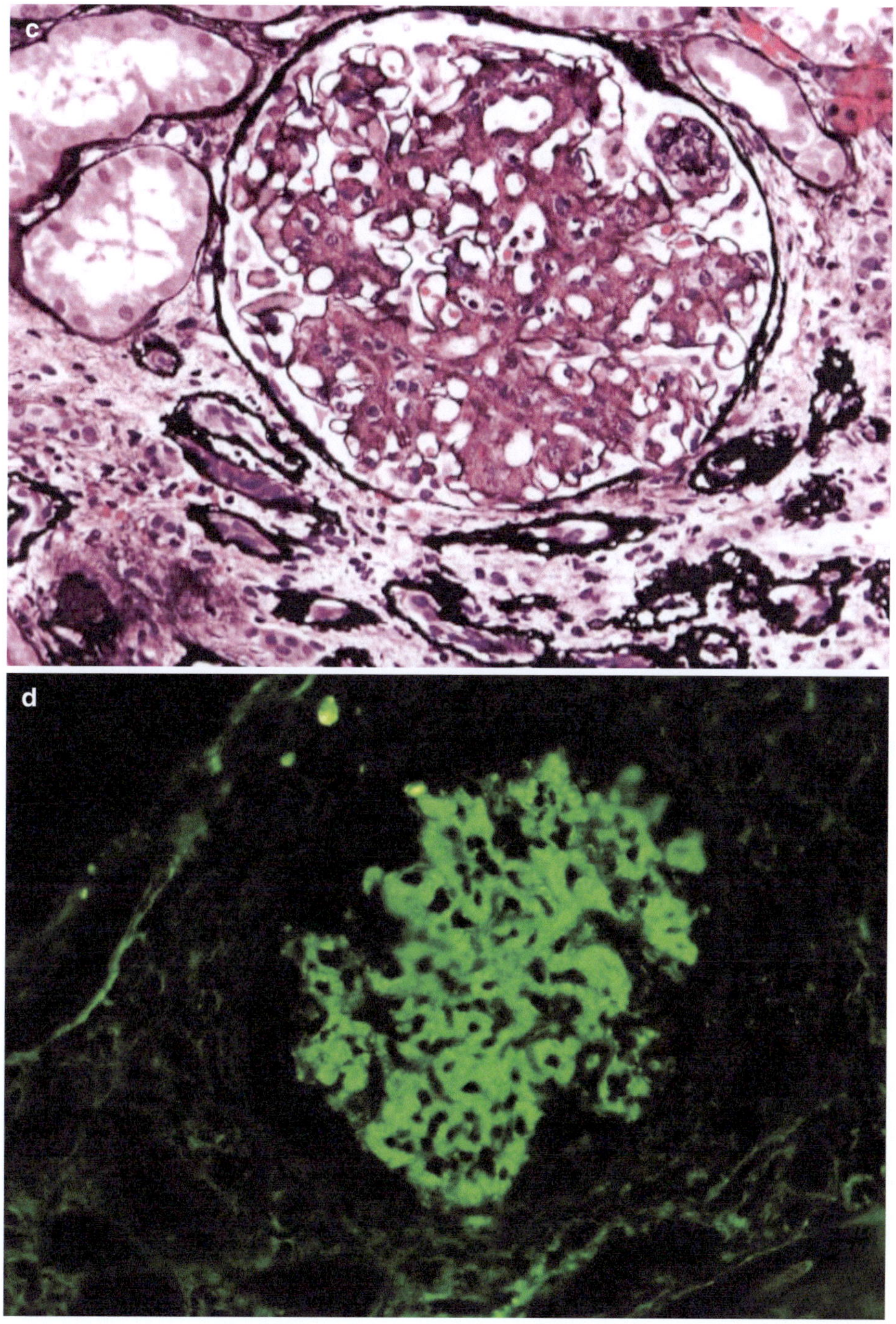

Fig. 19.2 (continued)

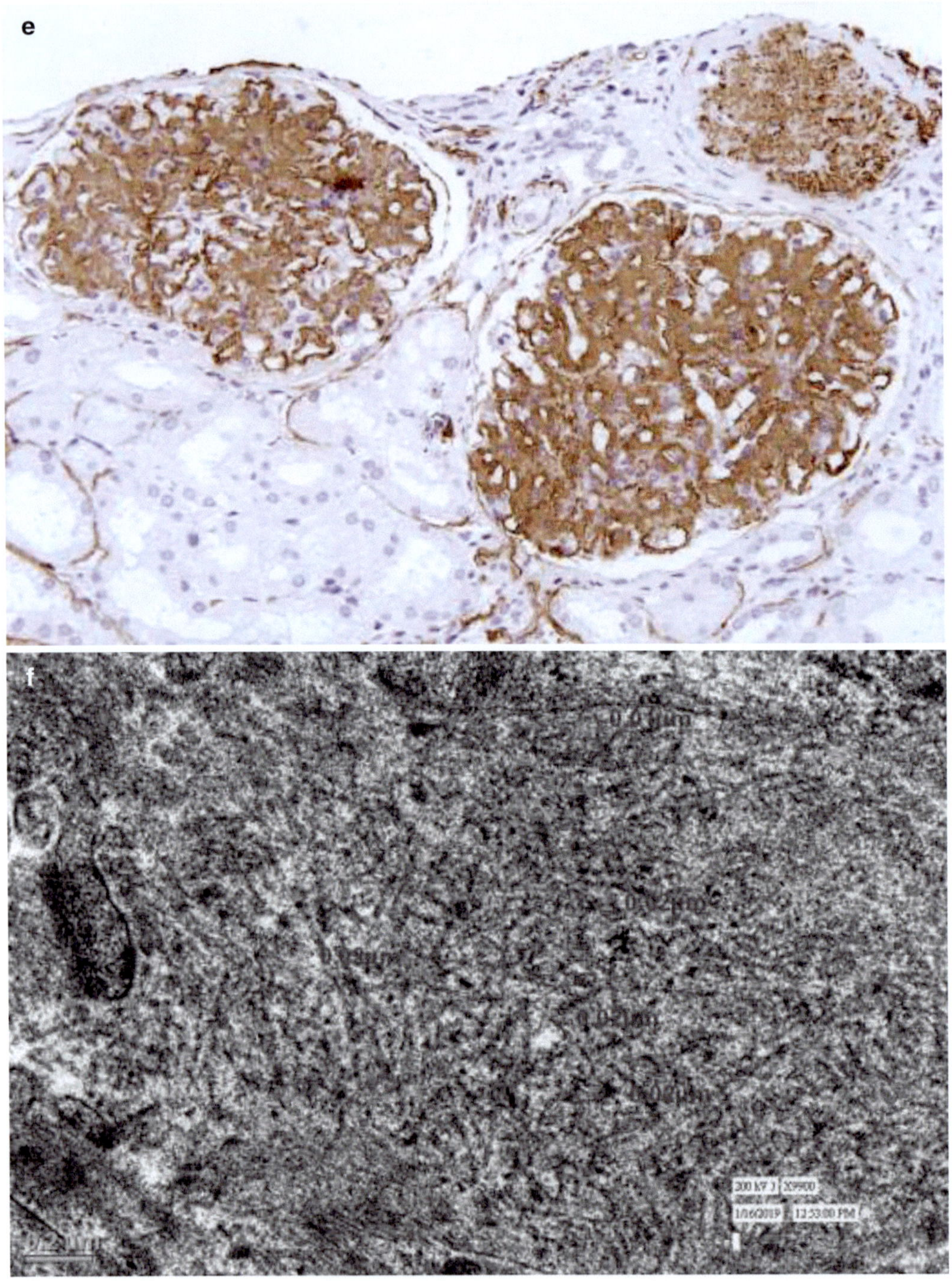

Fig. 19.2 (continued)

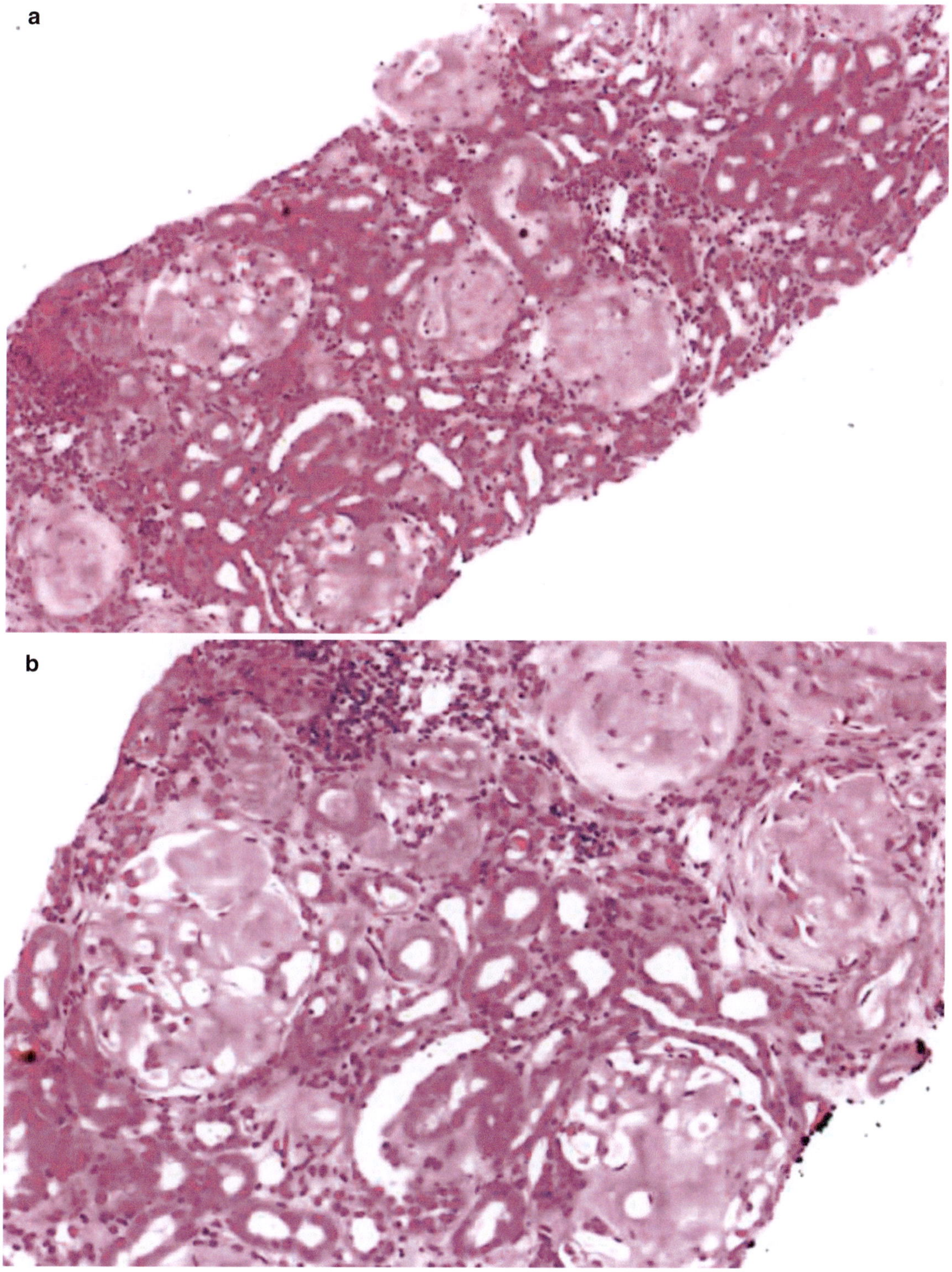

Fig. 19.3 Fibrillary Glomerulonephritis A 38-years male patient without any comorbidities, presented with uremic symptoms for the past 6 days. Renal biopsy revealed 18 glomeruli, all of them showed global deposition of extracellular amorphous eosinophilic material. Similar deposition was seen in the wall of blood vessels. Moderate tubular atrophy with moderate interstitial fibrosis was present. The deposits were congored negative. Polarizing microscopy did not show any apple green birefringence. IF showed smudgy positivity for IgG, kappa and lambda. EM showed randomly oriented fibrils measuring 15–20 nm in greater diameter and the cross-section of fibrillary deposits showed absent central lucencies (white arrow). (**a**) HE × 100, (**b**) HE × 200, (**c**) PAS × 400, (**d**) PSM × 400, (**e**) Polarizing microscopy, (**f**, **g**) EM (Contributor: Dr. V. Gnanapriya, Assistant Professor, Department of Pathology, St. John's Medical College, Bangalore)

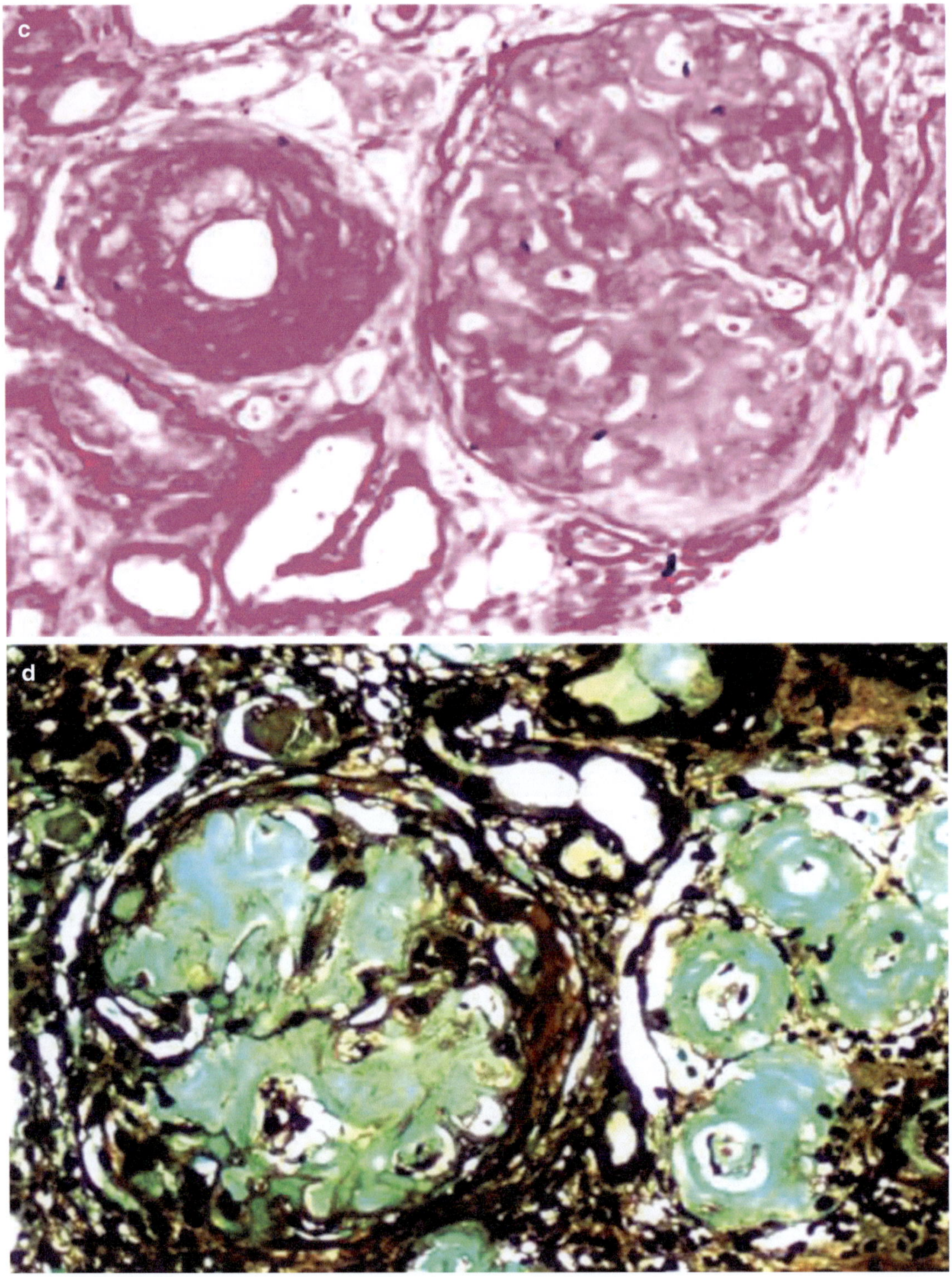

Fig. 19.3 (continued)

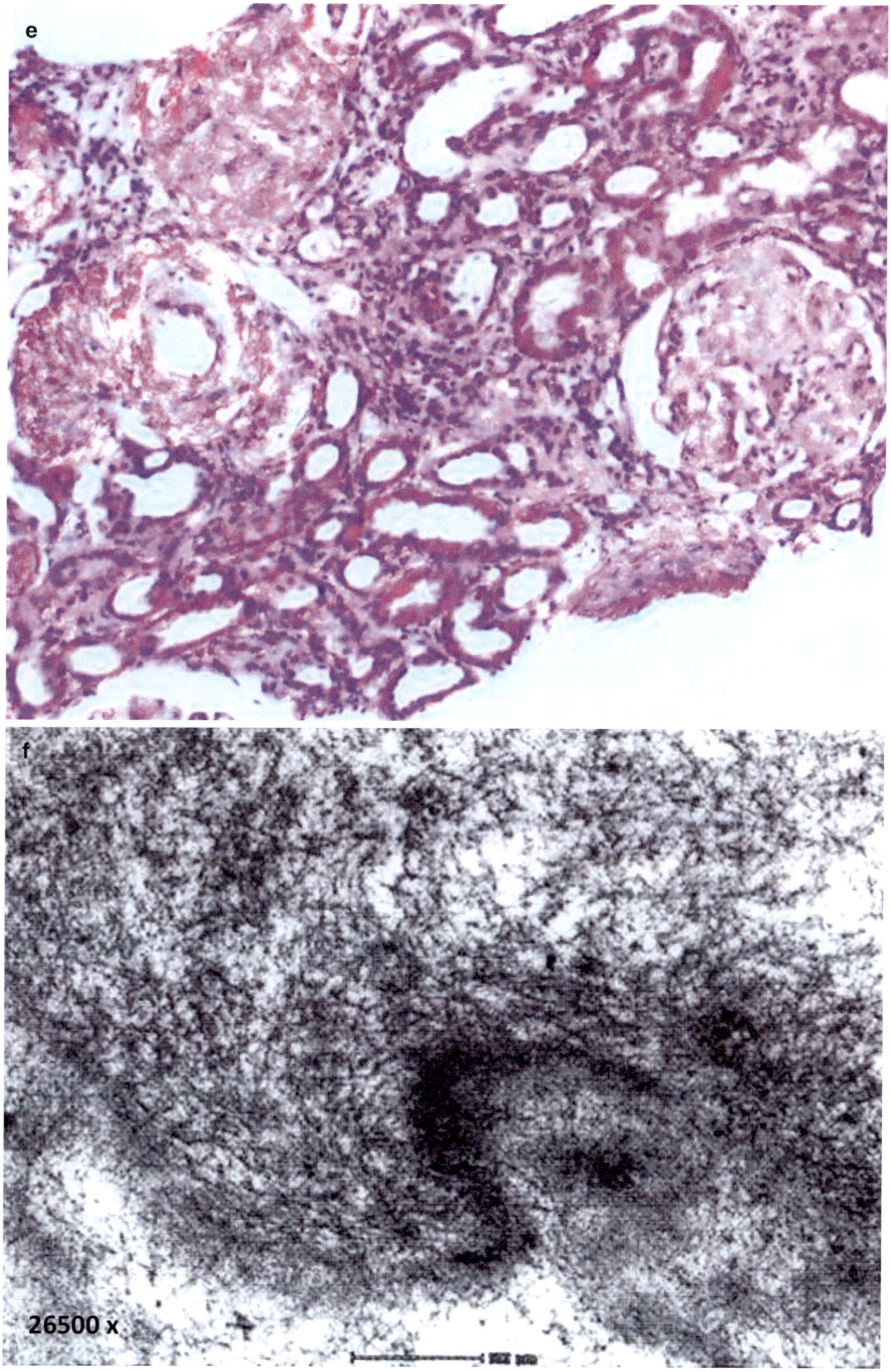

Fig. 19.3 (continued)

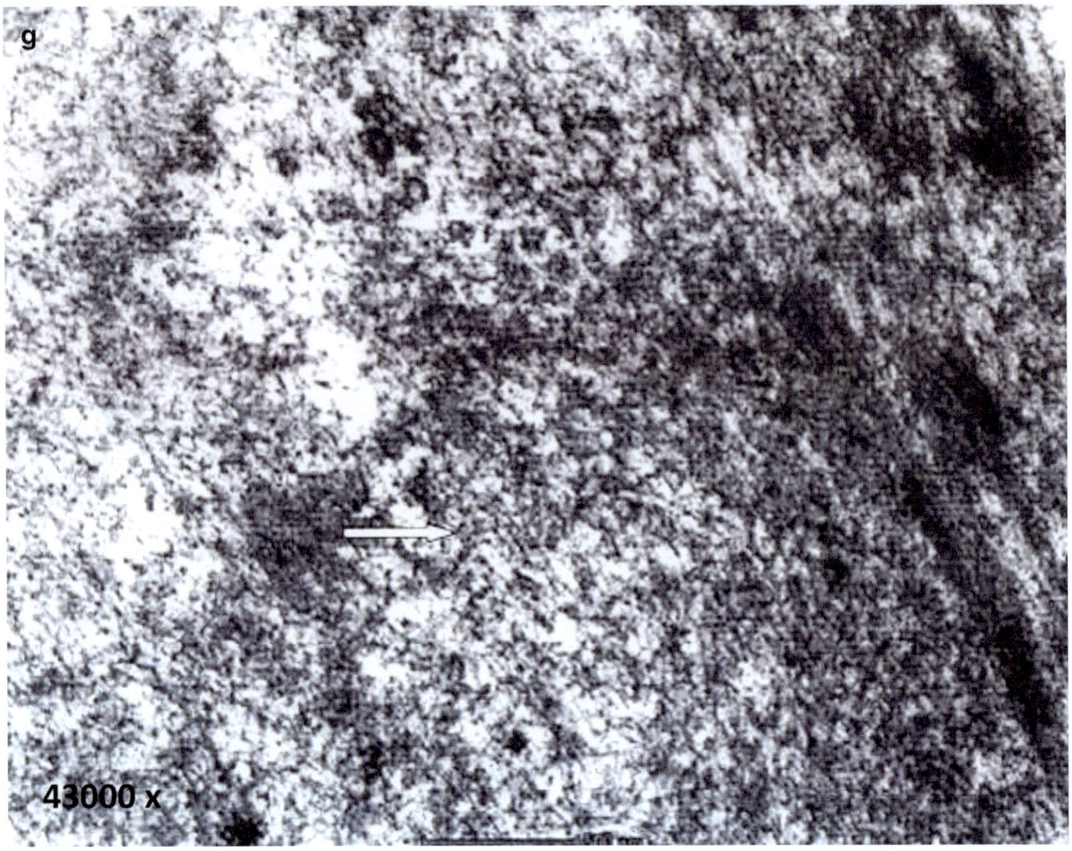

Fig. 19.3 (continued)

19.3 Collagenofibrotic Glomerulopathy

It is a rare glomerulopathy characterized by the deposition of type III collagen in the mesangial and subendothelial compartment of glomeruli. Normal kidney shows the deposition of type III collagen only in the blood vessels and renal interstitium. This disorder appears to be sporadic in adults, whereas it has autosomal recessive inheritance in children. Patients present with proteinuria, microscopic hematuria with or without hypertension. Nail Patella syndrome also shows the deposition of type III collagen in lamina densa of glomerular capillary basement membrane along with extra renal manifestations in the form of nail and patella deformities. Nail may appear split, discolored, or may even be absent. Patella can be displaced, small, or irregular in shape and in some cases can be absent. Mutation in the LMX1B has been described in these patients.

On light microscopy diffuse mesangial expansion by PAS and Congo red negative material is seen. Glomerular capillary double contours can also been seen. The collagenous nature of the material can be highlighted by Masson's trichrome stain. Nodular mesangial expansion can also be noted. Immunohistochemistry for type III collagen is positive in the glomerular deposits whereas staining for immunoglobulin, complements, and light chains is negative on immunofluorescence. Electron microscopy shows flocculent subendothelial and mesangial curved and banded fibrillary collagenous material. Lamina densa is spared. There is no definite therapy for this disease. Progressive decline in renal function is seen in these patients and patients often progress to ESRD. Recently a case of collagenofibrotic glomerulopathy has also been described in renal transplant recipient. A case of Collgenofibrotic Glomerulopathy is illustrated in (Fig. 19.4).

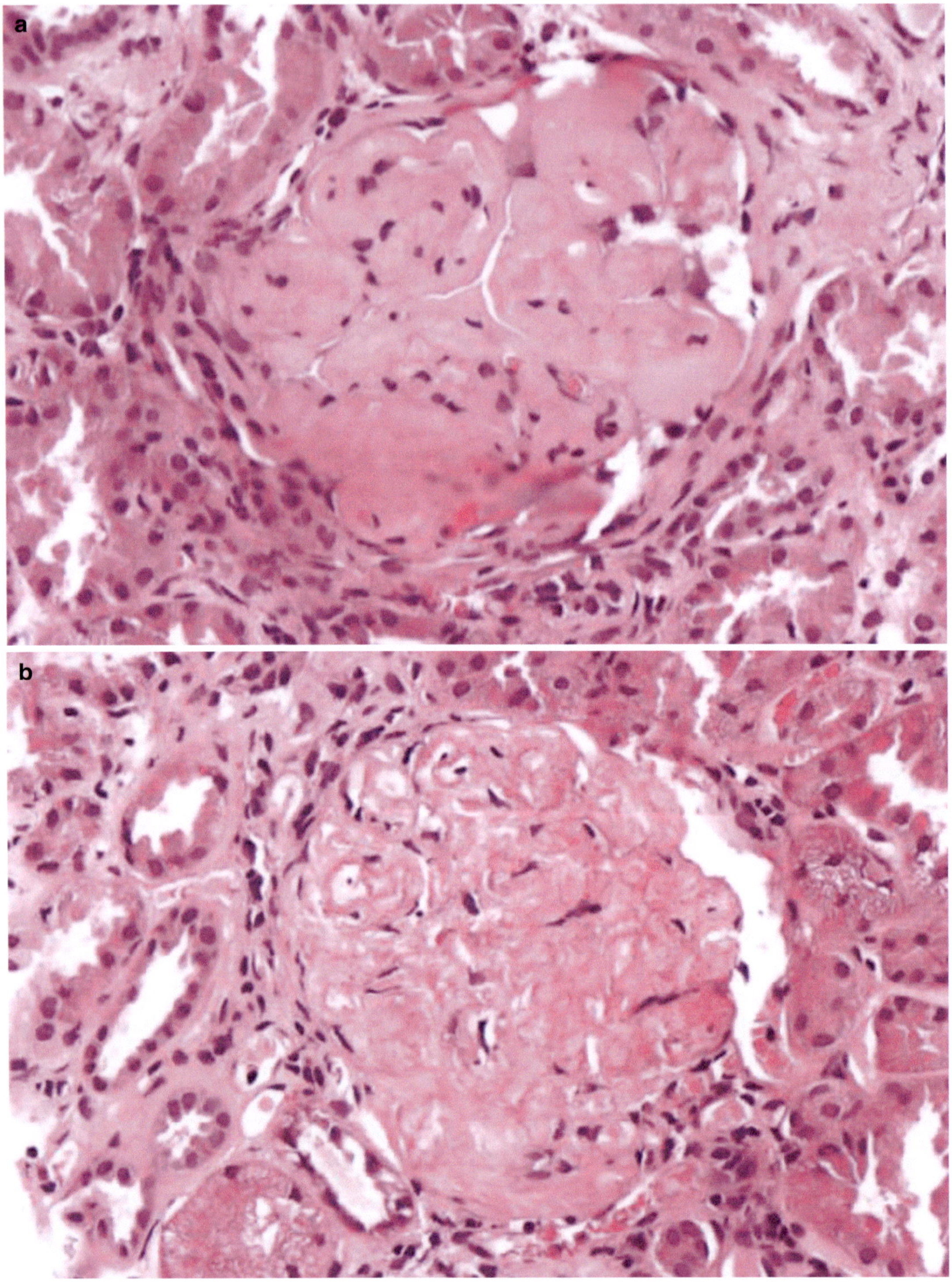

Fig. 19.4 Collagenofibrotic Glomerulopathy A 42 years female patient known to have nephrotic syndrome since last 5 years, was initially on wysolone and then tacrolimus followed by rituximab. Now the patient presented with proteinuria of 11 g/24 h. Urine analysis showed albumin 4+, pus cells 2–4, and RBC 1–2/hpf. Serum creatinine was 1.3 mg/dl and the serum electrolytes were wnl. Serum complements were also wnl and serology for HBsAg and HCV was negative. Renal biopsy revealed 14 glomeruli, all showed mesangial expansion by eosinophilic material (which was PAS, PSM and Congo red negative) with thickening and reduplication of capillary basement membrane. IHC for collagen Type III was positive in glomerular deposits. EM showed focal effacement of foot processes of visceral epithelial cells and massive expansion of mesangial and subendothelial regions by irregular bundles of fibrillary material with banded appearance and periodicity of about 30–60 nm. (**a**, **b**) HE × 400, (**c**) PAS × 400, (**d**) PSM × 400 and (**e**) MT × 400. (**f**) IHC for collagen 3b × 400, (**g**, **h**) EM (identity of the patient has been concealed)

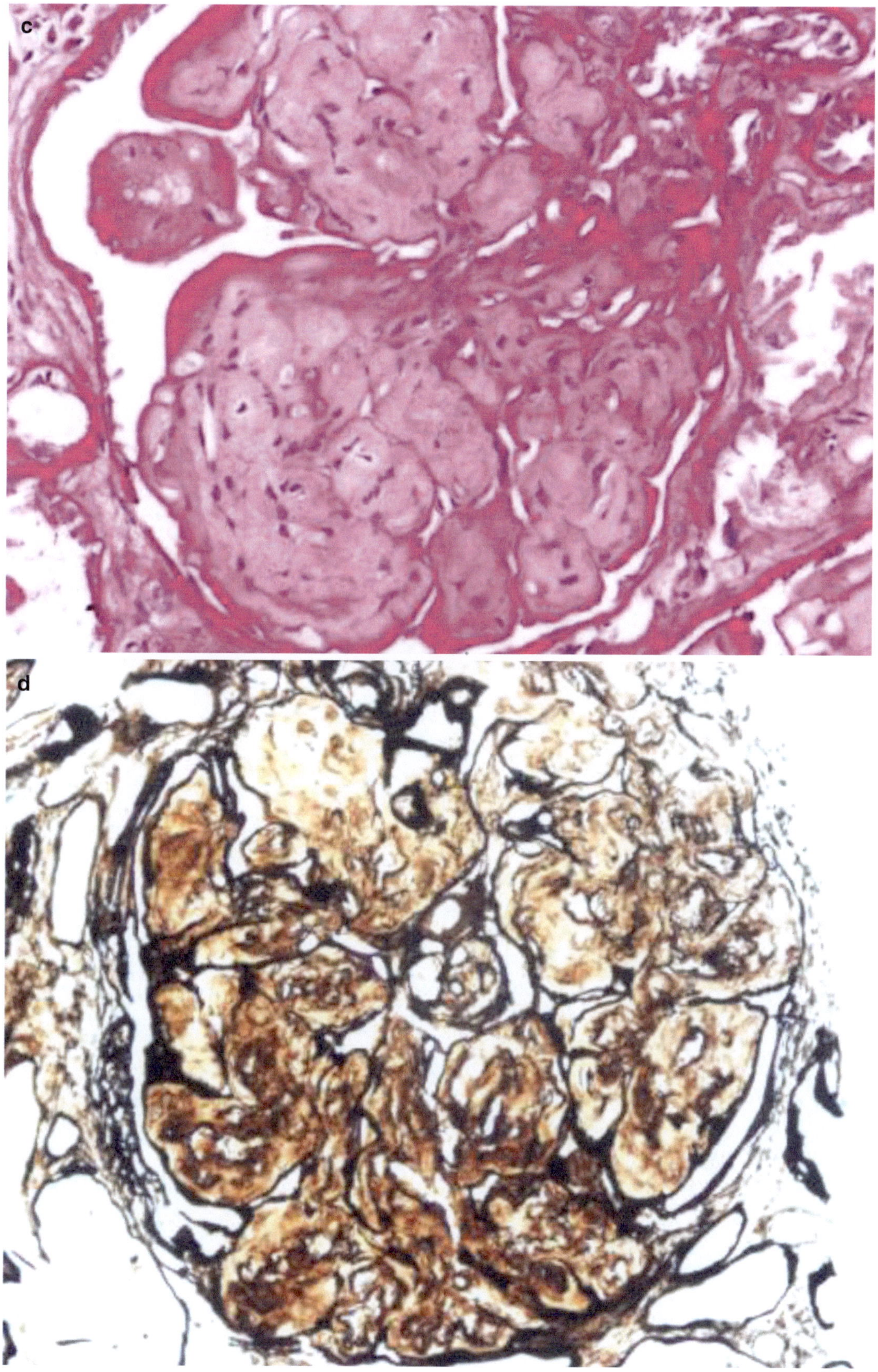

Fig. 19.4 (continued)

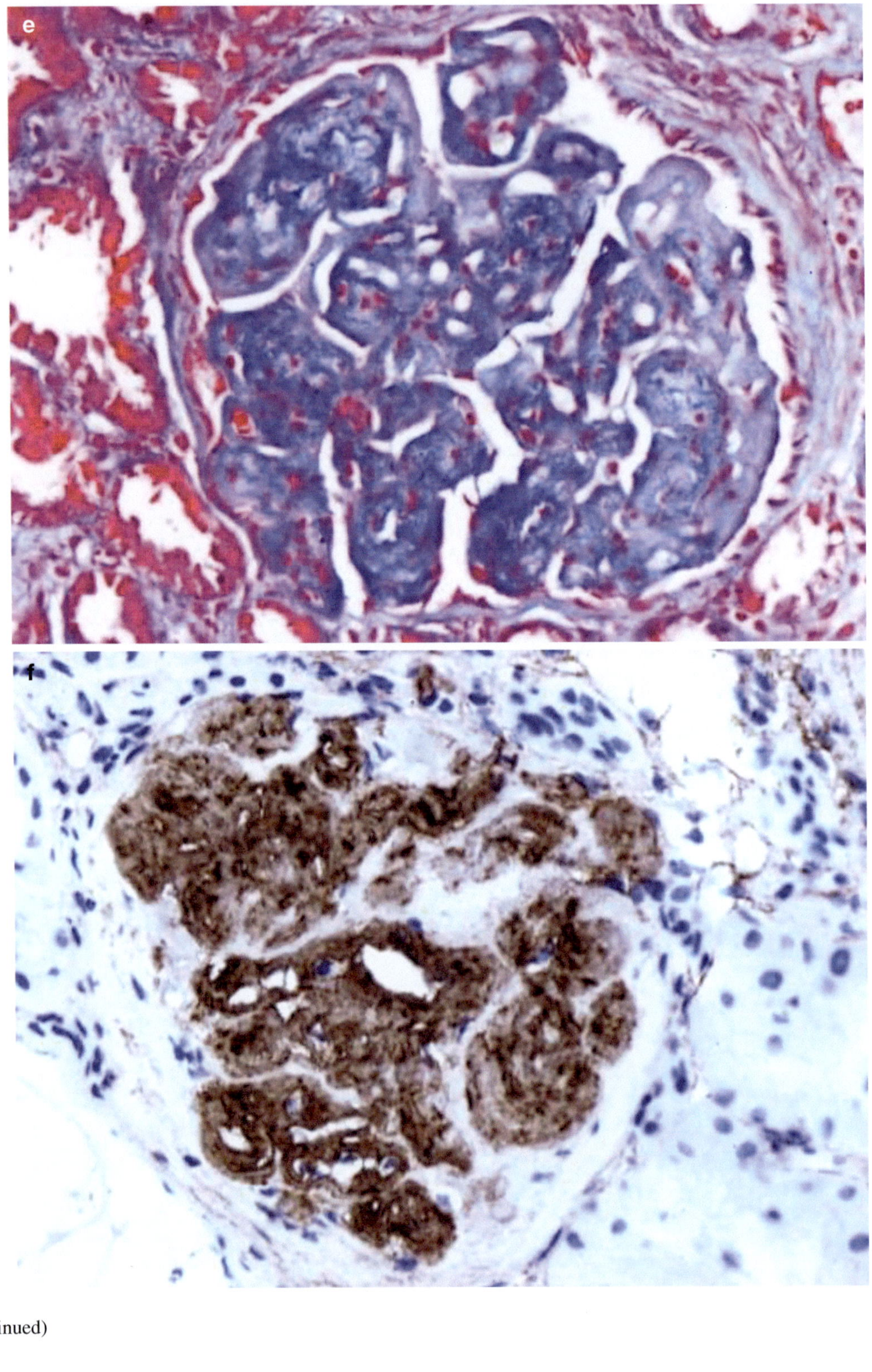

Fig. 19.4 (continued)

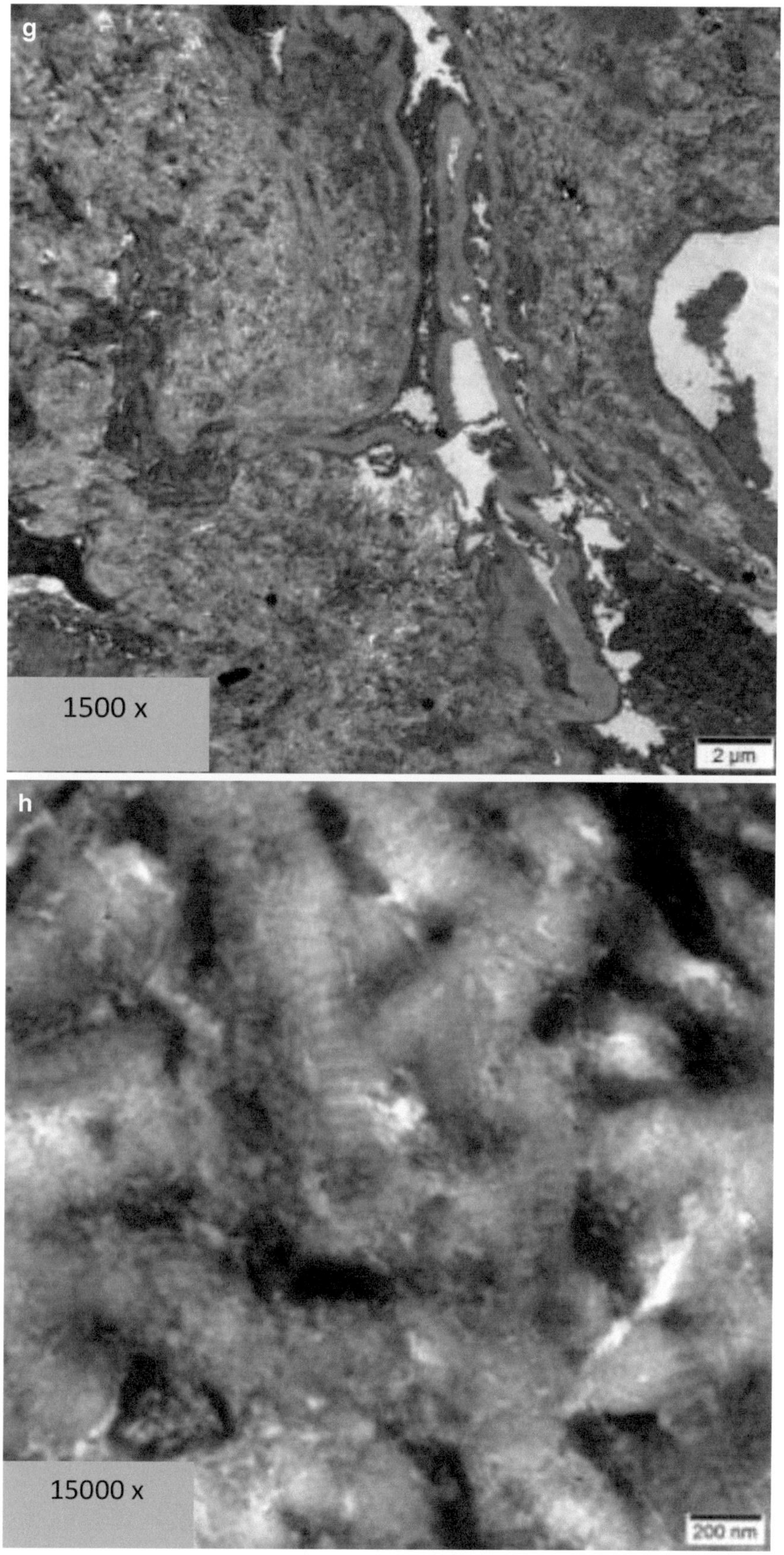

Fig. 19.4 (continued)

Further Reading

Cryoglobulinemic Glomerulonephritis

Li C, Li H, Su W, Wen YB, Ye W, Ye WL, Cai JF, Qin XZ, Li XM, Li XW. Clinicopathological study of mixed cryoglobulinemic glomerulonephritis secondary to hepatitis B virus infection. BMC Nephrol. 2020;21:395.

Motwani SS, Herlitz L, Monga D, Jhaveri KD, Lam AQ, American Society of Nephrology Onco-Nephrology Forum. Paraprotein-related kidney disease: glomerular diseases associated with paraproteinemias. Clin J Am Soc Nephrol. 2016;7(11):2260–72.

Obrişcă B, Jurubiţă R, Sorohan B, Iliescu L, Baston C, Bobeică R, Andronesi A, Leca N, Ismail G. Clinical outcome of HCV-associated cryoglobulinemic glomerulonephritis following treatment with direct acting antiviral agents: a case-based review. Clin Rheumatol. 2019;38:3677–87.

Rossi D, Sciascia S, Fenoglio R, Ferro M, Baldovino S, Kamgaing J, Ventrella F, Kalikatzaros I, Viziello L, Solfietti L, Barreca A, Roccatello D. Cryoglobulinemic glomerulonephritis: clinical presentation and histological features, diagnostic pitfalls, and controversies in the management. State of the art and the experience on a large monocentric cohort treated with B cell depletion therapy. Minerva Med. 2020;112(2):162–74. https://doi.org/10.23736/S0026-4806.20.07076-7.

Silva F, Pinto C, Barbosa A, Borges T, Dias C, Almeida J. New insights in cryoglobulinemic vasculitis. J Autoimmun. 2019;105:102313.

Fibrillary Glomerulonephritis

Nasr SH, Valeri AM, Cornell LD, Fidler ME, Sethi S, Leung N, Fervenza FC. Fibrillary glomerulonephritis: a report of 66 cases from a single institution. Clin J Am Soc Nephrol. 2011;6:775–84.

Nasr SH, Vrana JA, Dasari S. DNAJB9 is a specific immunohistochemical marker for fibrillary glomerulonephritis. Kidney Int Rep. 2018;3:56–64.

Rosenstock JL, Markowitz GS, Valeri AM. Fibrillary and immunotactoid glomerulonephritis: distinct entities with different clinical and pathologic features. Kidney Int. 2003;63:1450–61.

Rosenstock JL, Markowitz GS. Fibrillary glomerulonephritis: an update. Kidney Int Rep. 2019;4:917–22.

Collagenofibrotic Glomerulopathy

Alchi B, Nishi S, Narita I, Gejyo F. Collagenofibrotic glomerulopathy: clinicopathologic overview of a rare glomerular disease. Am J Kidney Dis. 2007;49:499–506.

Gubler MC, Dommergues JP, Foulard M, et al. Collagen type III glomerulopathy: a new type of hereditary nephropathy. Pediatr Nephrol. 1993;7:354–60.

Jdiaa SS, Moeckel GW, Kfoury HM, Medawar WA, Abu-Alfa AK. Collagenofibrotic glomerulopathy in a kidney transplant recipient: a first report. Am J Transplant. 2021;21:1948–52.

Kurien AA, Larsen CP, Cossey LN. Collagenofibrotic glomerulopathy. Clin Kidney J. 2015;8:543–7.

Manocha A, Gupta P. Collagenofibrotic glomerulopathy: a rare diagnosis and seldom thought of differential for nodular glomerular mesangial expansion. J Clin Diagn Res. 2020;14:ED01–2.

Miyake M, Katayama K, Ehara T, Sado Y, Nawa S, Murata T, Mizutani Y, Joh K, Ito M, Dohi K. Collagenofibrotic Glomerulopathy. Intern Med. 2021;60:911–5.

20 Renal Involvement in Lysosomal Storage Disorders (Fabry's Disease, Niemann–Pick Disease) and LCAT Deficiency

20.1 Fabry's Disease

It is a rare X-linked lysosomal storage disorder caused by deficiency of lysosomal enzyme α-galactosidase A. This results in the accumulation of glycosphingolipid in endothelial cells in the kidney, brain, heart, and skin and results in endothelial dysfunction. Patients can have systemic manifestations in the form of angiokeratoma, acroparesthesia, hypohydria, facial dysmorphism, corneal opacities, hypertrophic cardiomyopathy, and gastrointestinal symptoms. Renal function can be normal without any significant proteinuria at presentation but eventually the patient will develop progressive renal disease and can progress to ESRD.

On light microscopy, glomeruli will show enlarged podocytes with a vacuolated appearance of cytoplasm. In addition, mesangial cell, endothelial cell, and parietal epithelial cell cytoplasm may also show vacuolation. Endothelial cells of the blood vessels can also show similar vacuolated appearance. Interstitium can show the presence of foam cells. Later with the progression of disease, segmental sclerosis can be seen along with tubular atrophy and interstitial fibrosis.

Immunofluorescence is non-contributory as it does not show any specific deposits of immunoglobulin(s) and complement(s).

Electron microscopy is diagnostic and shows the presence of cytoplasmic intralysosomal lamellated membranous structures in the form of parallel dense zebra bodies. They are commonly seen in podocytes and distal tubular epithelial cells but can also be demonstrated in vascular myocytes, parietal epithelial cells, and mesangial cells. A case of Fabry's disease is illustrated (Fig. 20.1).

P. Gupta, R. K. Gupta, *Pathology of Glomerular Diseases*, https://doi.org/10.1007/978-981-19-1430-0_20

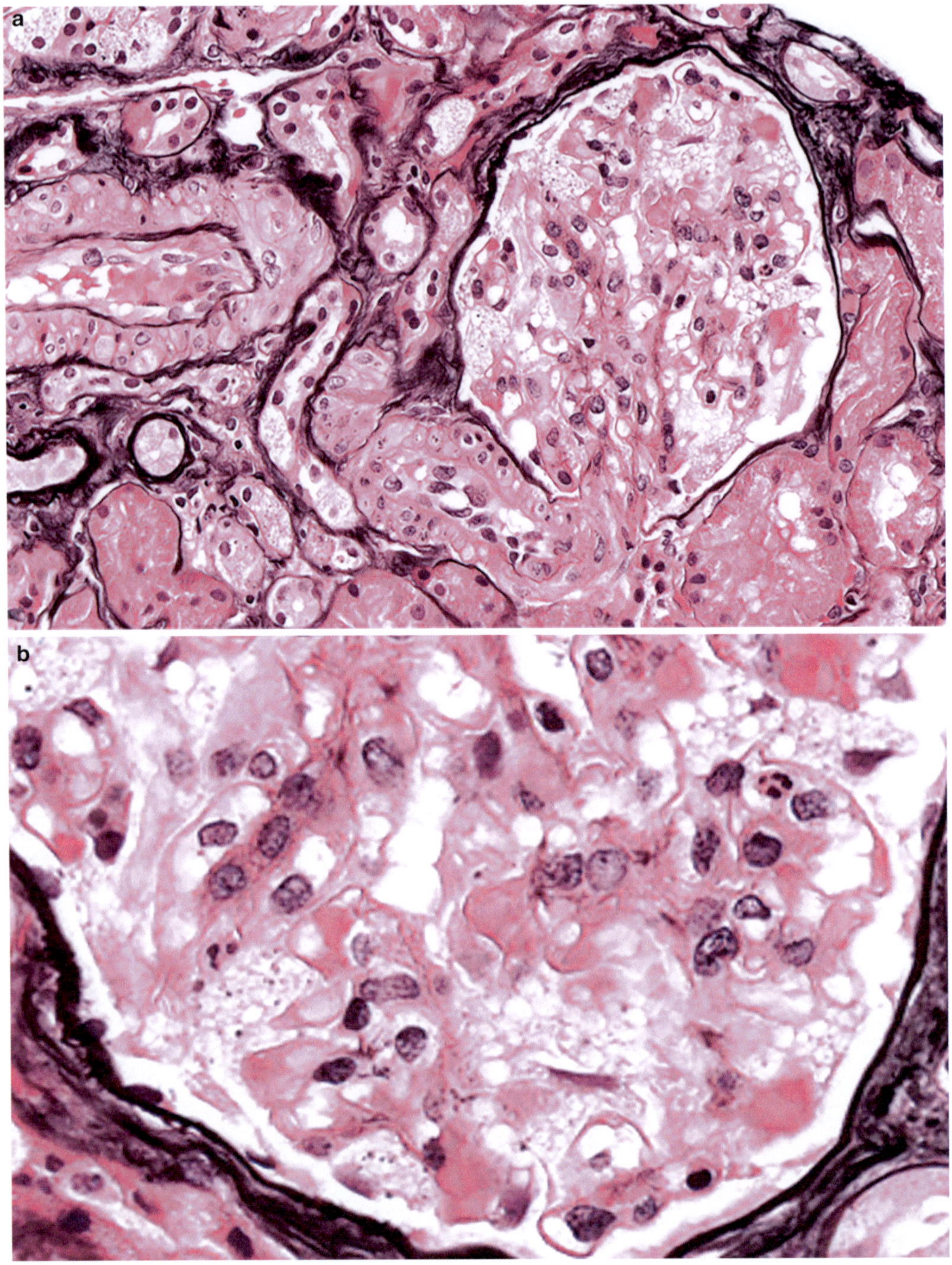

Fig. 20.1 **Fabry's Disease** A 25-years male patient presented with slowly increasing pedal edema and fatigue. Urine analysis revealed albuminuria 5.7 g/24 h without any active sediment. Serum creatinine was 138 μmol/l and serum albumin was 28 g/L. Renal biopsy showed normocellular glomeruli with inconspicuous mesangial areas. Podocytes showed hypertrophy and appeared swollen; arterioles also showed swollen endothelial cells. IF was negative. EM revealed extensive intracytoplasmic inclusions of concentric lamellated myelin bodies in podocytes; these zebra bodies displayed a periodicity of approx. 6 nm. Tubular epithelium and endothelial cells of peritubular capillaries also showed similar inclusions. (**a**) Jones × 400, (**b**) Jones × 1000, and (**c–f**) EM (Contributor—Dr. Joris J. Roelofs, Department of Pathology, Amsterdam University Medical Centers, Amsterdam, The Netherlands)

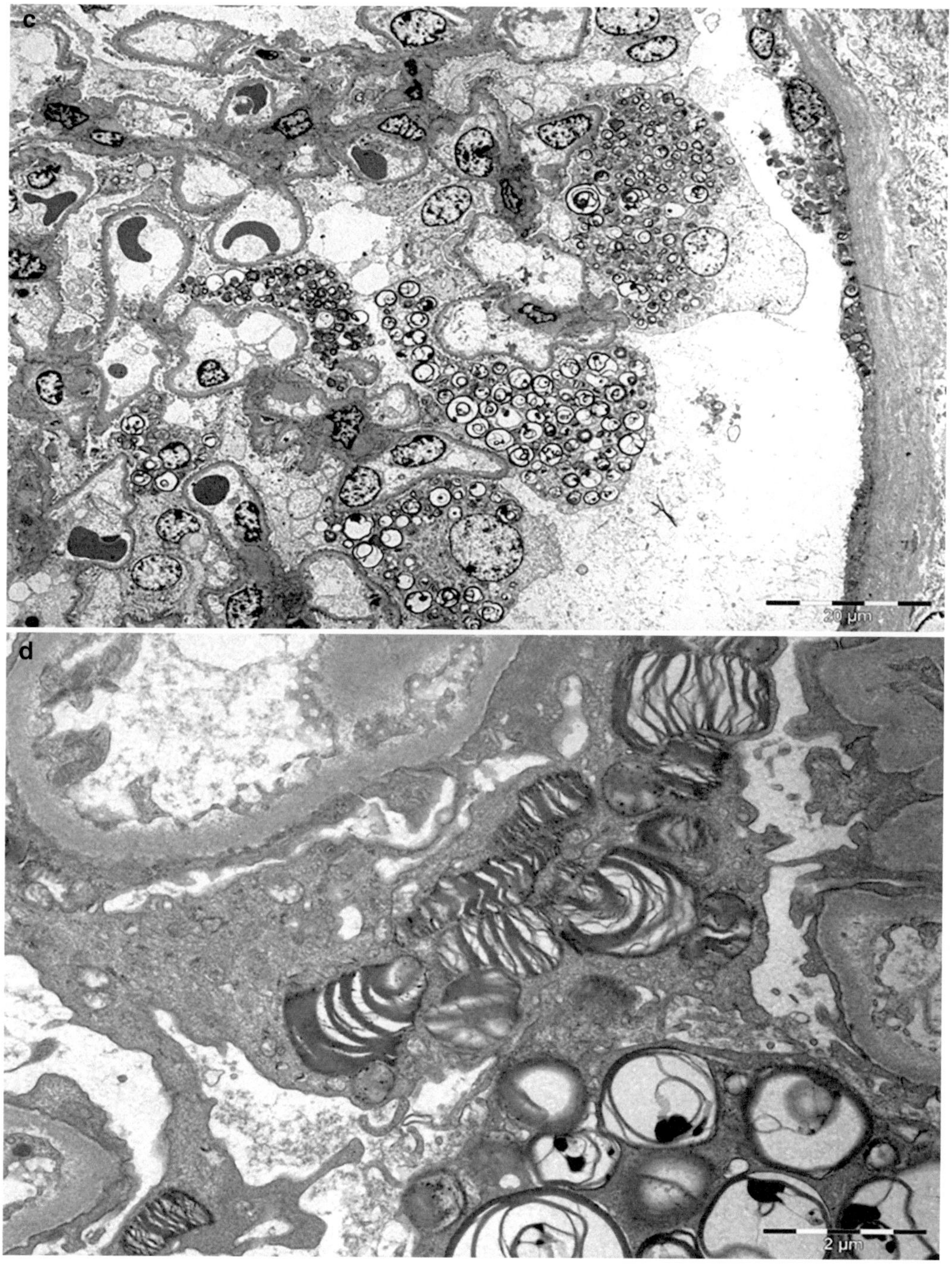

Fig. 20.1 (continued)

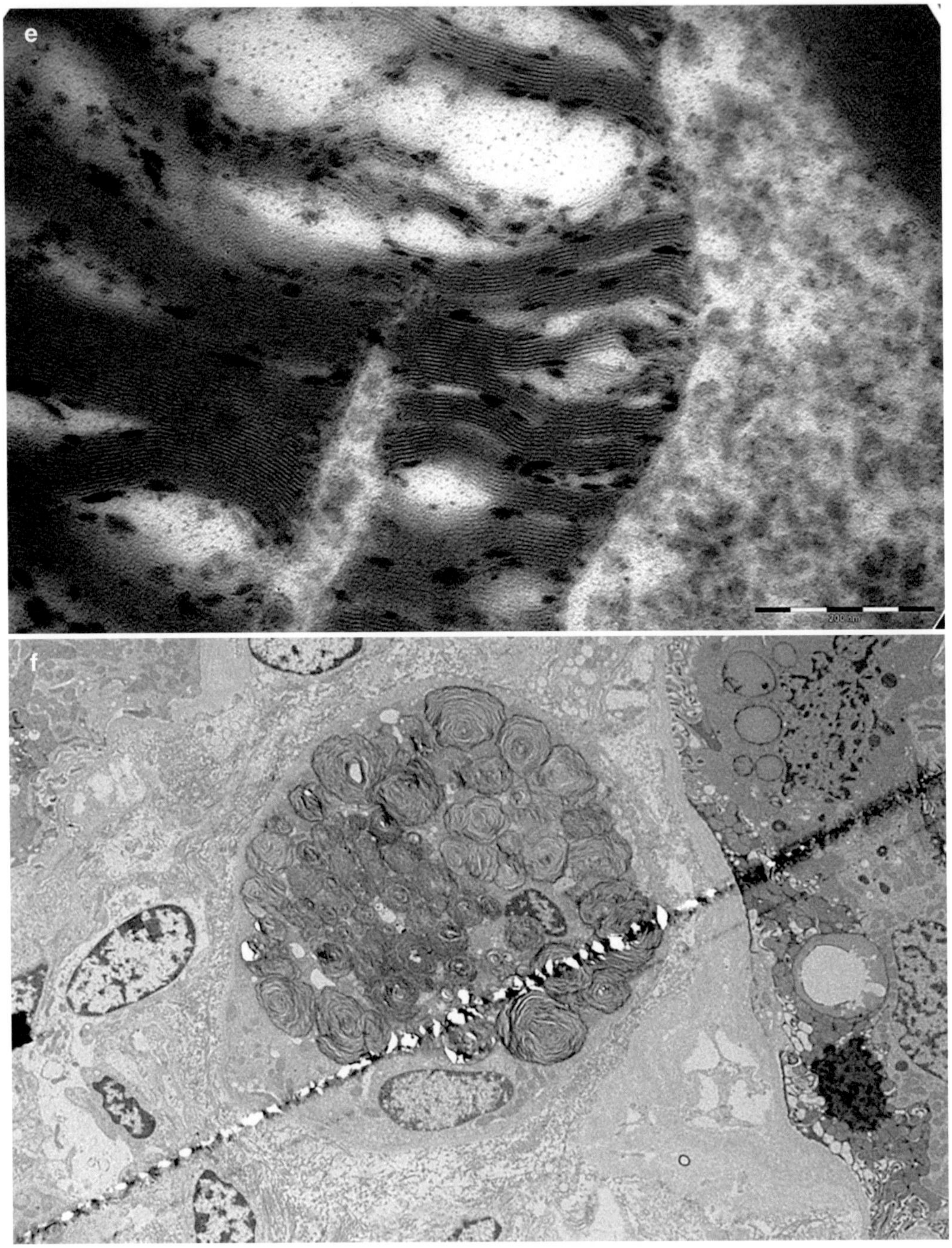

Fig. 20.1 (continued)

20.2 Niemann–Pick Disease

Niemann–Pick disease is an autosomal recessive lysosomal storage disorder characterized by a deficiency of sphingomyelinase resulting in accumulation of sphingomyelin in tissue and toxic injury to the affected organs. It can be of three types.

Type A has early onset with severe brain damage along with hepatosplenomegaly and lymphadenopathy. Children usually do not survive beyond 18 months.

Type B juvenile onset and patient have hepatosplenomegaly with lung involvement and peripheral neuropathy. Brain involvement is usually not seen.

Type C is caused by deficiency of NPC 1 or 2 proteins resulting in a defect in cholesterol transport. The patients have variable age at presentation and can present with hepatosplenomegaly with hearing impairment and loss of vision. Severe brain damage may be observed in these patients as well.

Renal involvement is rare in Niemann–Pick disease type B and type C and has been described as rare case reports. It is in the form of small uniform cytoplasmic vacuoles within the cytoplasm of podocytes, distal and proximal tubular epithelial cells, endothelial cells of blood vessels and interstitial foam cells. Some authors have described the MPGN pattern of glomerular morphology. Occasional case reports of thrombotic microangiopathy have also been described. Immunofluorescence does not show any immunoglobulin or complement deposit. Electron microscopy shows myelin-like inclusions (lipidic deposits) in the cytoplasm of endothelial cells and podocytes. A case of Niemen-Pick disease is illustrated (Fig. 20.2).

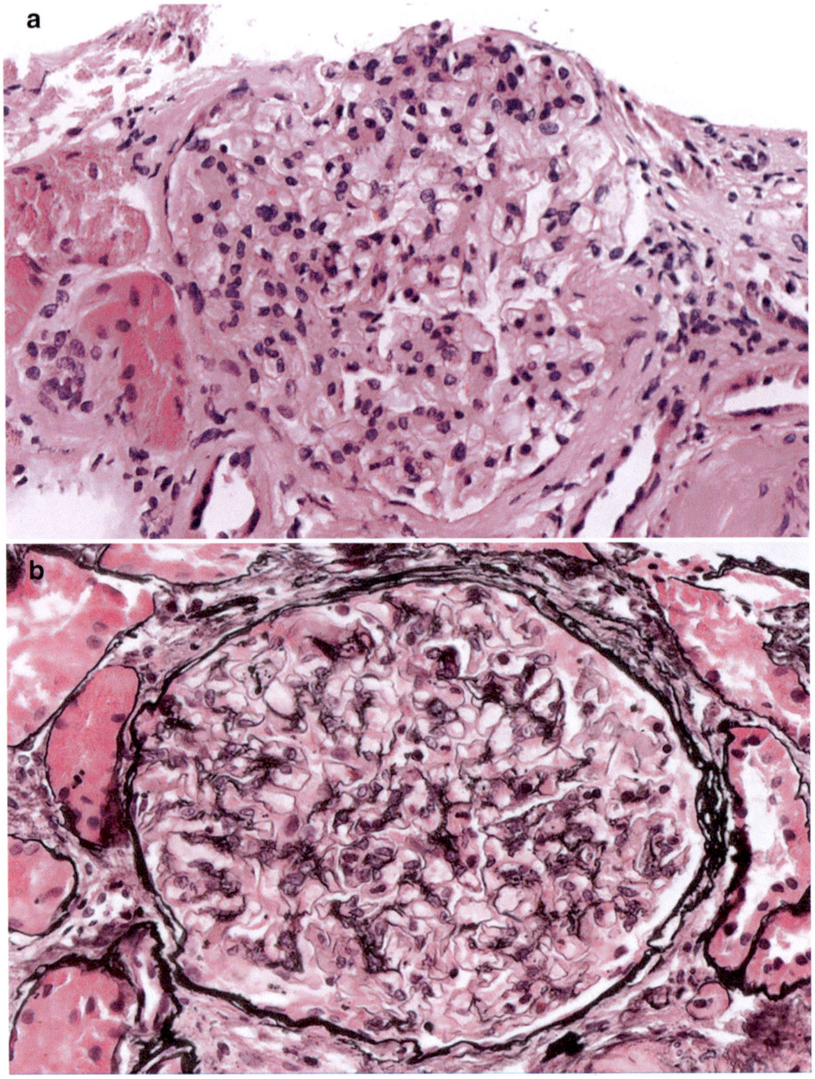

Fig. 20.2 **Niemann Pick Disease** A 49-years male patient presented with gradually developing nephrotic range proteinuria and decline in renal function; eGFR being 46 ml/min. During childhood, he had been diagnosed with type B Niemann–Pick disease. Renal biopsy had only 4 glomeruli which showed mild endocapillary hypercellularity with presence of few foam cells within the capillary lumen; none of the glomeruli were sclerosed. Interstitium showed chronic damage consisting of tubular atrophy and interstitial fibrosis in about 70% of the biopsy. Oil-Red-O staining on fresh frozen section showed lipid accumulation within the glomerular foam cells, tubular epithelial cells, and arteriolar endothelium. IF was negative. EM showed moderate effacement of podocyte foot processes and numerous intralysosomal myelin figures, within podocytes, glomerular macrophages/foam cells, mesangial cells, endothelial cells, and tubular epithelial cells. (**a**) HE × 400, (**b**) Jones × 400, (**c**) Oil-Red-O × 400, (**d, e**) EM (Contributor—Dr. Joris J. Roelofs, Department of Pathology, Amsterdam University Medical Centers, Amsterdam, The Netherlands)

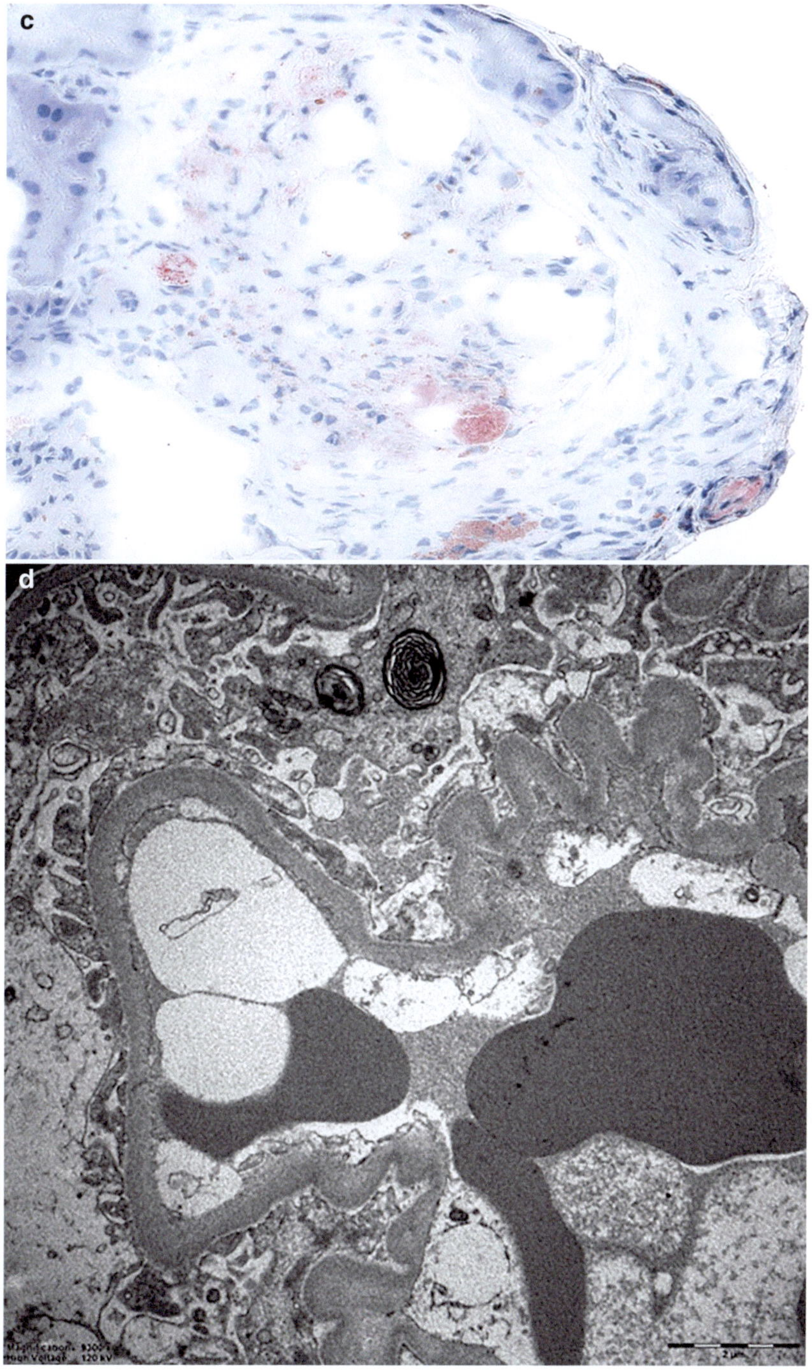

Fig. 20.2 (continued)

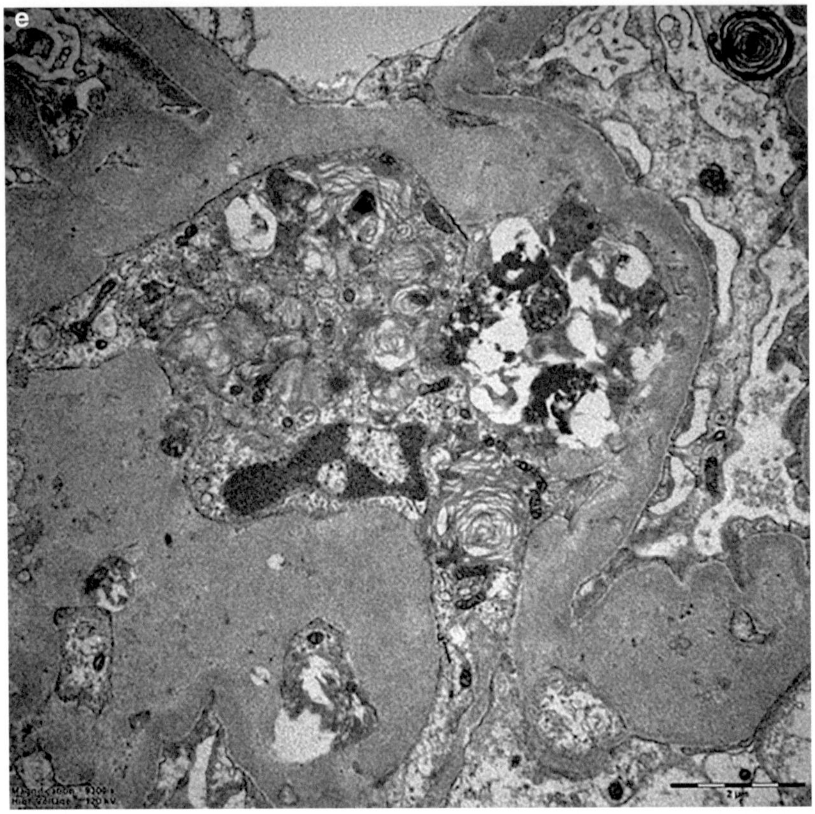

Fig. 20.2 (continued)

20.3 LCAT Deficiency

Lecithin cholesterol acyltransferase is an enzyme synthesized in liver and is responsible for reverse cholesterol transport from the peripheral tissues to the liver by esterification of free cholesterol. LCAT gene is located on chromosome 16 q21-22.

LCAT deficiency is an autosomal recessive disorder; patients will have a loss or decrease of LCAT activity in serum. More than 80 mutations have been recognized in the LCAT gene. These patients will have increased serum free cholesterol, and increase in serum Apo E levels. They will also show decrease in Apolipoprotein A-I and A-II. Low serum HDL is most important finding in these patients and there is lack of maturation of nascent HDL. This can be observed under an electron microscope as rouleaux formation.

Patients with LCAT deficiency show normochromic anemia, renal manifestations in the form of proteinuria and corneal opacities are present as initial clinical manifestations. These manifestations result from the deposition of free cholesterol and phospholipid on RBC, cornea, and kidney.

Renal pathology shows glomeruli with expanded mesangium having foamy appearance. Glomerular capillary basement membrane is thickened with a bubbly vacuolated appearance and spikes and GBM double contour can be seen. Wall of the blood vessels can also show a bubbly, vacuolated appearance. On immunofluorescence, no immune deposit is seen.

Electron microscopic findings show mesangial, subendothelial, intramembranous, and epimembranous rounded lamellar deposits along with vacuolations of varying sizes. Similar deposits can also be observed in the endothelium of the vessel wall. A case of LCAT deficiency is illustrated (Fig. 20.3).

These patients can show a progression to ESRD and may require renal replacement therapy in the form of dialysis or renal transplantation.

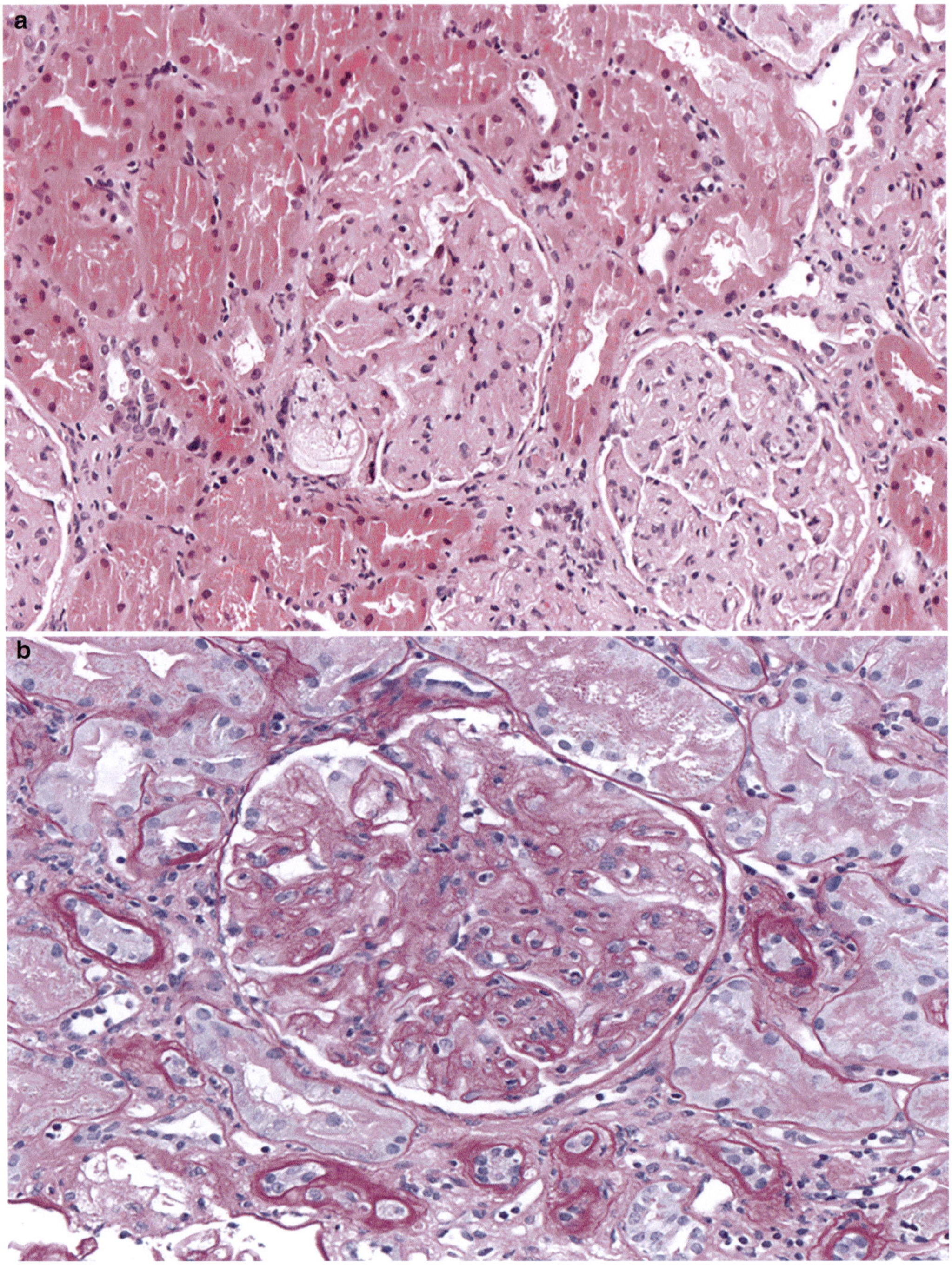

Fig. 20.3 **LCAT deficiency** A 56-years male patient, a known case of lecithin cholesterol (LCAT) deficiency, gradually developed end-stage kidney disease, for which he received renal allograft 2 years ago. Now presented with allograft dysfunction. Renal biopsy showed mesangial hypercellularity and endocapillary hypercellularity with GBM duplication. On IF C4d was negative in PTC; IgG, IgM, IgA, C3, C1q and kappa and lambda were all negative. EM showed extensive presence of myeline bodies in glomerular endocapillary cells, capillary endothelial cells as well as within the double contours of GBM, within the wall of peritubular capillaries and along the tubular basement membrane. (**a**) HE × 200, (**b**) PAS × 200, (**c**) Jones × 400, (**d**) IF × 200 and (**e**–**i**) EM (Contributor—Dr. Joris J. Roelofs, Department of Pathology, Amsterdam University Medical Centers, Amsterdam, The Netherlands)

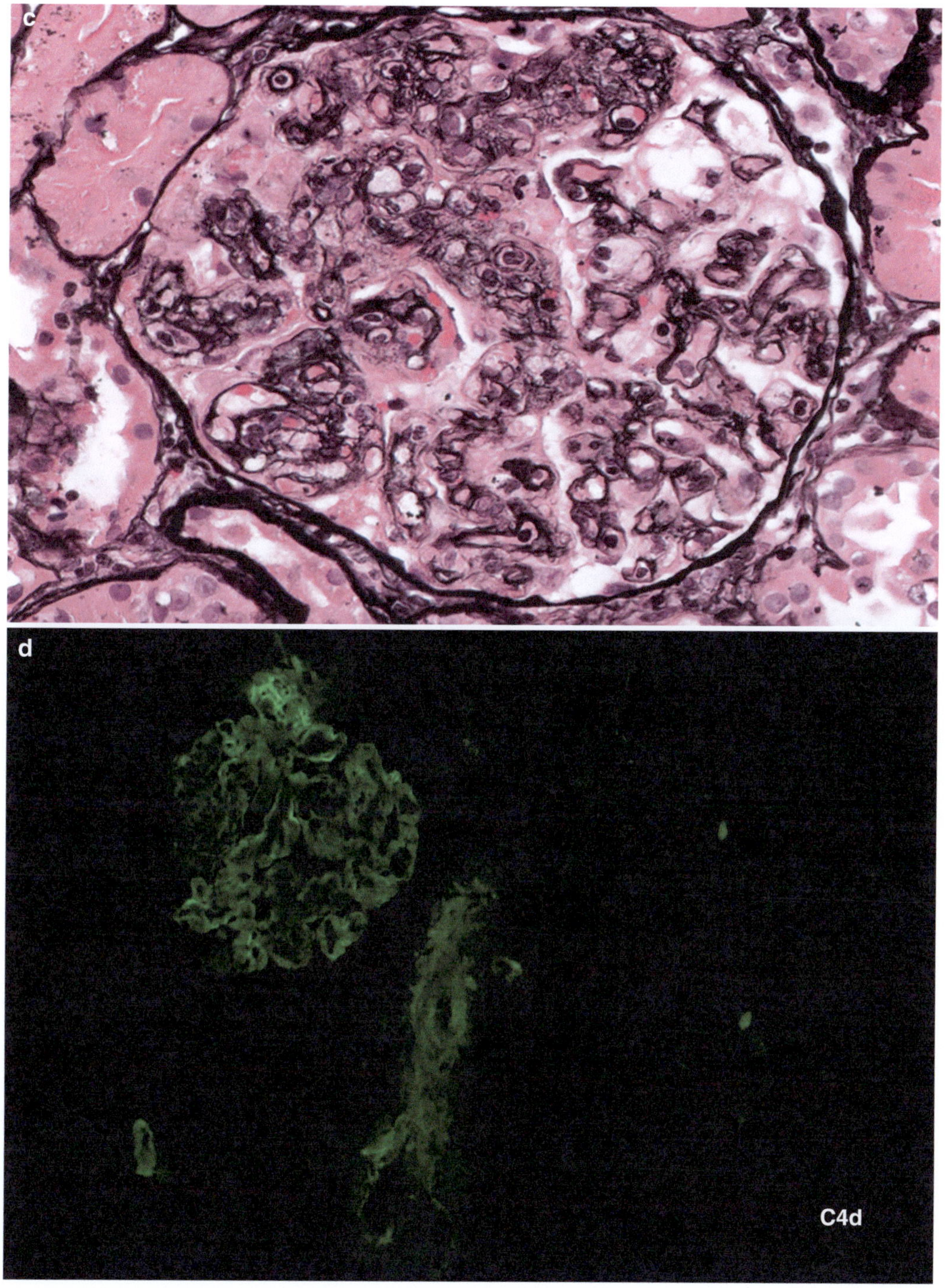

Fig. 20.3 (continued)

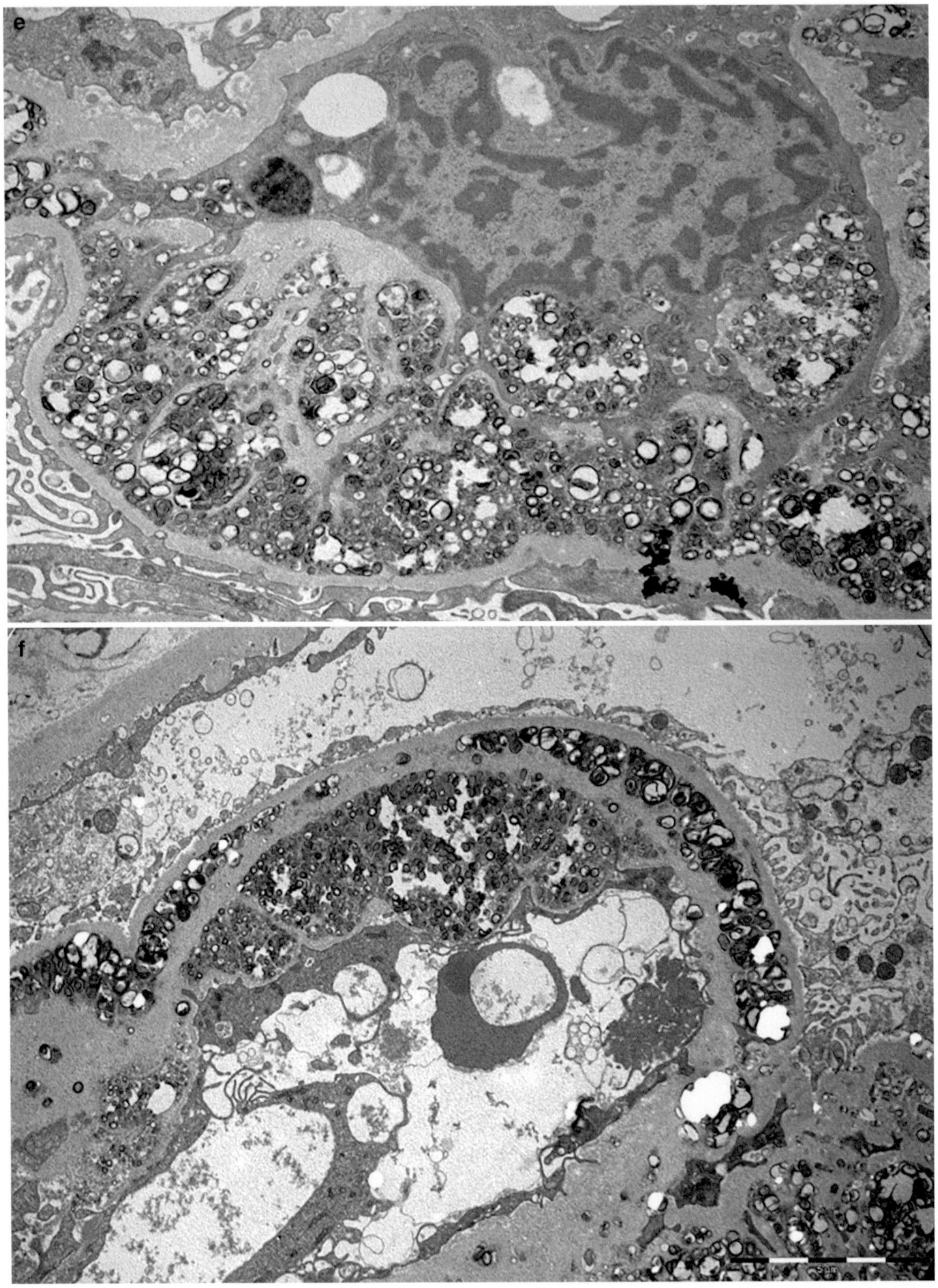

Fig. 20.3 (continued)

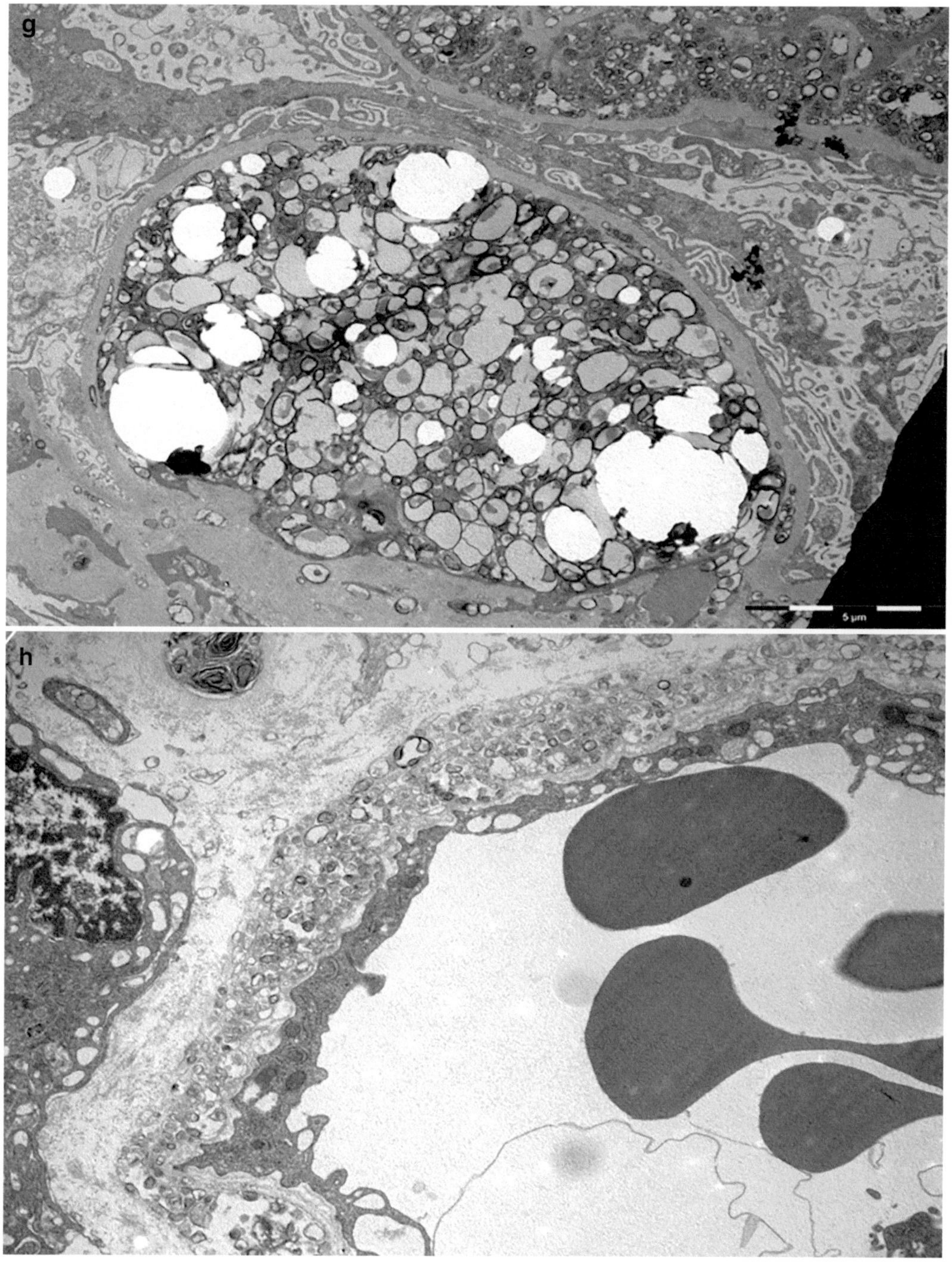

Fig. 20.3 (continued)

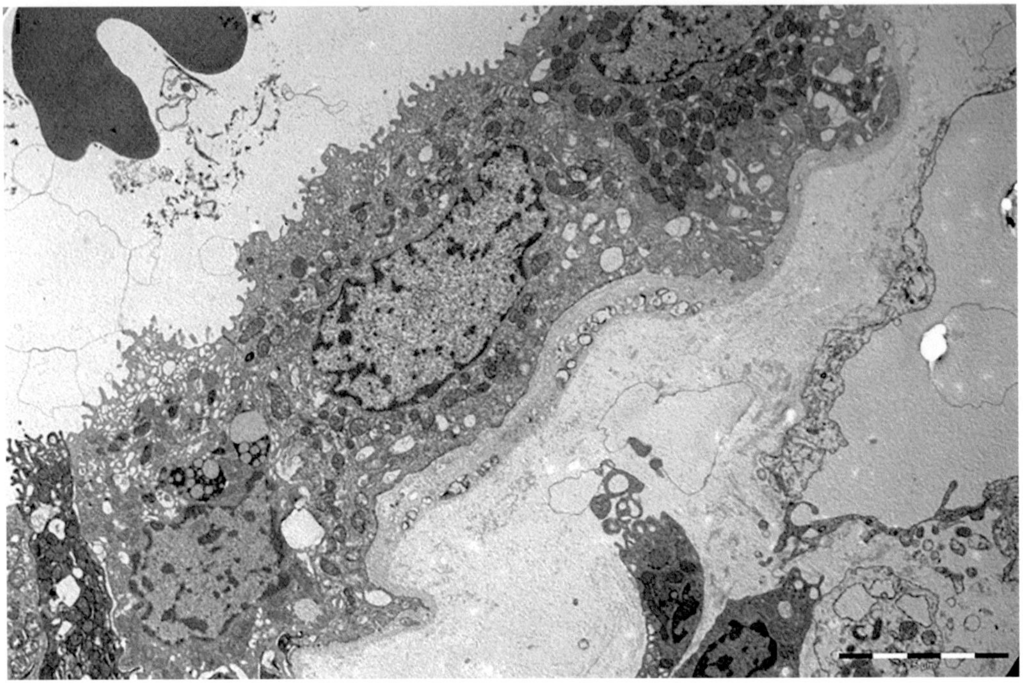

Fig. 20.3 (continued)

Further Reading

Fabry's Disease

Abensur H, Reis MA. Renal involvement in Fabry disease. J Bras Nefrol. 2016;38:245–54.
Chan B, Adam DN. A review of Fabry disease. Skin Therapy Lett. 2018;23:4–6.
Jennette JC, Olson JL, Silva FG, D'agati VD. Heptinstall's pathology of the Kidney. 7th ed. Philadelphia: Wolters Kluwer; 2014.
Kantola IM. Renal involvement in Fabry disease. Nephrol Dial Transplant. 2019;34:1435–7.
Okuda S. Renal involvement in Fabry's disease. Intern Med. 2000;39:601–2.

LCAT Deficiency Glomerulopathy

Hirashio S, Ueno T, Naito T, Masaki T. Characteristic kidney pathology, gene abnormality and treatments in LCAT deficiency. Clin Exp Nephrol. 2014;18:189–93.
Morales E, Alonso M, Sarmiento B, Morales M. LCAT deficiency as a cause of proteinuria and corneal opacification. BMJ Case Rep. 2018;13:bcr2017224129.
Pavanello C, Calabresi L. Genetic, biochemical, and clinical features of LCAT deficiency: update for 2020. Curr Opin Lipidol. 2020;31(4):232–7.

Niemann Pick Disease

Jennette JC, Olson JL, Silva FG, D'agati VD. Heptinstall's pathology of the Kidney. 7th ed. Philadelphia: Wolters Kluwer; 2014.
Jerbi M, Sayhi M, Gaied H, et al. Renal thrombotique microangiopathy: an unusual renal involvement in Niemann-Pick disease type B. Clin Case Rep. 2020;8:3316–21.
Lidove O, Belmatoug N, Froissart R, et al. Acid sphingomyelinase deficiency (Niemann-Pick disease type B) in adulthood: a retrospective multicentric study of 28 adult cases. Rev Med Intern. 2017;38:291–9.
Philit JB, Queffeulou G, Walker F, Gubler MC, Dupuis E, Vrtovsnik F, Mignon F. Membranoproliferative glomerulonephritis type II and Niemann-Pick disease type C. Nephrol Dial Transplant. 2002;17:1829–31.
Zheng Z, Cheng C, Zhao W, Feng Q, Li C, Lou T. Renal failure and ascites in a patient with Niemann-Pick disease: case report and literature review. Int J Clin Exp Med. 2016;9:4800–4.

21 Hypertensive Nephrosclerosis

21.1 Benign Nephrosclerosis

Renal involvement in hypertensive patients is seen long time after the onset of systemic hypertension. These patients are initially asymptomatic but have a gradual progressive rise in serum creatinine with mild proteinuria. In some cases, nephrotic range proteinuria may be seen.

On light microscopy, the renal cortex shows glomeruli with wrinkling of glomerular capillary basement membrane. Shrinking or collapse of glomerular capillary tuft can be seen with fibrous occlusion (collagenization) of the Bowman's space starting at the hilar pole. Later focal segmental glomerulosclerosis and obsolescent solidified glomeruli can be seen. Glomerular hyalinosis and mesangial widening can also be seen. Tubular atrophy and interstitial fibrosis of varying degree accompany glomerulosclerosis. The arterioles and smaller arteries show hyalinosis (glassy eosinophilic appearance on PAS) with narrowing of lumen and medial thickening and interlobular arteries show fibrointimal hyperplasia and reduplication of the elastic lamina which can be better visualized on Verhoeff's elastic stain or Verhoeff's Van Gieson stain. Arcuate and larger arteries also show fibrointimal thickening.

On immunofluorescence, arterioles show deposition of IgM and C3. Other immunoglobulins and complements are absent both within glomeruli as well as blood vessels.

Electron microscopy confirms the light microscopy findings with wrinkling and thickening of glomerular capillary basement membrane and collagen fibrils in Bowman's space. Myofibroblastic nature of the cells in thickened intima of large blood vessels is also confirmed. A case of benign nephrosclerosis is illustrated (Fig. 21.1).

P. Gupta, R. K. Gupta, *Pathology of Glomerular Diseases*, https://doi.org/10.1007/978-981-19-1430-0_21

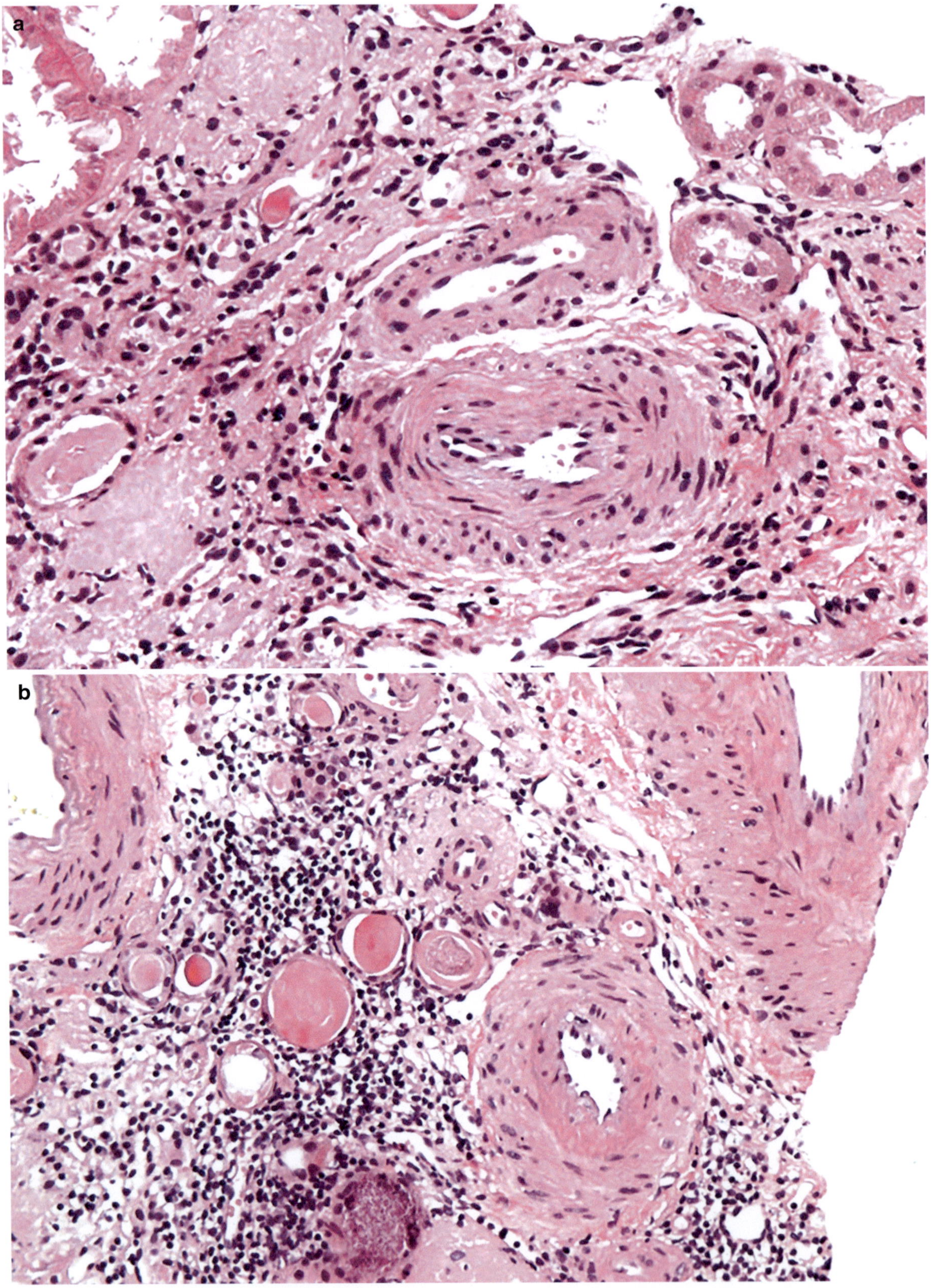

Fig. 21.1 **Benign Nephroscleoris** A 56-years male patient known to be hypertensive for last 10 years, presented with rise in serum creatinine and proteinuria for 6 months. USG showed that the right kidney was 9.0 × 3.7 cm and the left kidney was 9.0 × 4.1 cm; CMD was lost with increased cortical echogenecity. Laboratory workup revealed urinary proteinuria 2+ with bland urinary sediments; PC ratio was 1.8. Hemoglobin was 10.5 g/dl. BUN was 93 mg/dl and the serum creatinine was 3.8 mg/dl. Renal biopsy had 8 glomeruli, six of which were globally sclerosed, thickening and wrinkling of glomerular basement membrane was seen in remaining glomeruli. Moderate tubular atrophy with interstitial fibrosis was seen and the blood vessels showed arteriosclerosis with reduplication of internal elastic lamina. IF for IgG, IgM, IgA, C3, C1q, kappa and lambda was negative. (**a–c**) HE × 200, (**d**) PAS × 200, (**e**) PSM × 200, and (**f**) Orcein × 400

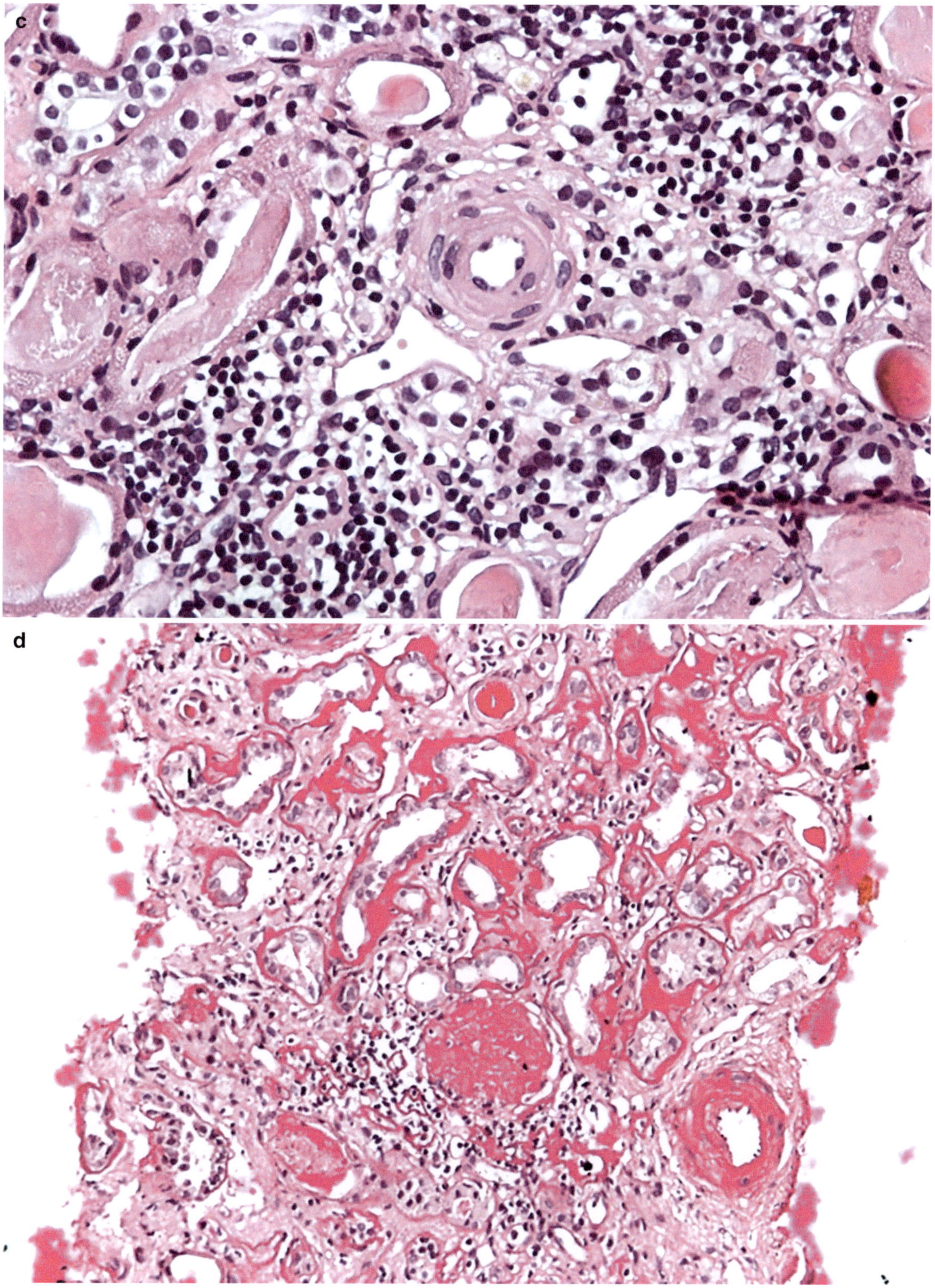

Fig. 21.1 (continued)

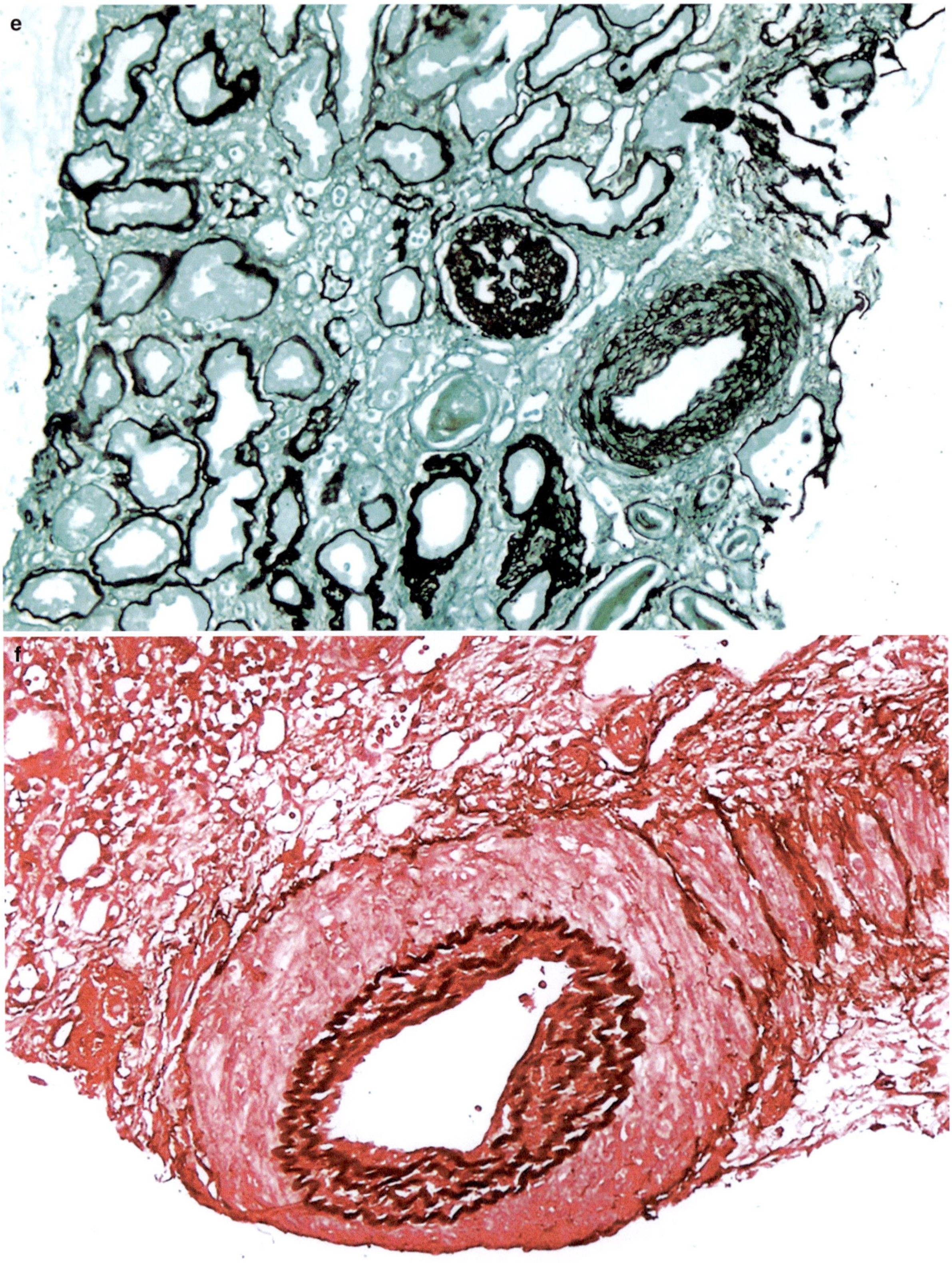

Fig. 21.1 (continued)

21.2 Malignant Nephrosclerosis

It can be seen in patients with accelerated phase of essential hypertension or in patients with de novo malignant hypertension. These patients frequently have bilateral retinal hemorrhage with or without accompanying papilloedema. Frequently these patients present with thrombotic microangiopathy.

Light microscopy appearances can be similar to that seen in other causes of thrombotic microangiopathy. Cases who do not have TMA can show wrinkling and collapse of glomerular capillary tuft. Both ischemic and solidified patterns of glomerular obsolescence can be seen. Patients can have focal global glomerulosclerosis. Tubules will show varying degree of tubular atrophy accompanied by interstitial fibrosis and inflammatory cell infiltrate. Most prominent findings are seen in the blood vessels. Larger arteries can show arteriosclerosis, narrowing of lumen, and disruption of elastic lamina. Arcuate arteries can show fibrointimal hyperplasia and reduplication of elastic lamina. Smaller arteries can show mucoid intimal hyperplasia, fibrinoid necrosis, and onion skin concentric thickening. Arterioles can show medial hypertrophy, hyalinosis, and segmental fibrinoid necrosis.

On immunofluorescence similar to its benign counterpart arterioles can show deposition of IgM and C3. Fibrinogen deposits can be seen in the wall of arterioles and arteries with fibrinoid necrosis or within glomeruli in patients with thrombotic microangiopathy.

Electron microscopy shows wrinkling and thickening of glomerular capillary basement membrane with a widened subendothelial zone. Collagen fibrils filling the bowman's space can be seen. A case of malignant nephrosclerosis is illustrated (Fig. 21.2).

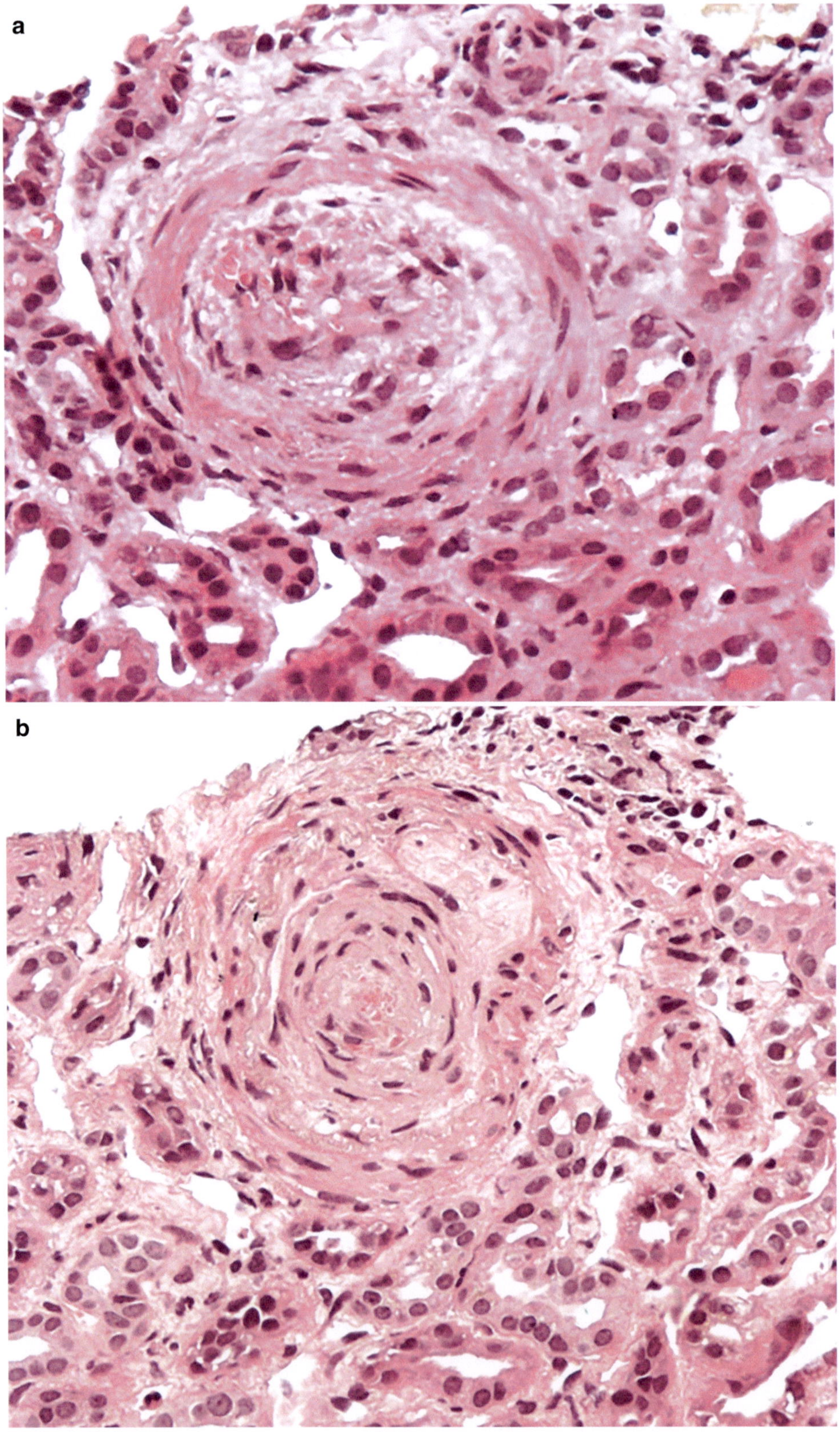

Fig. 21.2 Maliganant Nephrosclerosis A 45-years female patient presented with nausea and vomiting for past 1 month. Hypertension was detected in recent past but patient was not taking any medication for it. No history of fever or hematuria. On examination, there was no pedal edema. Blood pressure was 180/110 mm Hg. 24 h urine output was 900–1000 ml. Urine analysis showed absence of protein, RBC 3–5/hpf, WBC 0–2/hpf; PC ratio was 0.37. C3 and C4 were wnl. ANA was negative. Renal biopsy had 8 glomeruli, 1 was globally sclerosed, remaining showed mild thickening and wrinkling of glomerular capillary basement membrane with collapsed tuft in few of them. Tubules were unremarkable, and no interstitial infiltrate was seen. Blood vessels showed intimal mucoid edema with reduplication and break in elastic lamina and arterioles showed concentric thickening (onion skin appearance) of arteriolar wall. EM showed wrinkling of the glomerular capillary basement membrane and prominent subendothelial electron-lucent zone. (**a**, **b**) HE × 200, (**c**) PAS × 200, (**d**) Orcein × 400 and (**e**) EM (identity of the patient has been concealed)

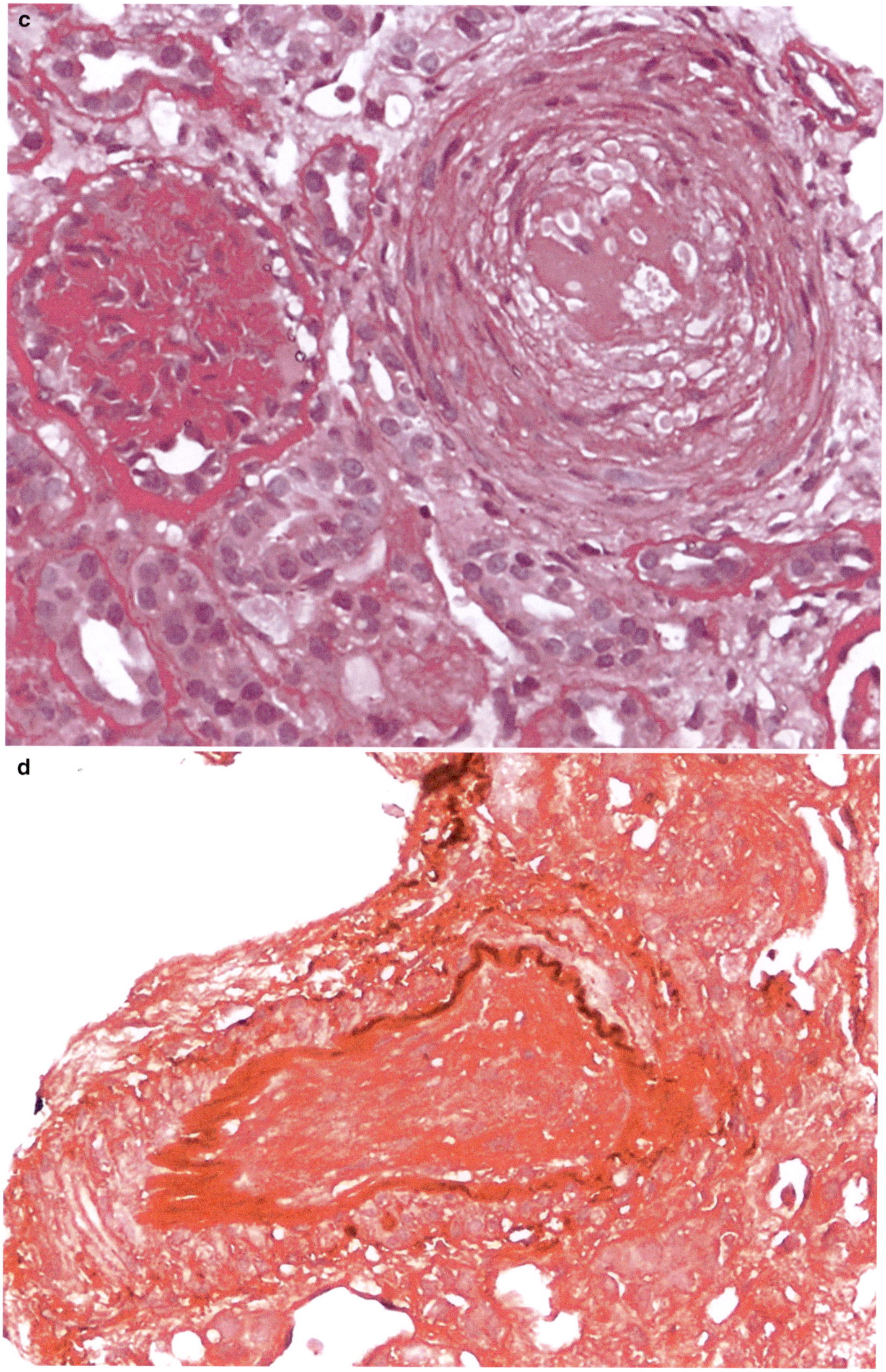

Fig. 21.2 (continued)

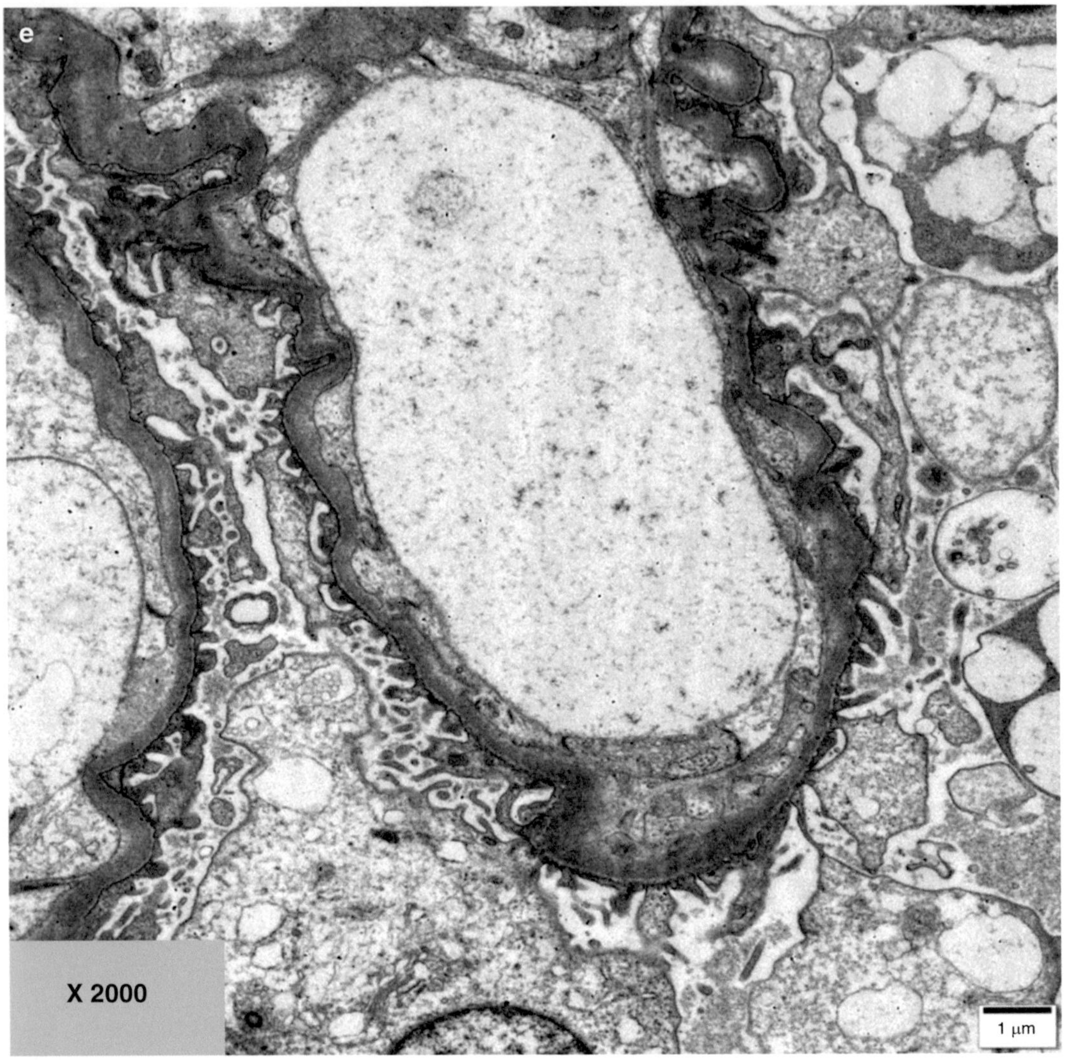

Fig. 21.2 (continued)

Further Reading

Bonsib SM. Non neoplastic diseases of the kidney, Chapter 5. In: Genitourinary pathology. New York: Elsevier; 2007. p. 225–80.

Liang S, Le W, Liang D, Chen H, Xu F, Chen H, Liu Z, Zeng C. Clinicopathological characteristics and outcomes of patients with biopsy-proven hypertensive nephrosclerosis: a retrospective cohort study. BMC Nephrol. 2016;17:42.

Shantsila A, Lip GYH. Malignant hypertension revisited-does this still exist? Am J Hypertens. 2017;30:543–9.

Sumida K, Hoshino J, Ueno T, Mise K, Hayami N, Suwabe T, Kawada M, Imafuku A, Hiramatsu R, Hasegawa E, Yamanouchi M, Sawa N, Fujii T, Ohashi K, Takaichi K, Ubara Y. Effect of proteinuria and glomerular filtration rate on renal outcome in patients with biopsy-provenbenign nephrosclerosis. PLoS One. 2016;11:e0147690.

Takebayashi S, Kiyoshi Y, Hisano S, Uesugi N, Sasatomi Y, Meng J, Sakata N. Benign nephrosclerosis: incidence, morphology and prognosis. Clin Nephrol. 2001;55:349–56.

22 Renal Sarcoidosis

Patients with renal sarcoidosis present with acute renal failure, hypercalcemia, and hypercalciuria. On histology interstitial granulomatous inflammation is common. The granulomas are non-necrotizing and discrete. A varying degree of interstitial fibrosis and tubular atrophy may be seen. Secondary glomerular involvement in the form of IgA nephropathy or membranous nephropathy can be seen. Rarely these patients can have AA amyloidosis. Nephrolithiasis and nephrocalcinosis have also been observed in these patients (Fig. 22.1).

P. Gupta, R. K. Gupta, *Pathology of Glomerular Diseases*, https://doi.org/10.1007/978-981-19-1430-0_22

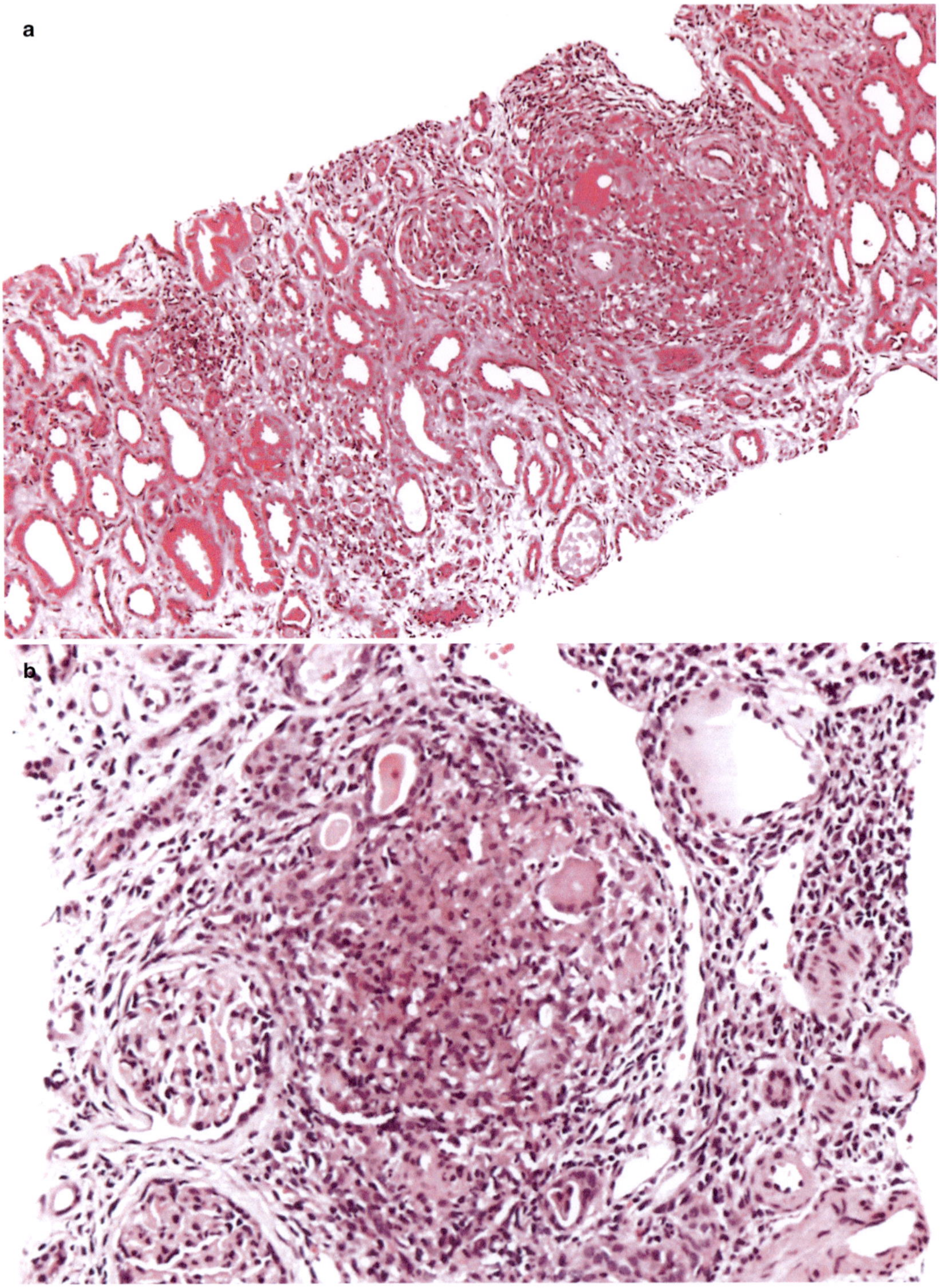

Fig. 22.1 **Renal Sarcoidosis** A 12-years male patient presented with joint pains for 1 year. X-ray chest revealed hilar lymphadenopathy and the Montoux test was negative. On laboratory workup he was found to be anemic with a hemoglobin level of 9.6 g/dL, total WBC count of 3500/cu mm, and platelets 68,000/cu mm; observed ESR for the first hour was 18 mm (Westergren). Urine analysis was unremarkable and the microscopic examination revealed 5–10 WBC/hpf. His serum creatinine was 2.3 mg/dL and serum calcium 10.95 mg/dL, serum ACE levels were 128 U/L, serum complements were wnl. Both c-ANCA and p-ANCA were negative. Quantiferon gold and TB PCR were negative. Renal biopsy had 8 glomeruli. No segmental or global glomerulosclerosis was seen. Several non-caseating naked epithelioid cell granulomas without surrounding lymphoid cuff and with foreign body giant cells were seen closely associated with glomeruli as well as in the interstitium; some of these granulomas showed microcalcification; acute tubular injury was also apparent. (**a**) PAS × 100, (**b**) HE × 200, (**c**, **d**) HE × 400, (**e**, **f**) HE × 200

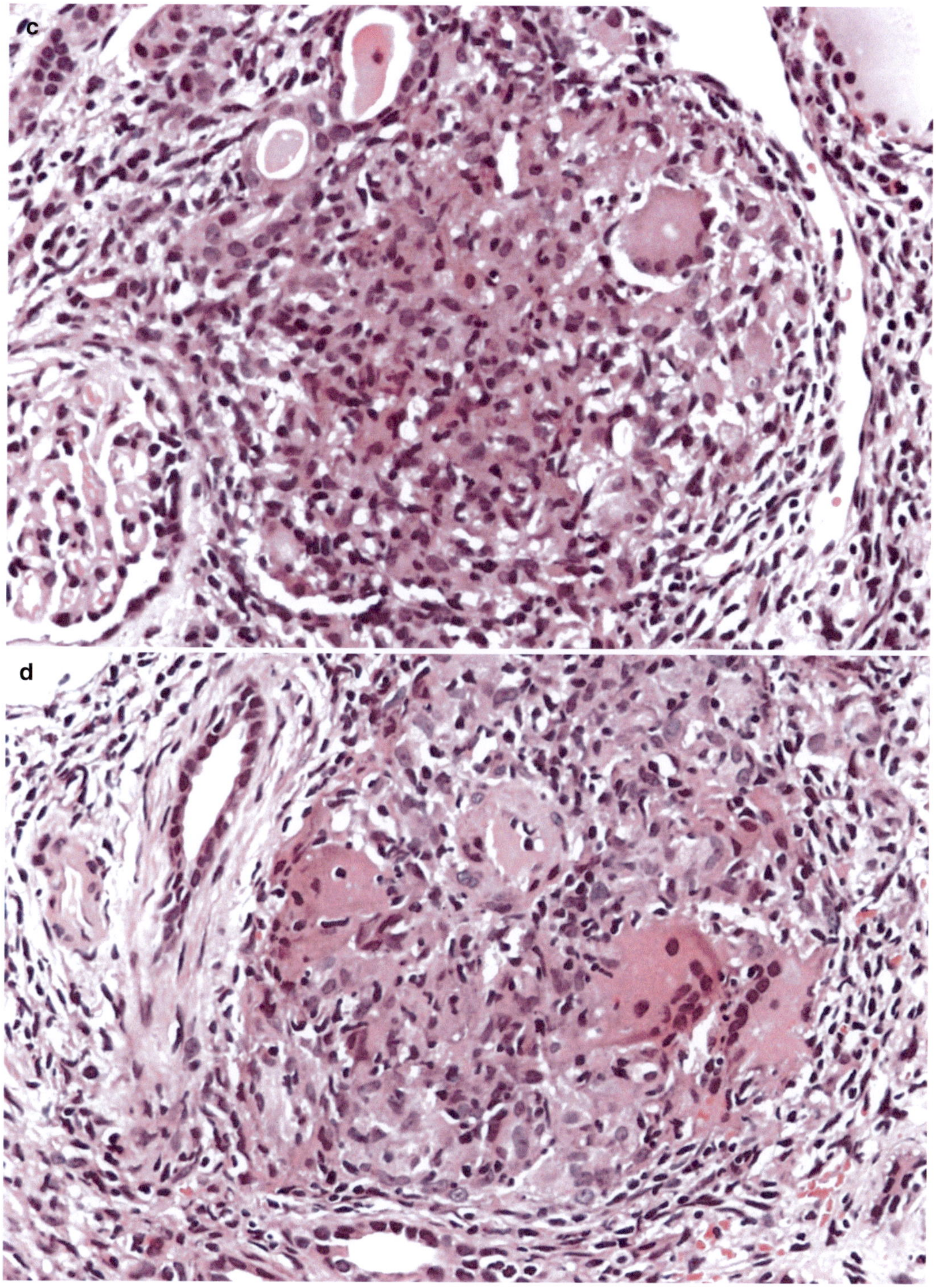

Fig. 22.1 (continued)

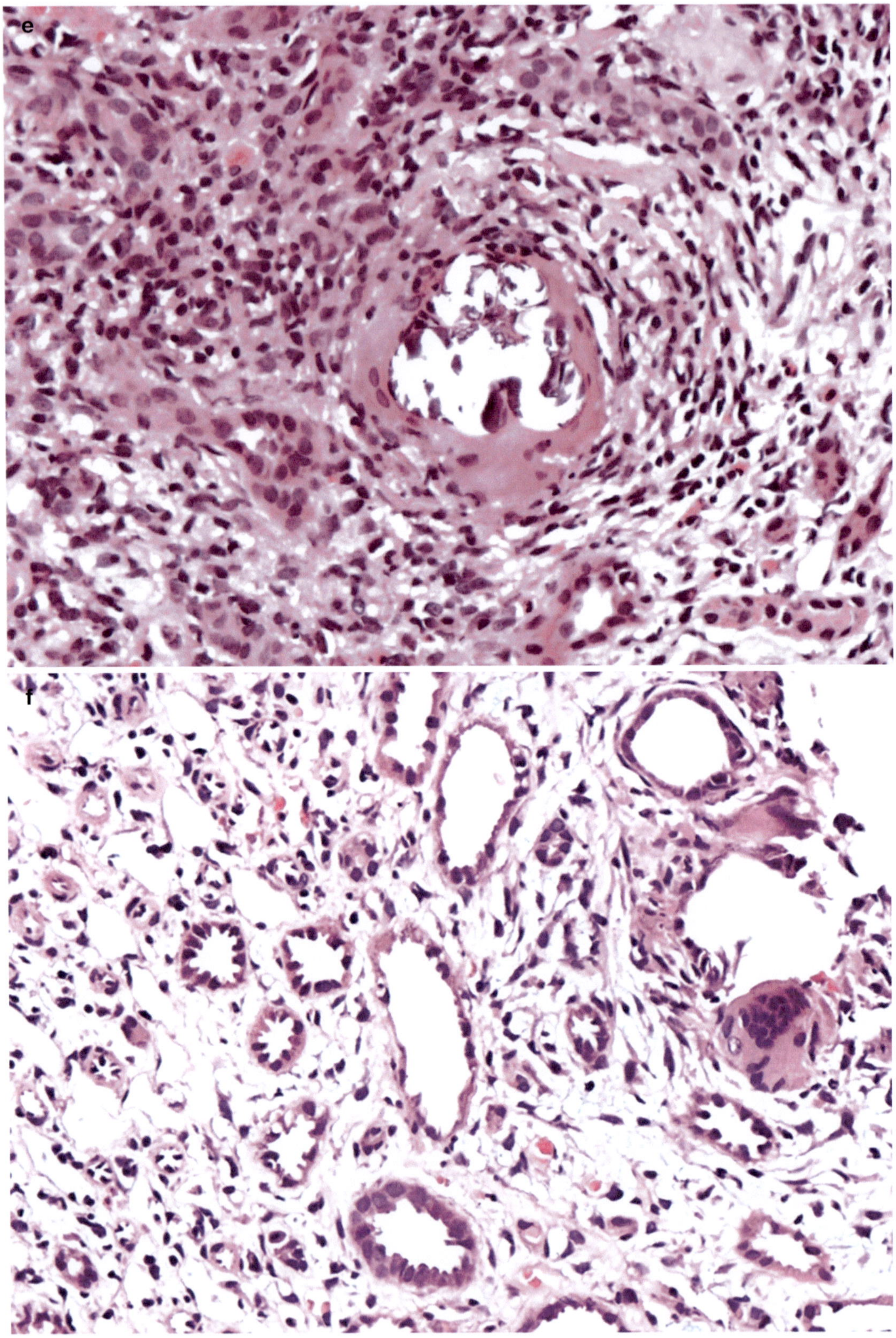

Fig. 22.1 (continued)

Further Reading

Bergner R, Löffler C. Renal sarcoidosis: approach to diagnosis and management. Curr Opin Pulm Med. 2018;24:513–20.

Correia FASC, Marchini GS, Torricelli FC, Danilovic A, Vicentini FC, Srougi M, Nahas WC, Mazzucchi E. Renal manifestations of sarcoidosis: from accurate diagnosis to specific treatment. Int Braz J Urol. 2020;46:15–25.

Hilderson I, Van Laecke S, Wauters A, Donck J. Treatment of renal sarcoidosis: is there a guideline? Overview of the different treatment options. Nephrol Dial Transplant. 2014;10:1841–7.

Menezes M, Patarata E. Renal sarcoidosis: a rare case. BMJ Case Rep. 2018;11:e227023.

23 Renal Involvement in HIV

23.1 HIVAN

The most common renal involvement in patients with HIV infection and AIDS is in the form of HIV-associated nephropathy (HIVAN); others being HIV associated immune complex-mediated glomerulonephritis (HIVIC) and noncollapsing focal segmental glomerulosclerosis. These patients usually have Cd4 counts <200 cells/cu mm. Clinically they present with significant proteinuria often in the nephrotic range and rapidly progressive renal failure.

On light microscopy, HIV-associated nephropathy has characteristic morphological findings in the form of collapsing pattern of focal segmental glomerulosclerosis. The glomerular capillary tuft is collapsed with wrinkling of the basement membrane. The podocytes show hypertrophy and hyperplasia often filling the Bowman's space to form pseudo crescents. These podocytes can have prominent nucleoli and mitosis may be seen. Tubules may be dilated and filled with proteinaceous material. Acute tubular injury can be seen. The interstitium can show edema, inflammation, and fibrosis.

On immunofluorescence IgM and C3 deposits can be seen in the collapsed tuft. IgG, IgA are negative.

On electron microscopy, tubuloreticular inclusions can be seen in the cytoplasm of endothelial cells. Wrinkling of glomerular capillary basement membrane can be seen along with hypertrophy of podocytes. Widespread and diffuse effacement of podocyte foot process and podocyte detachment can also be seen. A case of HIVAN is illustrated (Fig. 23.1).

P. Gupta, R. K. Gupta, *Pathology of Glomerular Diseases*, https://doi.org/10.1007/978-981-19-1430-0_23

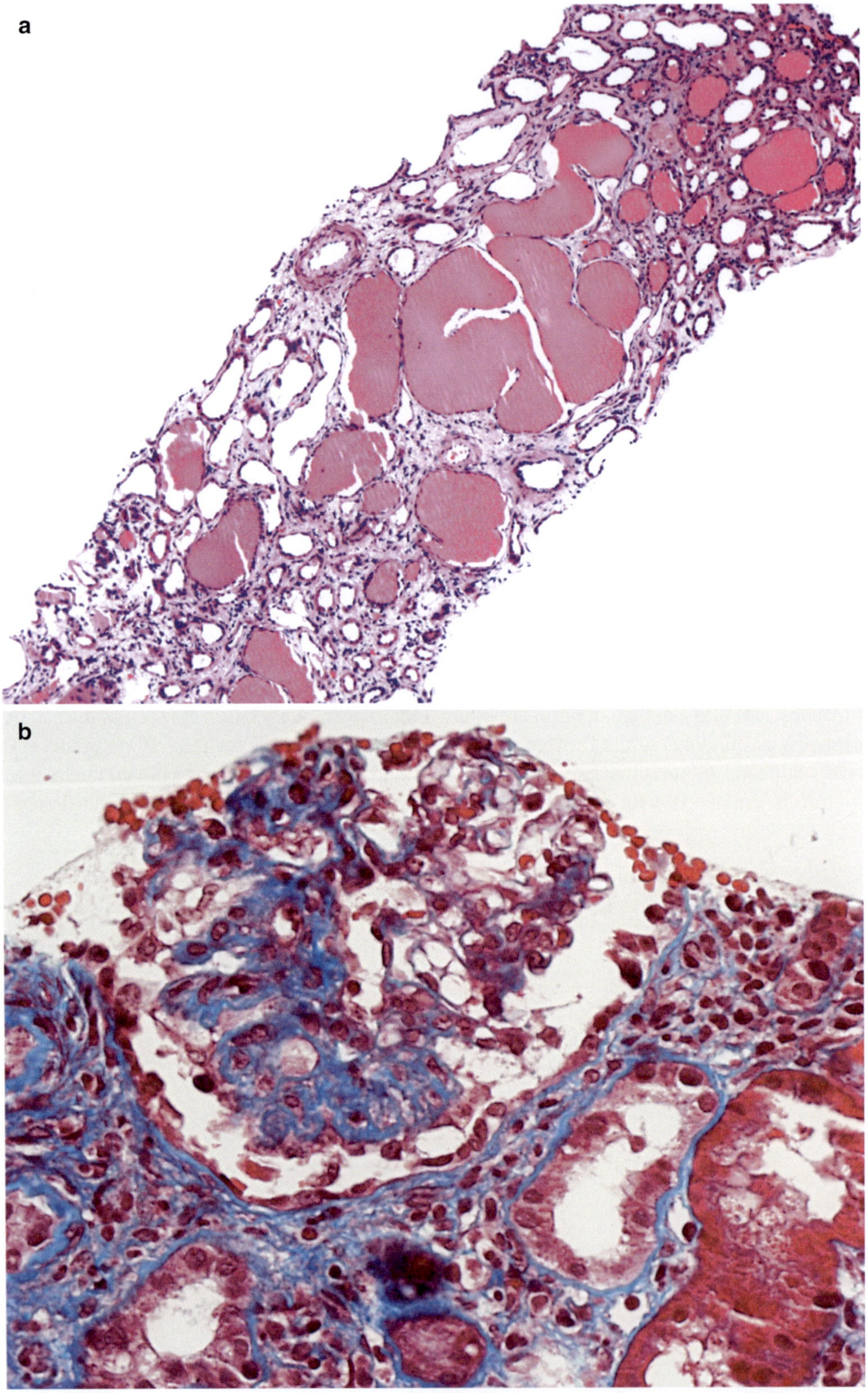

Fig. 23.1 **HIVAN** A 27-years African-American female patient presented with nephritic syndrome. She had proteinuria of 10 g/24 h, BUN was 26 mg/dl and the serum creatinine was 2.4 mg/dl. She was HIV-positive. Renal biopsy showed the collapse of glomerular tuft of capillaries with segmental sclerosis and hyperplasia of podocytes along with cystic dilatation of tubules. EM showed tubuloreticular inclusions within the cytoplasm of endothelial cells. (**a**) HE × 100, (**b**) MT × 200, (**c**) Jones × 200 and (**d**) EM. (Contributor—Dr. Helen Liapis, Professor of Pathology and Immunology and Internal Medicine (Renal) retired, Washington University School of Medicine, Saint Louis, MO, USA)

c

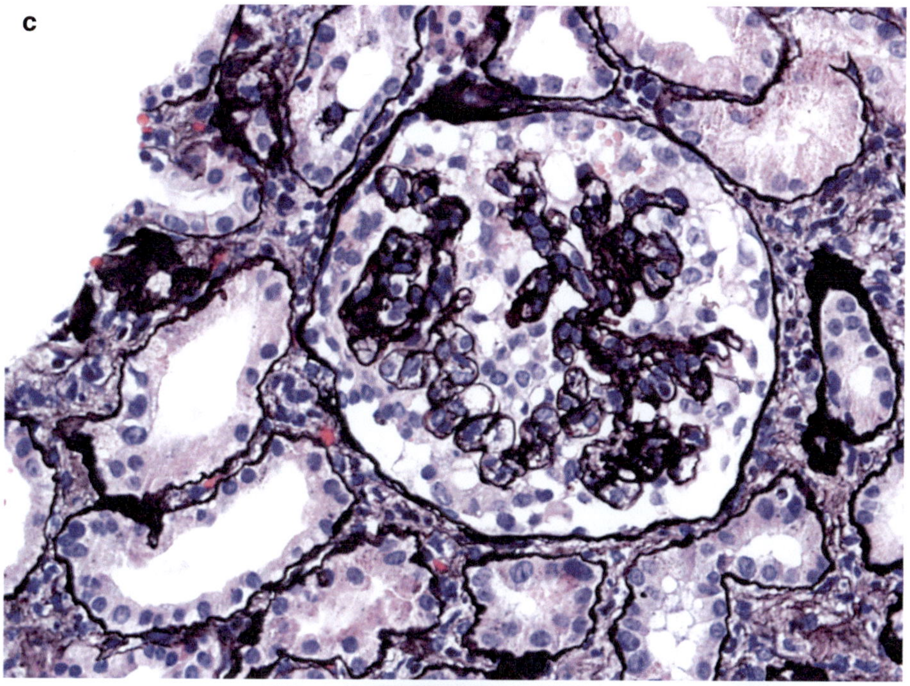

d

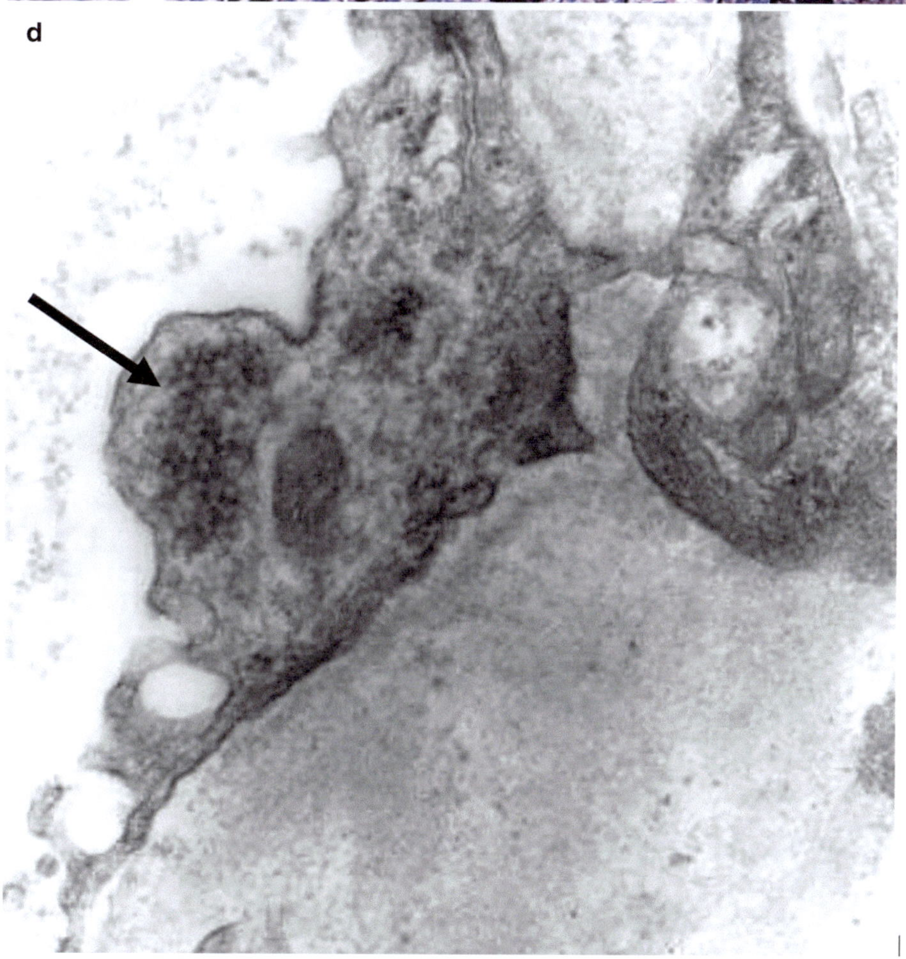

Fig. 23.1 (continued)

23.2 HIV-Associated Immune Complex (HIVIC) Mediated Kidney Disease

HIVAN the HIV-associated nephropathy was considered the most common glomerular disease in patients with HIV. After the introduction of HAART therapy classic FSGS emerged as a prominent glomerular disease in these patients. HIV associated immune complex-mediated glomerular disease (HIVIC) can account for up to 22–34% of cases of glomerular diseases in HIV-positive patients. Other glomerular diseases include minimal change disease, thrombotic microangiopathy, and crescentic glomerulonephritis. Patients with HIVIC present with renal dysfunction and proteinuria which can be in the nephrotic range. Hypertension can be observed at presentation in a few patients. HIVIC can have varied morphological appearances including mesangio-proliferative, MPGN or membranous patterns of glomerular involvement. These patients will have glomerular immune deposits visualized on immunofluorescence and electron microscopy. The clinical progression to ESRD is much lower in patients with HIVIC as compared to patients with HIVAN. A case of HIVIC presenting as crescentic glomerulonephritis is illustrated (Fig. 23.2).

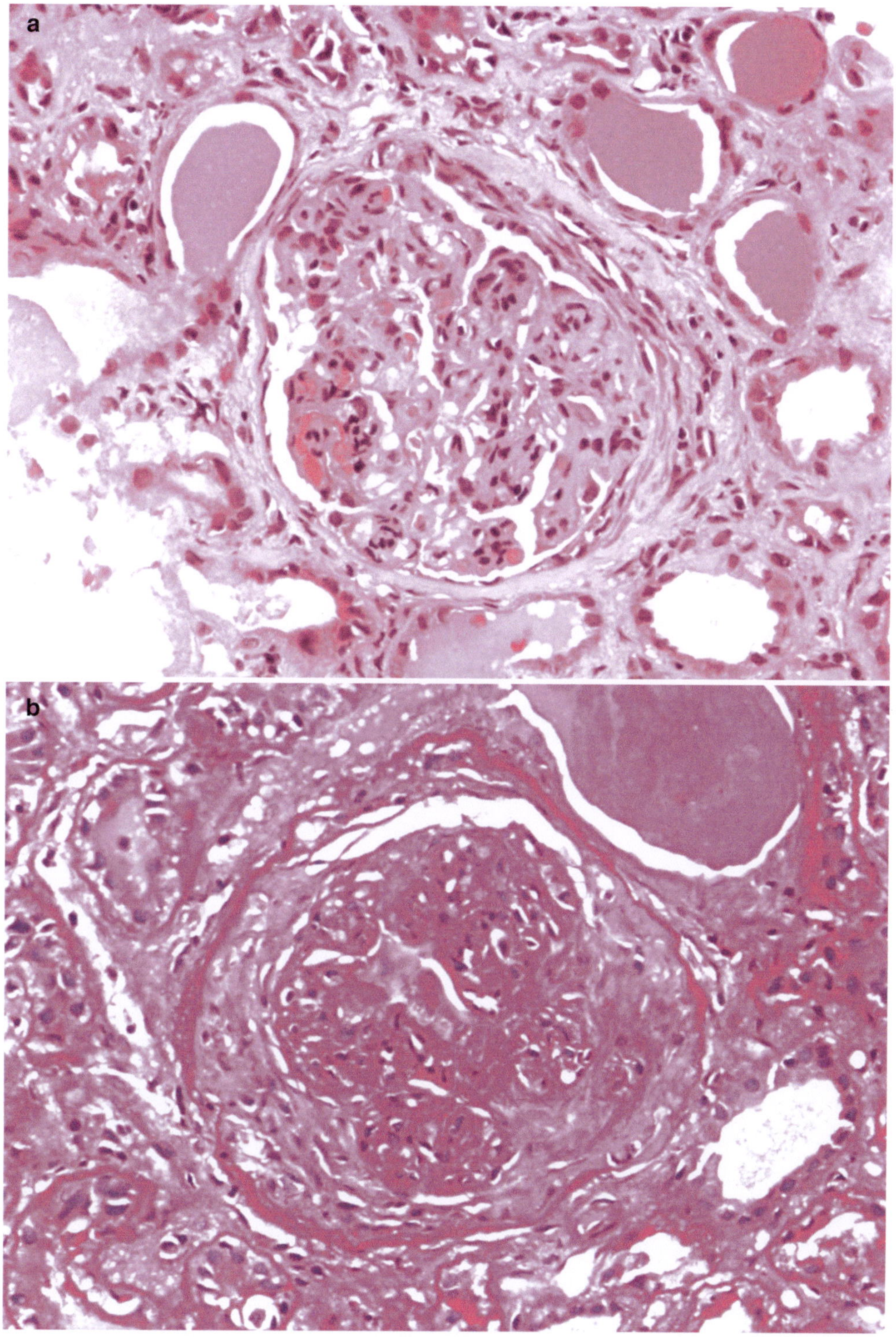

Fig. 23.2 **HIVIC** A 44-years male patient known to be seropositive for HIV, presented with fatigue, loss of weight, and appetite along with decreased urine output and generalized swelling over the body. His urine analysis showed protein 3+ with 15–20 RBC/hpf; urinary P/C ratio was 3.2. His serum creatinine was 13.2 mg/dl with low serum complement C3 (473 mg/L) and normal C4 levels. Renal biopsy contained 18 glomeruli, 16 of which had cellular to fibrocellular crescents with endocapillary and mesangial hyperplasia. Mild tubular atrophy along with moderate interstitial inflammation and fibrosis was seen. IF showed granular to smudgy mesangial and capillary wall deposits of IgG, IgM, C3, C1q, kappa and lambda. IgA was negative. Electron microscopy showed several subepithelial deposits and humps along with scattered subendothelial and mesangial deposits. (**a**) HE × 400, (**b**) PAS × 400, (**c**) PAS × 200, (**d**–**f**) IF × 400, and (**g**) EM

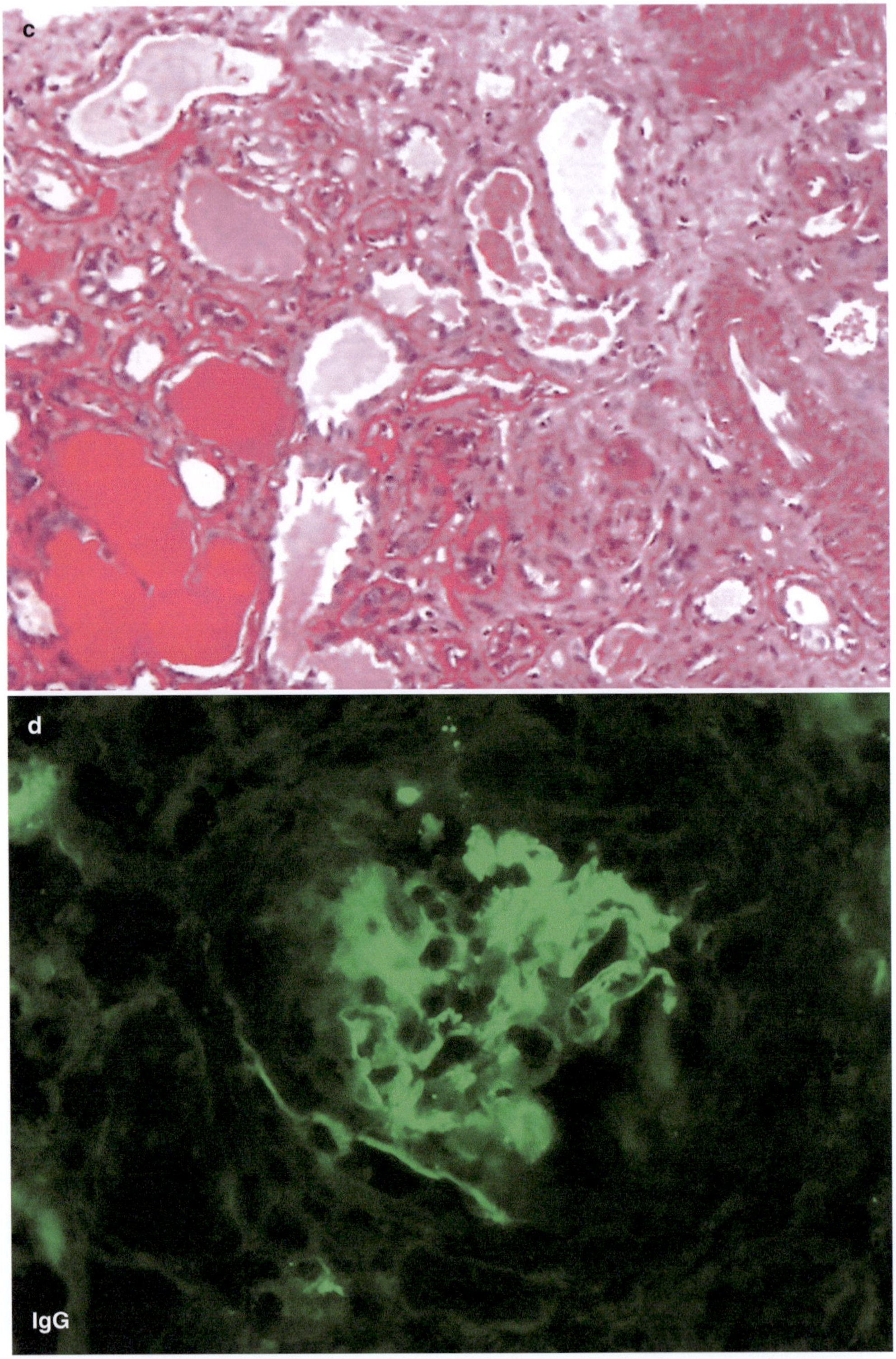

Fig. 23.2 (continued)

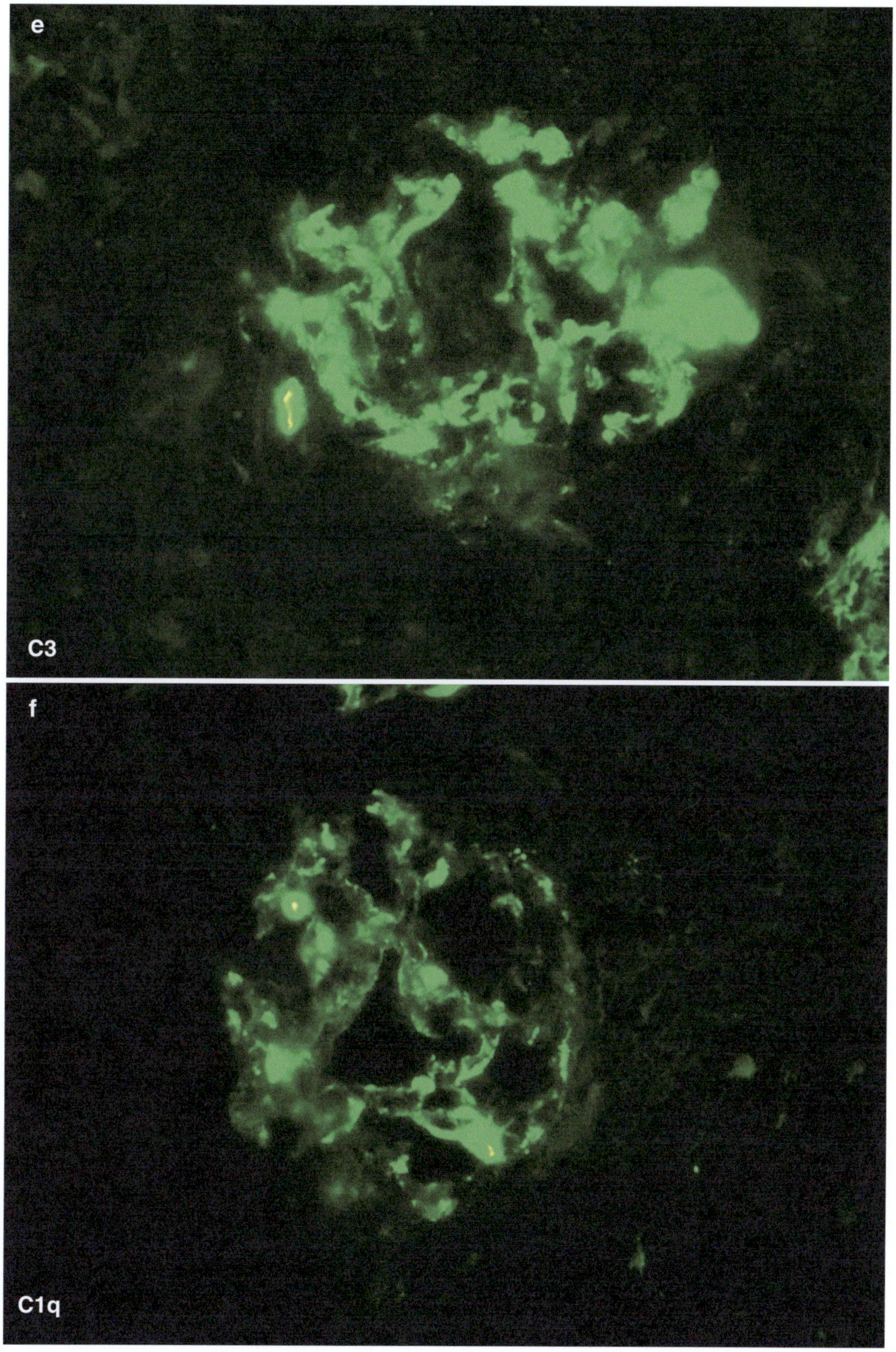

Fig. 23.2 (continued)

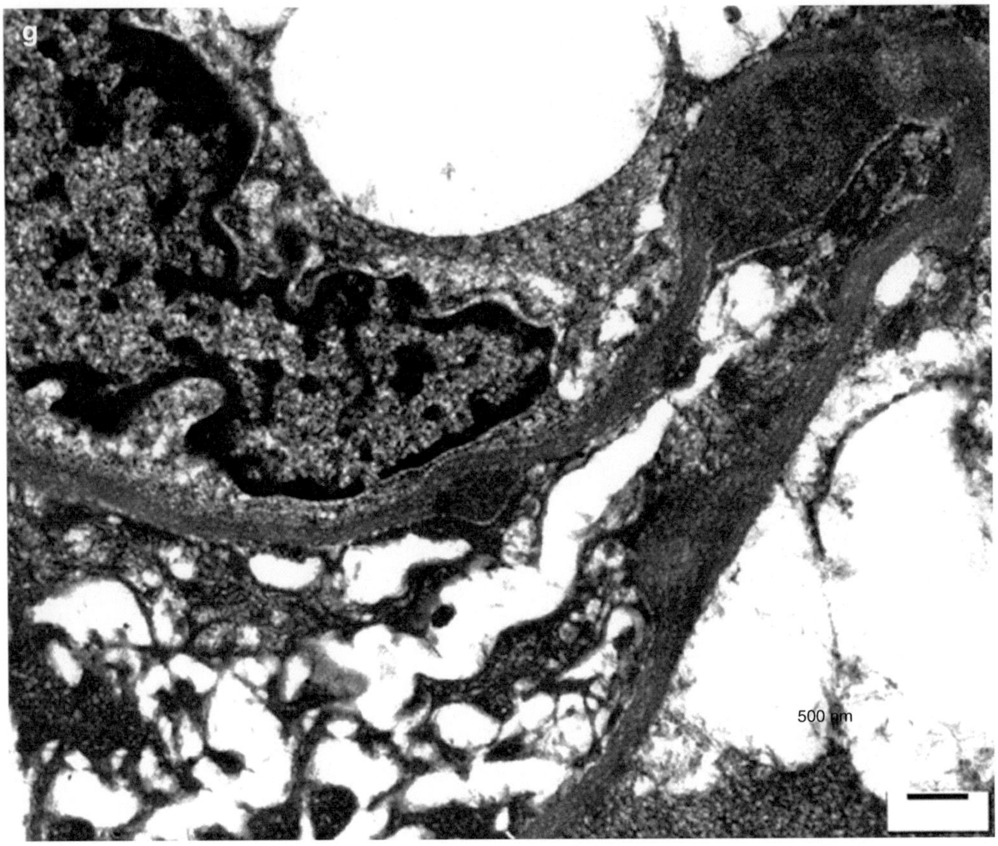

Fig. 23.2 (continued)

Further Reading

HIVAN

Khan S, Haragsim L, Laszik ZG. HIV-associated nephropathy. Adv Chronic Kidney Dis. 2006;13:307–13.

Kopp JB, Heymann J, Winkler CA. APOL1 renal risk variants: fertile soil for HIV-associated nephropathy. Semin Nephrol. 2017;37:514–9.

Swanepoel CR, Atta MG, D'Agati VD, Estrella MM, Fogo AB, Naicker S, Post FA, Wearne N, Winkler CA, Cheung M, Wheeler DC, Winkelmayer WC, Wyatt CM, Conference Participants. Kidney disease in the setting of HIV infection: conclusions from a kidney disease: improving global outcomes (KDIGO) controversies conference. Kidney Int. 2018;93:545–59.

Wyatt CM, Klotman PE, D'Agati VD. HIV-associated nephropathy: clinical presentation, pathology and epidemiology in the era of antiretroviral therapy. Semin Nephrol. 2008;28:513–22.

HIV Associated Crescentic Glomerulonephritis (Immune Complex Mediated)

Booth JW, Hamzah L, Jose S, Horsfield C, O'Donnell P, McAdoo S, Kumar EA, Turner-Stokes T, Khatib N, Das P, Naftalin C, Mackie N, Kingdon E, Williams D, Hendry BM, Sabin C, Jones R, Levy J, Hilton R, Connolly J, Post FA, HIV/CKD Study and the UK CHIC Study. Clinical characteristics and outcomes of HIV-associated immune complex kidney disease. Nephrol Dial Transplant. 2016;31:2099–107.

Lescure FX, Flateau C, Pacanowski J, Brocheriou I, Rondeau E, Girard PM, Ronco P, Pialoux G, Plaisier E. HIV-associated kidney glomerular diseases: changes with time and HAART. Nephrol Dial Transplant. 2012;27:2349–55.

Nobakht E, Cohen SD, Rosenberg AZ, Kimmel PL. HIV-associated immune complex kidney disease. Nat Rev Nephrol. 2016;12:291–300.

Wyatt CM. Kidney disease and HIV infection. Top Antivir Med. 2017;25:13–6.

24 Renal Involvement in Scleroderma

Scleroderma can be a localized disease with skin thickening or diffuse disease in which skin manifestations are accompanied by Reynaud phenomenon, arthralgia, fatigue, and involvement of other systems including lungs, gastrointestinal tract, heart, and kidneys. Sometimes overlap with other systemic disorders like SLE can be seen.

Scleroderma renal crisis is seen in <20% of scleroderma patients and is a serious complication manifesting as raised blood pressure, renal dysfunction, proteinuria, hematuria and can also show manifestations of thrombotic microangiopathy (hemolytic anemia, thrombocytopenia and raised reticulocyte count).

Renal pathology changes involve predominantly the blood vessels. Glomerular changes are similar to those seen in thrombotic microangiopathy of other etiologies. It is characterized by acute manifestation in the form of endothelial cell swelling, detachment from the basement membrane, fibrin thrombi within glomerular capillaries, and fragmented red blood cells. Chronic changes include mesangiolysis, double contour of GBM (MPGN pattern), segmental sclerosis, and widening of subendothelial space with electron-lucent material. Vascular manifestations include arterial intimal mucoid edema, fibrin thrombi, fibrointimal hyperplasia, and luminal narrowing. Organization of fibrin thrombi within the vascular lumen can be seen.

The presence of HLA-DRB1*0407 and *1304 are associated with an increased risk of scleroderma renal crisis. Anticentromere antibodies, anti-RNA polymerase III antibodies, and diffuse scleroderma are also associated with an increased risk of developing renal crisis.

Patient survival in scleroderma renal crisis is between 70% and 80% at 1 year. A case of renal involvement in scleroderma has been illustrated (Fig. 24.1).

P. Gupta, R. K. Gupta, *Pathology of Glomerular Diseases*, https://doi.org/10.1007/978-981-19-1430-0_24

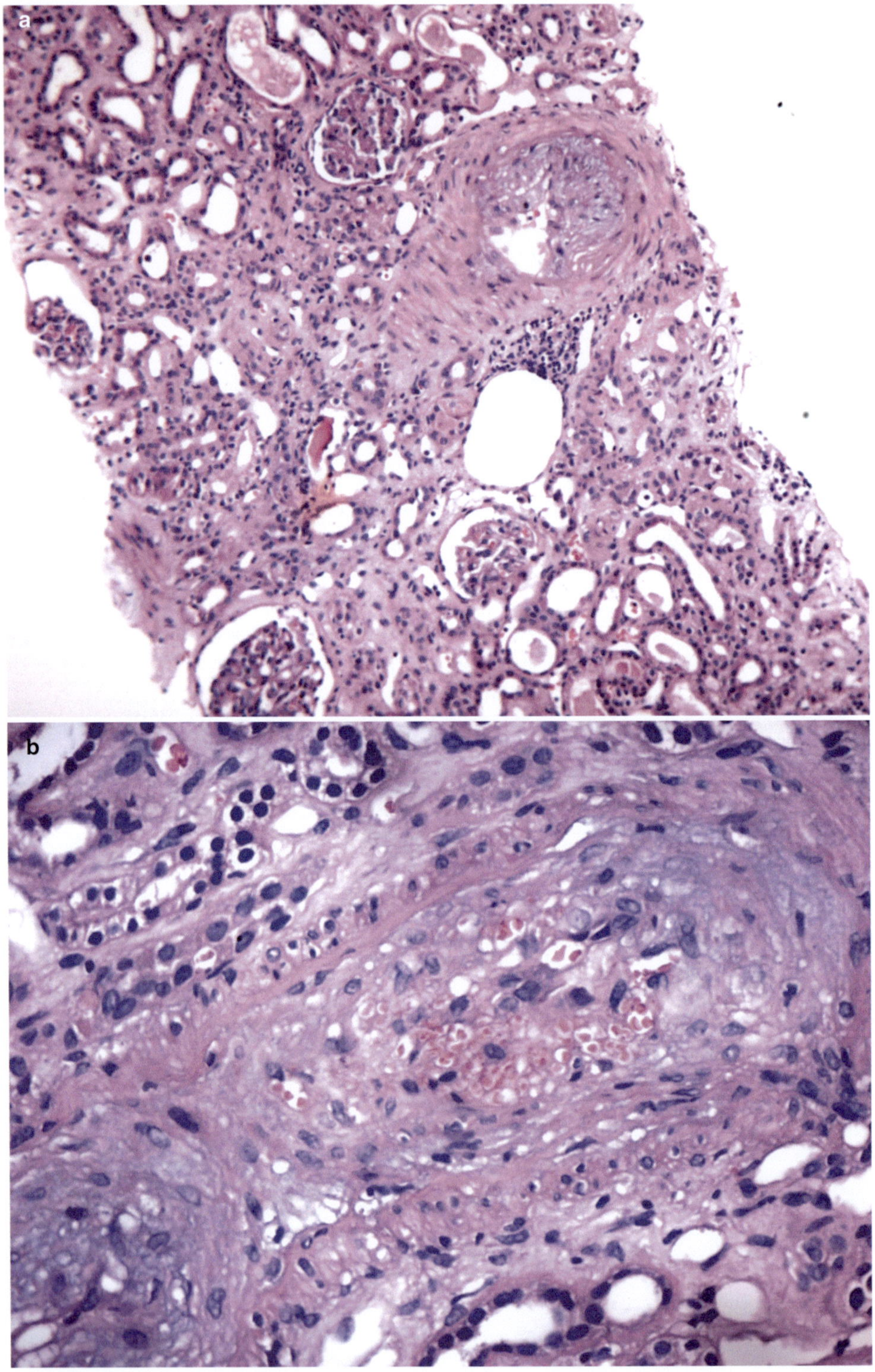

Fig. 24.1 **Renal involvement in Scleroderma** A 45-years female patient presented with thickening of skin, Reynaud's phenomena, ischaemic pits in multiple fingers for the past 7–8 years. Four years back she developed gangrene of distal phalanx of third finger of left hand, for which amputation had to be done. Three months back she was detected to have hypertension (200/110 mm/Hg). She also had watery and foul-smelling diarrhea, vomiting, and generalized weakness. CBC showed hemoglobin of 12.4 g%, TLC of 15,500/cu mm with 70% neutrophils. Platelets were 353,000/cu mm. Twenty-four hour urinary protein was 15.7 mg/dl. Serum creatinine was 3.1 mg/dl; ANA, DsDNA and serum complements were wnl. Single-core renal biopsy revealed 12 glomeruli which showed wrinkling of capillary basement membrane with no increase in endomesangial cellularity and matrix. Few foci of tubular atrophy and interstitial edema were evident. Blood vessels showed fibrointimal hyperplasia with intimal mucoid edema and occlusion of lumen. IF was non-contributory. (**a**, **b**) HE × 200 and (**c**, **d**) Masson's Trichrome × 400. (Contributor: Dr. Bhavna Asit Mehta, Senior Consultant Histoanatomic and Nephropathologist, Head of Histoanatomic Pathology Department, Supratech Micropath Laboratory (A Neuberg Associate), Neuberg Supratech Reference Laboratory, Ahmedabad-380006. Gujarat, India)

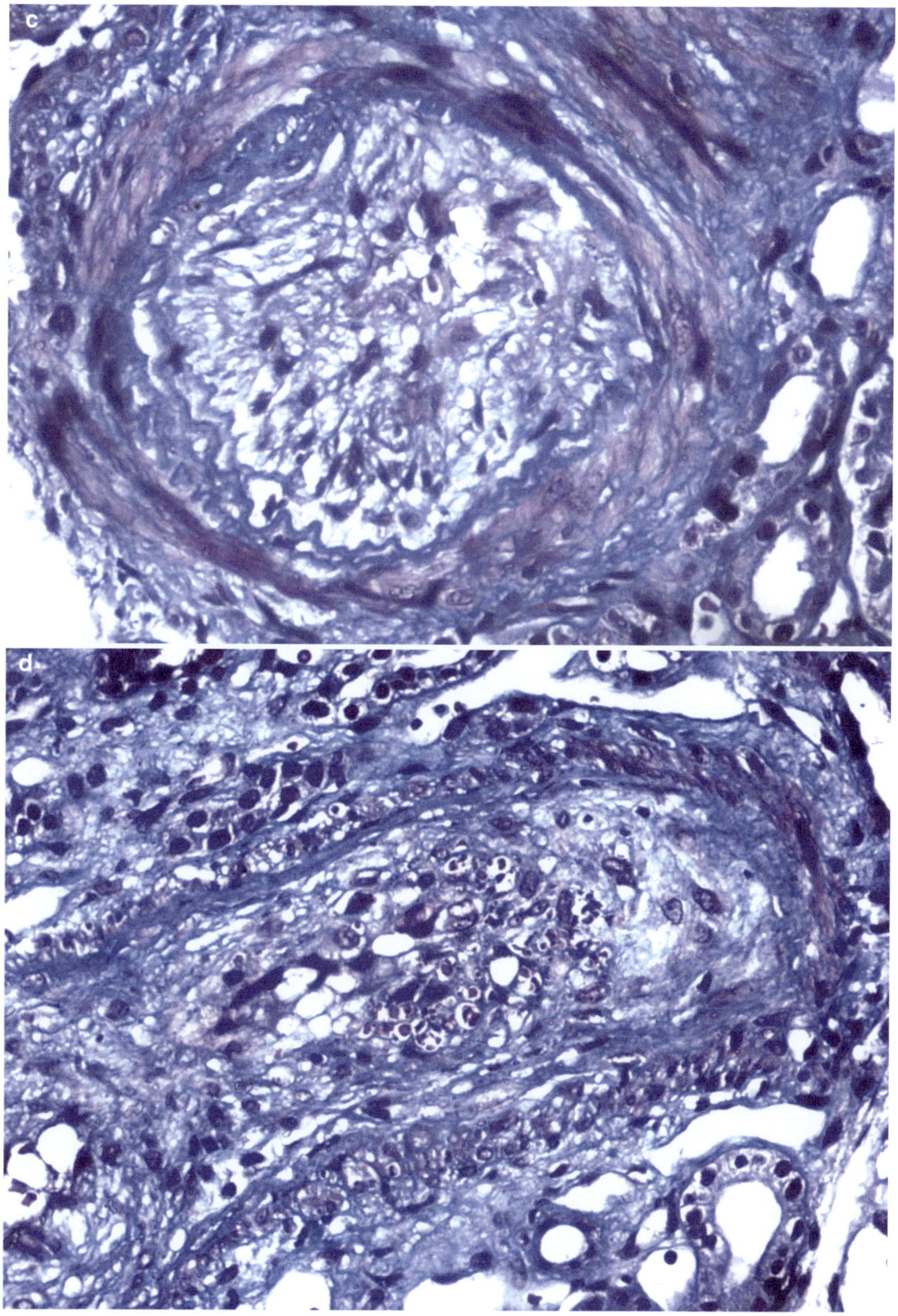

Fig. 24.1 (continued)

Further Reading

Bose N, Chiesa-Vottero A, Chatterjee S. Scleroderma renal crisis. Semin Arthritis Rheum. 2015;44:687–94.

Nagaraja V. Management of scleroderma renal crisis. Curr Opin Rheumatol. 2019;31:223–30.

Woodworth TG, Suliman YA, Li W, Furst DE, Clements P. Scleroderma renal crisis and renal involvement in systemic sclerosis. Nat Rev Nephrol. 2016;12:678–91.

Yamashita H, Kamei R, Kaneko H. Classifications of scleroderma renal crisis and reconsideration of its pathophysiology. Rheumatology (Oxford). 2019;58:2099–106.

Zanatta E, Polito P, Favaro M, Larosa M, Marson P, Cozzi F, Doria A. Therapy of scleroderma renal crisis: state of the art. Autoimmun Rev. 2018;17:882–9.

25 Warfarin-Induced Nephropathy

Warfarin-induced nephropathy is a type of acute kidney injury caused by excessive anticoagulation by anticoagulants such as warfarin. It is characterized by glomerular hemorrhage which manifests as RBCs in Bowman's space, acute tubular injury with RBCs and RBC casts in tubular lumen and interstitial nephritis. Anti-coagulant-related nephropathy can also be seen with other anticoagulants like acitrom, dabigatran, rivaroxaban, etc. These patients frequently have deranged INR. In these patients, many red blood cells get filtered through glomerulus with accumulation in Bowman's space along with red cell lysis resulting in free radical damage to tubular lining. Although complete recovery can be seen, some patients can progress to end-stage renal disease and may require renal replacement therapy. A case of warfarin induced nephropathy is illustrated (Fig. 25.1).

P. Gupta, R. K. Gupta, *Pathology of Glomerular Diseases*, https://doi.org/10.1007/978-981-19-1430-0_25

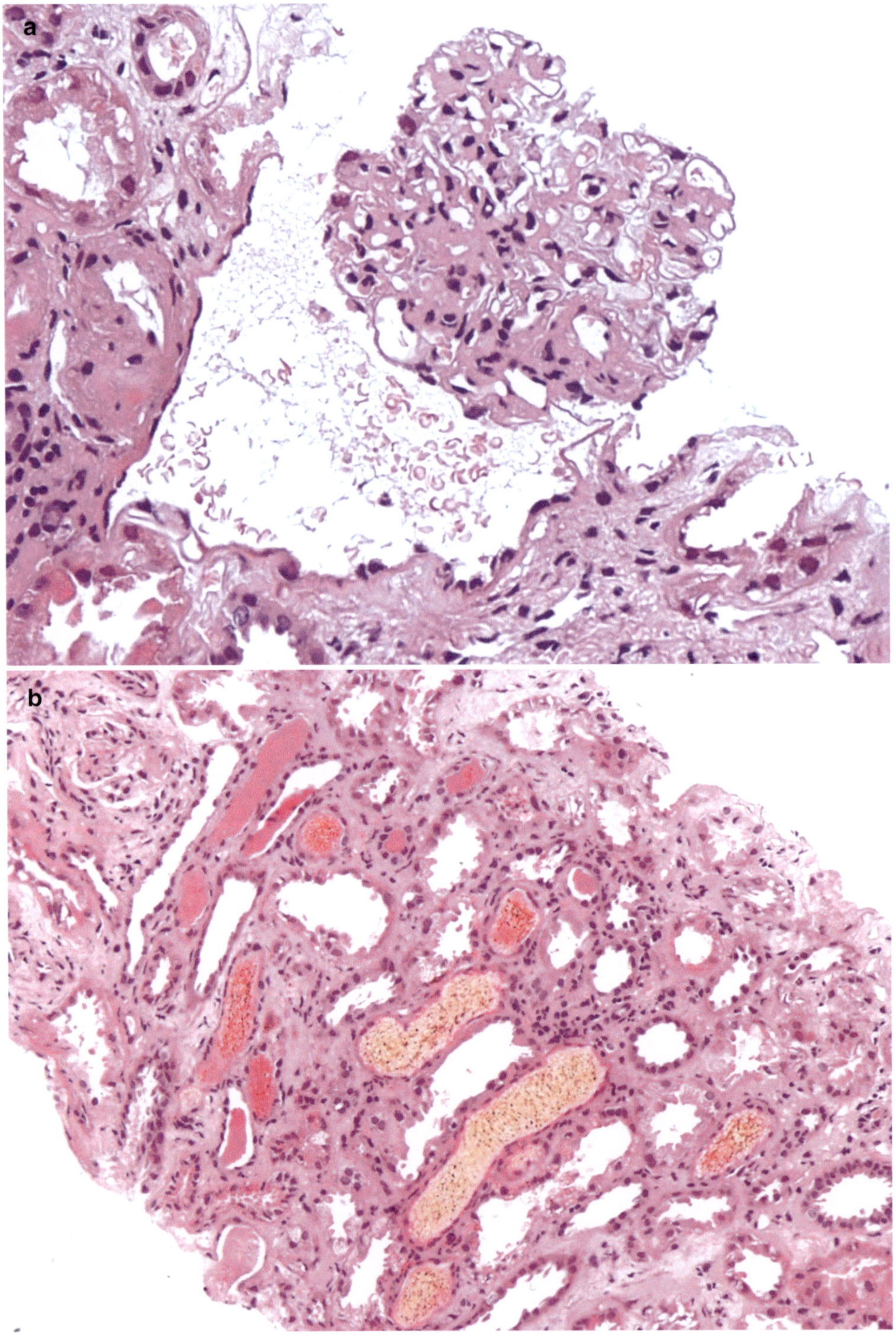

Fig. 25.1 **Warfarin Nephropathy** A 54-years male patient was known to be hypertensive. He had been suffering from rheumatic heart disease and had undergone aortic valve replacement. He was on warfarin 3 mg once daily dose. He presented with decreased urine output (<500 ml/day) and hematuria for 1 week. He had no h/o fever, sore throat, shortness of breath, headache, or visual disturbances. There was no history of any other medication intake. He had deranged renal function with serum creatinine of 8.00 mg/dl and coagulopathy with INR of 6.2. Other lab investigations revealed hemoglobin 9.2 g/dl; total and differential WBC were wnl and the blood platelets were 190,000/cu mm. Urine analysis revealed albumin 2+ and glucose was negative; urinary sediments had plenty of RBC with numerous RBC cast and 10–12 WBC/hpf. ANA and ANCA were negative. He was put on hemodialysis. Warfarin was discontinued and he was put on low molecular weight heparin and oral steroids 1 mg/kg, which was tapered off within 1 month. Patient had improved urine output and became dialysis independent. Renal biopsy had eight glomeruli, one glomerulus showed expansion of Bowman's space with the presence of plenty of RBC. Renal tubules showed presence of RBC and RBC cast with presence of hemosiderin pigment in renal tubules. Renal tubules also showed features of acute tubular injury; interstitium had mild lymphocytic infiltrate with presence of few polymorphs and eosinophils. IF for IgG, IgM, IgA, complement C3 and C4 and kappa and lambda light chains was negative. (**a**, **b**) HE × 200 and (**c**) Persian blue × 200

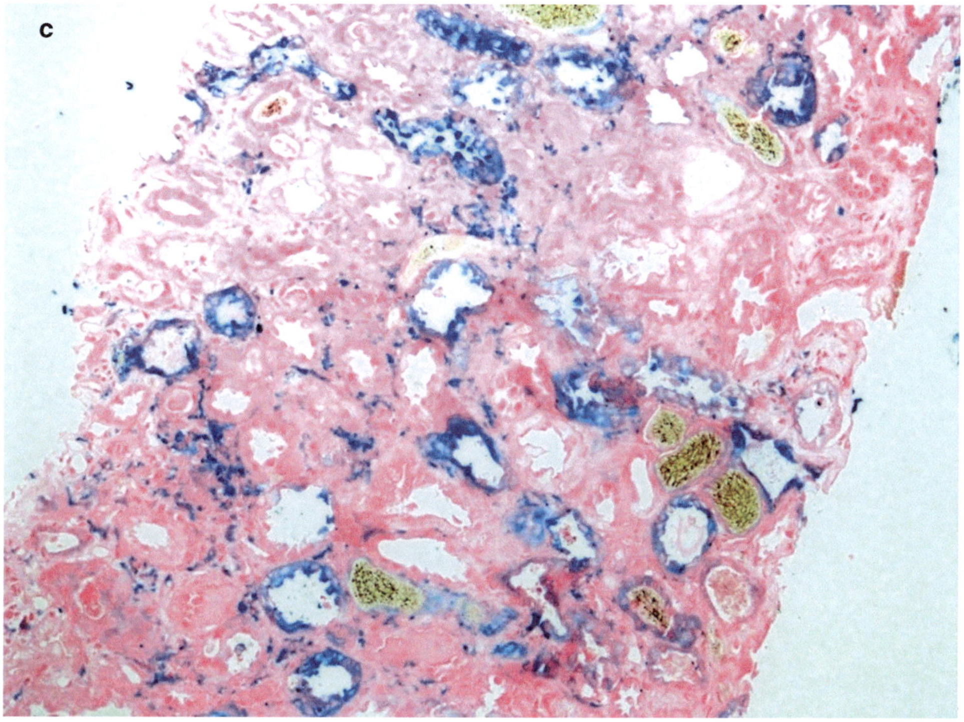

Fig. 25.1 (continued)

Further Reading

Brodsky S, Eikelboom J, Hebert LA. Anticoagulant-related nephropathy. J Am Soc Nephrol. 2018;29:2787–93.

De Aquino Moura KB, Behrens PMP, Pirolli R, Sauer A, Melamed D, Veronese FV, et al. Anticoagulant-related nephropathy: systematic review and meta-analysis. Clin Kid J. 2019;12:400–7.

Ryan M, Ware K, Qamri Z, Satoskar A, Wu H, Nadasdy G, et al. Warfarin-related nephropathy is the tip of the iceberg: direct thrombin inhibitor dabigatran induces glomerular hemorrhage with acute kidney injury in rats. Nephrol Dial Transplant. 2014;29:2228–34.

Piran S, Traquair H, Chan N, Robinson M, Schulman S. Incidence and risk factors for acute kidney injury in patients with excessive anticoagulation on warfarin: a retrospective study. J Thromb Thrombolysis. 2018 May;1(45):557–61.

Appendices

Appendix 1: Staining Procedures

Hematoxylin and Eosin (HE) Stain

Reagents

1. Mayer's Hematoxylin
2. 0.3% acid alcohol
3. 2% aqueous Eosin

Procedure

1. Sections are deparaffinized.
2. Sections are hydrated with distilled water.
3. Stain with Mayer's hematoxylin for 5 min.
4. Stain is rinsed with smoothly running tap water.
5. Differentiate with 0.3% acid alcohol for bluing till the background becomes colorless.
6. Stain is rinsed in smoothly running tap water.
7. Stain with eosin for 2 min.
8. Wash excesses eosin in running tap water.
9. Dehydrate, clear and mount using DPX and a clean coverslip.

Interpretation

1. Nuclei are stained blue.
2. The cytoplasm and extracellular matrix have varying degrees of pink staining.

   Nucleoli also appear pink.

Periodic Acid Schiff (PAS) Stain

Reagents

1. Periodic acid 1%
2. Schiff Reagent: dissolve 1 g basic fuchsin in 200 ml of boiling distilled water. Allow the solution to cool to 50 °C and add 2 g potassium metabisulphite with mixing. Allow to cool to room temperature and add 2 ml conc. HCl. Mix and add 2 g activated charcoal and leave overnight in the dark at room temperature. Filter through Whatman's no.1 filter paper. Store in a dark container at 4 °C.

Procedure

1. Deparaffinize and bring sections to water
2. Treat with 1% periodic acid—5 min.
3. Wash well with several changes of distilled water.
4. Cover with Schiff reagent—30 min.
5. Wash in running water—5–10 min.
6. Stain nuclei with Harris hematoxylin
7. Differentiate in 1% acid alcohol and blue as usual
8. Wash in water.
9. Dehydrate, clear and mount in DPX using a clean coverslip.

Interpretation

1. PAS-positive structures—magenta pink
2. Nuclei-blue

Masson's Trichrome Stain (MT Stain)

Reagents

1. Harris Hematoxylin
2. Gomori trichrome stain. It is prepared by mixing
   - Chromotrope 2R 0.6 g
   - Fast green FCF 0.3 g
   - Phosphotungstic acid 0.6 g
   - Deionized water 100 ml
   - Acetic acid, glacial 1.0 ml
   - Adjust pH of the mixture to 3.4 using 1 N NaOH
   - Store at room temperature, prepare weekly
3. Acetic Acid—0.2%

P. Gupta, R. K. Gupta, *Pathology of Glomerular Diseases*, https://doi.org/10.1007/978-981-19-1430-0

Procedure

1. After deparaffinization sections are hydrated using distilled water
2. Sections are Immersed in Harris hematoxylin for 5 min.
3. Wash with tap water until the water is clear.
4. Immerse sections in Gomori trichrome stain for 10 min.
5. Differentiate using 0.2% acetic acid (a few dips are sufficient).
6. Dehydrate using 95% alcohol (×2) followed by absolute alcohol (×2).
7. Clear with xylene (×3–4).
8. Mount using DPX and clean coverslip.

Interpretation

1. Nuclei—purple
2. Normal muscle myofibrils—red
3. Intermyofibrillar muscle membranes—magenta red
4. Immune deposits—magenta red
5. Interstitial collagen—green

Periodic Acid Silver Methenamine (PSM) Stain

Reagents

1. Periodic Schiff 0.5% solution
2. Stock solution of 5% silver nitrate 5 ml + 3% hexamine (silver methenamine solution)
3. 5% borax solution
4. 3% sodium thiosulphate
5. 0.2% light green
6. 1% sodium or potassium metabisulphite
7. Working solution of silver methenamine is freshly prepared by mixing stock solution of
   - Silver methenamine—5 ml
   - Borax solution 5%—3 ml
   - Distilled water—8 ml

Procedure

1. Deparaffinize the sections.
2. Hydrate the sections with distilled water.
3. Rinse in 1% sodium or potassium metabisulphite.
4. Wash in running water.
5. Incubate in freshly prepared silver methenamine working solution at 58–60 °C for 30–60 min.
6. Rinse in distilled water.
7. Rinse with sodium thiosulphate.
8. Wash in distilled water.
9. Counterstain with light green.
10. Dehydrate, clear and mount in DPX using a clean coverslip

Interpretation

1. Silver stains basement membrane—black
2. Background—pale green

Jones Methenamine Silver Stain

Reagents

1. 0.5% Periodic acid solution
2. 0.5% Thiosemicarbazide solution
3. 5.0% Silver nitrate solution
4. 3.0% Methenamine solution
   - Hexamethyleneteteraamine (Methenamine)—12.0 g
   - Distilled water—375 ml
   - Ethylene Glycol—25 ml
5. Methenamine-Silver Nitrate Solution
   - Silver Nitrate 5% solution—20 ml
   - Methenamine 3% solution—400 ml
6. 3% Sodium Borate (Borax) solution
7. Methenamine-Silver Nitrate working solution (freshly prepared)
   - Methenamine-Silver Nitrate stock solution—20 ml
   - Distilled water—20 ml
   - Sodium Borate 3% solution—2 ml
8. 1% Gold Chloride solution in distilled water (stock)
9. 0.2% Gold Chloride working solution in distilled water
10. 2% Sodium Thiosulfate solution in distilled water
11. Hematoxylin stain
12. Eosin stain

Procedure

1. Deparaffinize and hydrate
2. Place in 0.5% periodic aid solution—10 min.
3. Rinse in distilled water (×4).
4. Place in 0.5% thiosemicarbazide—5 min.
5. Rinse in distilled water (×4).
6. Place in working methenamine-silver nitrate solution at 43 °C water bath for 2 min.
7. Then transfer to 58 °C water bath for 15 min.
8. Rinse in distilled water (×4).
9. Tone with 0.2% gold chloride for 1 min.
10. Rinse in distilled water (×2).
11. Place in 2% sodium thiosulphate solution for 1 min.
12. Rinse in distilled water (×4).
13. Counterstain with hematoxylin for 3 min.
14. Acid Rinse, bluing and wash in distilled water
15. Counterstain with eosin.

16. Dehydrate, clear and mount in DPX using a clean coverslip.

Interpretation

1. Basement membranes of glomeruli, Bowman's capsule, tubular basement membrane—black
2. Nuclei—blue
3. Background—pink

Orcein Stain

Reagents

1. 0.3% Acidified potassium permanganate (stock)

- Potassium permanganate—0.3 g
- Distilled water—100 ml
- Sulphuric acid conc.—0.2 ml
- For use dilute with equal parts of distilled water

2. 1.0% Oxalic Acid Solution in distilled water
3. 1.0% Orcein Solution (To be stored at room temperature for 1 week before use)

- Orcein—1 g
- Alcohol 70%—100 ml
- Hydrochloric acid (conc.)—1.0 ml

Procedure

1. Deparaffinize and hydrate.
2. Place in dilute acidified potassium permanganate solution for 5 min.
3. Rinse in distilled water (×2).
4. Place in 1% oxalic acid solution for 2 min.
5. Wash in running tap water for 1 min.
6. Rinse in distilled water (×2).
7. Dip several times in 70% alcohol.
8. Place in orcein solution in a Coplin jar and microwave at power for 1 min, transfer to 37 °C water bath for 2 h.
9. Rinse in distilled water (×4).
10. Dehydrate, clear and mount in DPX using a clean coverslip.

Interpretation

1. Hepatitis B surface antigen (HbsAg)—brown, diffuse cytoplasmic
2. Copper binding protein—brown, fine cytoplasmic granules
3. Elastic fibers—brown

Congored Stain

Reagents

1. Modified Weigert's Iron Hematoxylin
2. 0.5% acid alcohol solution
3. Sodium chloride-alcohol solution
   - Sodium chloride—2.5 g
   - Distilled water—50 ml
   - Absolute alcohol—50 ml
4. 1% Potassium hydroxide
5. Congo red solution
   - Sodium chloride alcohol solution—50 ml
   - Congo red—0.1 g
   - 1% Potassium hydroxide—0.5 ml

Procedure

1. Paraffin sections are cut at 6 microns.
2. Sections are deparaffinized and hydrated.
3. Place in modified Weigert's iron hematoxylin for 10 s.
4. Wash briefly in running tap water and rinse in distilled water (×2).
5. Place in acid alcohol solution for 5 s.
6. Wash in running tap water for 1 min.
7. Place in 95% alcohol for 5 s.
8. Stained with Congo Red working solution—20 min.
9. Rinse in distilled water.
10. Differentiated quickly (5–10 dips) in alkaline alcohol solution.
11. Rinse in tap water.
12. Dehydrate, clear and mount in DPX using a clean coverslip.

Interpretation

1. Amyloid—pink or red
2. Nuclei—black
3. Erythrocytes—pale orange
4. Eosinophil granules—reddish orange
5. Polarization microscopy—apple green birefringence

Thyoflavin-T Staining

Reagents

1. 1.0% Thioflavin S aqueous solution
2. 1.0% Thioflavin T aqueous solution
3. Modified Weigert's Iron Hematoxylin

4. 0.5% Acid alcohol solution
5. 1.0% Acetic acid solution

Procedure

1. 6–8 μm sections are deparaffinized and hydrated.
2. Place in modified Weigert's iron hematoxylin solution for 15 s.
3. Rinse in distilled water (×3).
4. Place in 0.5% acid alcohol solution for 5 s.
5. Rinse in distilled water (×4).
6. Stain with 1% thioflavin T for 5 min (as per requirement).
7. Wash well in running water.
8. Place in 1.0% acetic acid for 15 min.
9. Rinse in distilled water (×3).
10. Dry in air, dip in Xylene and mount in DPX using a clean coverslip.

Interpretation

When visualized in fluorescence microscope:

1. Amyloid—Fluorescence
2. Background—Black

Perl's Prussian Blue Staining for Iron

Reagents

1. 20% Aqueous solution of Hydrochloric acid:
2. 10% Aqueous solution of Potassium ferrocyanide
3. Working solution—mix equal parts of 20% HCl and 10% Potassium ferrocyanide solution just before use.
4. 0.5% aqueous Neutral Red or 0.1 % aqueous Nuclear Fast Red Solution

Procedure

1. Deparaffinize and bring the sections to water.
2. Treat the sections with freshly prepared acid ferrocyanide solution for 10–30 min.
3. Wash in distilled water (×3).
4. Stain with 0.5% aqueous neutral red or 0.1% aqueous nuclear fast red solution for 5 min.
5. Wash in distilled water (×2)
6. Dehydrate, clear and mount in DPX using a clean coverslip.

Interpretation

1. Iron (ferric form)—bright blue
2. Nuclei—red
3. Cytoplasm—pink

Ziehl Neelsen Stain for Acid-Fast Bacilli

Reagents

Carbol fuschin solution

- 1 g basic fuschin is dissolved in 10 ml of absolute alcohol and 100 ml of 5%aqueous phenol is added. Mix well and filter.

1. 1.0% Acid alcohol solution
2. 1.0% aqueous methylene blue solution

Procedure

1. Sections are deparaffinized and hydrated
2. Stain in Coplin jar with filtered Carbol Fuschia at 60 °C temperature for 30—60 min.
3. Wash in running tap water.
4. Differentiate in 1% acid alcohol until the background staining is removed.
5. Wash in running tap water.
6. Counterstain nuclei with 1% methylene blue for 1 min.
7. Dehydrate, clear and mount in DPX using a clean coverslip.

Interpretation

1. Acid-fast organisms—magenta
2. Background—pale blue

Oil Red O Staining

Reagents

1. 0.5% oil red O solution
   - O.5 g oil red O
   - Propylene glycol 100%—100 ml
   - Heat gently until the solution reaches 95–100 °C.
   - Filter solution through coarse filter paper.
   - Stored at room temperature
2. 85% Propylene glycol solution:
   - Propylene glycol 100%--------------85 ml
   - Distilled water------------------------15 ml
3. Mayer's Hematoxylin solution

Procedure

1. Fresh frozen 5–10 μm thick sections are mounted on slides.

2. Slides are air dried for 30–60 min at room temperature and then fixed in ice cold 10% formalin for 5–10 min. Air dried again for another 30–60 min.
3. Place in absolute propylene glycol for 2–5 min.
4. Stain in pre-warmed Oil Red O solution for 8–10 min in 60 °C oven.
5. Differentiate in 85% propylene glycol solution for 2–5 min.
6. Rinse in 2 changes of distilled water.
7. Stain with Mayer's hematoxylin for 30 s.
8. Wash thoroughly in running tap water for 3 min.
9. Place slides in distilled water.
10. Mount with glycerin jelly or other aqueous mounting media.

Results

1. Lipids—red
2. Nuclei—pale blue

Direct Immunofluorescence Staining on Frozen Sections

Procedure

1. Tissue received in normal saline is allowed to freeze in cryostat at −25°C for 10–15 min.
2. 2–3 μ sections at obtained on multiple slides.
3. Sections are fixed by air drying for 2–4 h.
4. Washed with PBS (one wash).
5. Add desired antibody conjugated with FITC (dilution 1:50).
6. Put the coverslip and keep for half an hour in a dark chamber.
7. Wash with PBS 6–7 times.
8. Mount in glycerine.
9. Examine under fluorescence microscope.
10. DIF intensity was scored semi-quantitatively on a scale of 0 (negative), (trace), 1+ (mild), 2+ (moderate) and 3+ (strong positivity).

IF on Formalin Fixed Paraffin Sections

Procedure

IF staining was performed after antigen retrieval using proteinase-K on FFPE tissues.

1. 3 μm sections were taken on poly-L-lysine coated slides.
2. Slides were incubated at 37 °C on slide warmer for 6 h.
3. Deparaffinization was done by giving two changes in xylene for 5 min each, one change in ethanol 100% for 5 min followed by changes in 70% and 50% alcohol for 5 min.
4. Slides were rehydrated by washing in distilled water and kept in Tris buffer (pH 9.0) at 37 °C for 20 min.
5. Incubation with proteinase-K, (Sigma Aldrich, P2308) 0.25 mg/ml at 37 °C for 15 min.
6. After washing with Tris buffer, (pH 9.0) slides were incubated at 4 °C for 20 min.
7. Fluorescein isothiocyanate (FITC) conjugated polyclonal antibodies directed for immunoglobulins (IgG, IgA, IgM), complements (C3, C1q), light chains (kappa, lambda) (Dako, USA) were used as per manufacturer instructions.
8. Incubation was performed for 2 h in a wet humidified chamber.
9. Finally, slides were rinsed in PBS and mounted with phosphate buffer glycerine.
10. DIF intensity was scored semi-quantitatively on a scale of 0 (negative), (trace), 1+ (mild), 2+ (moderate) and 3+ (strong positivity).

Immunostaining (IHC)

Procedure

1. 2–3 μ sections obtained on coated slides were deparaffinized and rehydrated (2 changes xylene for10 min each, 1 change 90% alcohol, 1 change 70% alcohol for 5 min each, rehydration in tap water for 2–5 min).
2. Antigen retrieval was done by boiling.
3. Boiling (manual): Citrate buffer (1 L) was taken in a pressure cooker. Slides were placed in a slide rack. Pressure cooker was heated for a while and allowed to cool to room temperature.
4. Slides are incubated in 3% hydrogen peroxide for 10 min and washed with phosphate buffer saline (PBS).
5. Slides were covered with protein block and allowed to incubate for 3–5 min.
6. Primary antibody was added and incubated for 30 min.
7. Slides were washed with phosphate buffer saline (PBS).
8. Post-primary antibody enhancer was added and left for 30 min. Slides were again washed with PBS.
9. HRP (Horseradish peroxidase) polymer added for 30 min and washed with PBS.
10. DAB (3,3'-diaminobenzidine) solution poured for 5 min and washed with PBS.
11. Counterstain with hematoxylin.
12. Dried and mounted with permanent mounting media (DPX) using a clean coverslip.

Transmission Electron Microscopy

Procedure

1. Tissue for ultra-structural analysis was fixed promptly in 3% glutaraldehyde with 0.1 mol/L phosphate buffer, pH 7.4 for 24 h.
2. Washed by phosphate buffer by two rinses of 30 min each.
3. Postfixed in buffered 1% osmium tetroxide for30 min.

4. Washed with buffer (as in step 2).
5. Dehydrated using increasing concentrations of ethanol (35%, 70%, 90%, 100%; each for 30 min twice).
6. Embedded in epoxy resin.
7. Semi-thin/"survey" sections of 0.5 to 1 micron thickness were reviewed on LM by staining with toluidine blue to identify glomeruli.
8. Area of interest trimmed out.
9. Thin sections of 70–90 nm were cut with diamond knives on a Reichert ultra-microtome.
10. Sections were mounted on carbon-coated copper grids.
11. Stained with 2% uranyl acetate for five min and lead citrate for 3 min.
12. Examined under electron microscope.

Appendix 2: Biological Reference Ranges

Parameters	Biological reference range	Method
Hematology		
Hemoglobin		
Male	14.0–16.0 g/dl	Photometry
Female	12.0–15.0 g/dl	
Total WBC Count	4.0–11.0/µl	Flow cytometry
DLC		
Polymorphs	53–68%	Flow cytometry
Lymphocytes	25–40%	Flow cytometry
Eosinophils	0–6%	Flow cytometry
Monocytes	3–7%	Flow cytometry
Platelets	150–450/µl	Flow cytometry
Observed ESR		
Male	0–15 mm/h	Westergren
Female	0–20 mm/h	
Prothrombin time	10.6–13.6 s	Electromagnetic mechanical clot detection
INR	0.8–1.4	Calculated
APTT	23.2–34.6 s	Electromagnetic mechanical clot detection
Clinical pathology		
Urine Albumin	Nil	Dipstick
Urine Microalbumin	0–30 mg/L	Particle Enhanced Turbidimetric Inhibition-Immuo Assay
Urine 24 h protein	0–149 mg/24 h	Pyrogallol Red
Urine Glucose	Nil	Dipstick
Urine P:C ratio	21–161 mg/g Creatinine	Calculated
Microscopic		
WBC	0–3/phf	Microscopy
RBC	Nil	
Cast	Nil	

Parameters	Biological reference range	Method
Biochemistry		
Serum Glucose (F)	74–99 mg/dL	Hexokinase
Serum Glucose (PP)	100–140 mg/dL	
HbA1C	3.0–6.4%	HPLC
Serum Cholesterol	140–200 mg/dL	DEA-Hcl/APP
Serum Triglyceride	50–150 mg/L	Enzymatic Assay Direct (PVS/PEGME)
Serum HDL	40–60 mg/dL	Precipitation and Trinder Reaction
Serum LDL	upto 100 mg/dL	Calculated
HDL:LDL Ratio	0–1.5	Calculated
Serum VLDL	0–30 mg/dL	Calculated
Serum total proteins	6.6–8.7	Rate Biuret Assay
Serum Albumin	3.5–5.0	BCP
Serum Globulins	1.8–3.6	Calculated
A:G Ratio	2:1	Calculated
Serum beta 2 Microglobulin	0.8–2.34 mg/L	CLIA
Serum Urea	5.0–23.0 mg/dl	Urease Kinetic
BUN	5.0–20 mg/dl	Urease GLDH
Serum Creatinine	0.6–1.3/60–110 µmol/L	Jaffe Kinetic (IDMS)
Serum Calcium	8.2–10.40 mg/dl	ISE (indirect)
Serum phosphorus	2.5–4.6	Phosphomolybdate UV
Serum Sodium	132–148 mEq/L	ISE (Indirect)
Serum Pottasium	3.5–5.5 mEq/L	ISE (Indirect)
Serum Chloride	98–108 mEq/L	ISE (Indirect)
Serum Bicarbonate	22–32 mmol/L	ISE (Indirect)
Serum ACE inhibitors	8.0 to 65.0 U/l	Enzymatic
Serum Procalcitonin	<0.5 ng/ml	ELFA
Serum Complement C3	1032–1495 mg/L	Immunoturbidimetry
Serum Complement C4	167–385 mg/L	Immunoturbidimetry
Serum CRP	<6 mg/l	Immunoturbidimetry
Serum IgG	6.10–16.16 g/L	Immunoturbidimetry
Serum IgM	0.35–2.42 g/L	Immunoturbidimetry
Serum IgA	0.84–4.99 g/L	Immunoturbidimetry
Serum-free kappa light chain	3.30–19.40 mg/L	Immunoturbidimetry
Serum-free lambda light chain	5.71–26.30 mg/L	Immunoturbidimetry

Parameters	Biological reference range	Method
kappa: lambda ratio	0.26–1.65	Calculated
Serum ANA	Negative	IIF
Serum ds-DNA	<20 IU/ml	Immunoenzymatic (ELISA)
Serum p-ANCA (Anti MPO)	<12 AU/ml	Immunoenzymatic (ELISA)
Serum c-ANCA (Anti PR3)	<12 AU/ml	Immunoenzymatic (ELISA)
Serum Anti-GBM Antibody	<18 U/mL	Immunoenzymatic (ELISA)
Serum ASO	<200	Agglutination

MIX
Papier aus verantwortungsvollen Quellen
Paper from responsible sources
FSC® C105338

FSC
www.fsc.org

If you have any concerns about our products,
you can contact us on
ProductSafety@springernature.com

In case Publisher is established outside the EU,
the EU authorized representative is:
Springer Nature Customer Service Center GmbH
Europaplatz 3, 69115 Heidelberg, Germany

Printed by Libri Plureos GmbH
in Hamburg, Germany